Feminism
and Nursing

Feminism and Nursing

An Historical Perspective on Power, Status, and Political Activism in the Nursing Profession

Joan I. Roberts
and Thetis M. Group

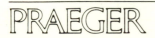

Westport, Connecticut
London

Library of Congress Cataloging-in-Publication Data

Roberts, Joan I.
    Feminism and nursing : an historical perspective on power,
status, and political activism in the nursing profession / Joan
I. Roberts and Thetis M. Group.
        p.   cm.
    Includes bibliographical references and index.
    ISBN: 0–275–94916–8 (alk. paper).—ISBN 0–275–95120–0 (pbk.)
    1. Nursing—Social aspects. 2. Feminism. 3. Nursing—Political
aspects. 4. Nurses—Political activity. 5. Nursing—History.
I. Group, Thetis M.   II. Title.
    [DNLM: 1. Nursing. 2. History of Nursing. 3. Women's Rights.
4. Nurses. 5. Politics. WY 16 R645f 1995]
RT86.5.R63 1995
610.73—dc20
DNLM/DLC   94–33756

British Library Cataloguing in Publication Data is available.

Library of Congress Catalog Card Number: 94–33756
ISBN: 0–275–94916–8
    0–275–95120–0 (pbk.)

First published in 1995

Praeger Publishers, 88 Post Road West, Westport, CT 06881
An imprint of Greenwood Publishing Group, Inc.

Printed in the United States of America

The paper used in this book complies with the
Permanent Paper Standard issued by the National
Information Standards Organization (Z39.48–1984).

10 9 8 7 6 5 4 3 2 1

Copyright Acknowledgment

Quotations from *Florence Nightingale and Her Era* by V. Bullough, B. Bullough,
and M. P. Stanton are reprinted by permission of Garland Publishing, Inc.
Copyright © 1990.

In memory of
Emily E. Anderson
1956–1991

One of our finest students, she received her BS and MS degrees in Nursing and Women's Studies.

Her untimely death has deprived the profession of a feminist nurse who shared in the discovery of nursing's place in women's history.

Contents

Acknowledgments   ix

Introduction   xi

Chapter 1:   "Awake, Ye Women, Awake!"
               Perspectives on Florence Nightingale   1

Chapter 2:   Nursing Leaders as Activists and Feminists   55

Chapter 3:   The Paradox: Nurses as Healers in "Men's
               Horrible Wars"   101

Chapter 4:   The Lively Debate: Nurses and Suffrage,
               the Equal Rights Amendment, and Social
               Reform   151

Chapter 5:   "What We May Become": The Sounds of
               Transition   171

Chapter 6:   The Turning Point: Nurses Connect with
               the Women's Movement   187

Chapter 7:   Poking Heads out of Their Apolitical Bonnets:
               Nurses Zero in on Gender, Power, and
               Leadership in the 1970s   221

Chapter 8:   "Ride the White Horse Yourself!" Women's
               Culture, Feminism, and Nursing in the 1980s   261

Contents

Chapter 9:   Where Will Nurses' Militancy Lead?   295

References   337

Index   357

Acknowledgments

This book originated in the many hours of dialogue our students have had with us over several years. Their determination and eagerness to discover feminist roots in nursing have sustained us throughout the writing of this text. Most notably, we are especially grateful to Emily E. Anderson, to whom this book is dedicated. She assisted us in our initial library research, coding of cross-era sources, and analysis of subject content. We are privileged to have known her and were deeply saddened by her untimely death. Other students, too, have given their valuable time in researching and coding sources and assisting in initial manuscript organization. We especially thank Linda Mueller for her invaluable help.

Close friends who shared in our vision and efforts deserve special thanks. Our dear friend, Shepard Holderby, gave to us many hours of her time and thought. Her early death deprived all feminist women of a true visionary who knew what a woman's world could be. We are especially grateful to our good friend and colleague Linda Cook. She has given many hours of her valuable time in checking for manuscript accuracy and contextual flow. Her constant support and encouragement are deeply appreciated.

Funding assistance for manuscript preparation has been provided by the Omicron Chapter of Sigma Theta Tau (Syracuse University College of Nursing), the Syracuse University Senate Research Committee, and the Syracuse University Small Grants Program, and Syracuse University Office of Research. Special thanks is extended to Ben Ware, Vice President of the Office of Research, who believed in our project and provided financial support throughout the manuscript revisions.

Finally, we wish to thank our manuscript typists, Irene Quinlan and Nancee Soule. We are especially grateful to Irene, who is not only a superb typist and formatter, but a contextual editor as well. She spent many hours helping prepare the manuscript for submission, always giving us invaluable assistance in critiquing meaning and consistency. We are fortunate indeed to have had her expertise in preparing this book for publication.

Joan I. Roberts
Thetis M. Group
Syracuse, New York, 1994

Introduction

Over the past three decades, significant changes have occurred in the nursing profession and in the conventional societal definitions of women and their roles. As the women's movement reemerged in the late 1960s and many women refused to uphold the traditional roles allocated to them, a parallel trend in nursing centered on the development of "expanded" roles for nurses—the "independent" practitioner, nurse clinician, and nurse practitioner. As these professional and societal trends gained momentum in the 1970s, the conflicts inherent in integrating professional and gender roles became overt and critically important. In nursing it became obvious that it would be improbable, if not impossible, to prepare assertive, independent nurse practitioners if they were socialized to be dependent females. Similarly, it is improbable, if not impossible, for female nurses to implement expanded roles if they are unaware of or unwilling to recognize the social constraints imposed on them because they are women. Indeed, the successes or failures of the nursing profession in its struggle to grow in stature and gain autonomy during its long history cannot be fully understood unless integrally linked to the relationship between gender and professional roles as these have changed over time.

Women in nursing have not consistently or systematically documented these interrelationships; thus, the analysis of nurses' perceptions of themselves as both women and nurses has only recently emerged. Ironically, nursing, one of the few occupations available to women in the industrial period, has seldom and only recently been the subject of woman's studies scholars. The absence of an extended dialogue between women scholars in the broader academic community and women in nursing has led to difficulties in understanding nursing as a predominantly woman's profession. On one hand, some feminists have advised women to enter medicine, believing nursing to be subservient—a model of professional domesticity. On the other hand, some women in nursing have seen the women's movement as peripheral to their long fight for independent professional status. Both inside and outside of nursing, women have too often neglected or misperceived each other because of a fundamental misunderstanding of the historical relationship of the nursing profession to the general societal subordination of women.

DOCUMENTING A LINEAGE OF CONCERN

In the summer of 1975 a preliminary bibliography, developed by the authors for a course on nursing and women's studies, produced scanty and sparse published materials on gender and professional roles of nurses; at that time, no centralized and comprehensive bibliographic sources related to this issue could be located. This contrasted sharply with more extensive bibliographic sources on women as physicians, women as health-care consumers, and the politics of sexism in the health-care system, all areas of considerable long-term interest to feminists. Indeed, the *Cumulative Index of Nursing and Allied Health Literature* (*CINAHL*) did not include the topics "sexism" (sex discrimination) and "women's rights" (feminism) until 1983, and it was not until 1984 that *CINAHL* was computerized. Thus, a painstaking review of all topics in the nursing literature was required, making our research task more complex.

Feminist scholars have documented the politics of sexism in medicine and health care in the 19th century and again in the 20th century with the reemergence of feminism. For example, Barbara Ehrenreich and Deirde English (1973) in *Complaints and Disorders: The Sexual Politics of Sickness*, Ellen Frankfort (1972) in *Vaginal Politics*, Germaine Greer (1971) in *The Female Eunuch*, and Barbara Seaman (1972) in *Free and Female* brought issues of discriminatory medical practices against women to the public's notice. From these earlier exposés, books documenting sexist practices in women's health care emerged; for example, Belita Cowan's (1977) *Women's Health Care*; Sheryl B. Ruzek's (1978) *The Women's Health Movement: Feminist Alternatives to Medical Control*; Diane K. Kjervik and Ida M. Martinson's (1979) *Women in Stress* and later (1986) in *Women in Health and Illness*; Helen I. Marieskind's (1980) *Women in the Health Delivery System: Patients, Providers and Programs*; Marguerite Sandelowski's (1980) *Women, Health and Choice*; Elizabeth Fee's (1983) *Women and Health: The Politics of Sex in Medicine*; Gena Corea's (1985) *The Hidden Malpractice*; Ellen Lewin's (1985) *Women, Health, and Healing*; Sue Fisher's (1986) *In the Patient's Best Interest*; Alexandra Todd's (1989) *Intimate Adversaries*; Clarice Feinman's (1992) *The Criminalization of a Woman's Body*; and Helen Roberts' (1992) *Women's Health Matters*. To his credit, Robert S. Mendelsohn (1982), one of the few male physicians to write on sexism and medicine, made a scathing indictment of current medical practices in *Malepractice: How Doctors Manipulate Women*.

Much more has been written on women in medicine from the view of sexism than on nurses. Four books of several published over the past three decades analyze the major problems: Carol Lopate's (1968) *Women in Medicine*; Margaret Campbell's (1974) *Why Should a Girl Go into Medicine?*; Mary Walsh's (1977) *Doctors Wanted: No Women Need Apply, Sexual Barriers in the Medical Profession, 1835–1975*; and Judith Lorber's (1984) *Women Physicians: Careers, Status, and Power*.

Even with the reemergence of feminism, fewer works appeared on sexism and nursing, but probably the earliest is *Witches, Midwives, and Nurses* (Ehrenreich & English, 1972). This was followed by the historical study of American nursing by Jo Ann Ashley (1976) in *Hospitals, Paternalism and the Role of the Nurse*, and the more sociological analysis, *WomanPower and Health Care*, by Marlene Grissum and Carol Spengler (1976). A later anthology by Janet Muff (1982), *Socialization, Sexism and Stereotyping*, focused on women's issues in nursing. Although only somewhat concerned with gender and sexism, some later histories on nursing have some relevance, such as *Ordered to Care* by Susan Reverby (1987b). Bonnie and Vern Bullough (e.g., 1978; 1984) have contributed most consistently to issues of sexism and gender in nursing from historical perspectives in a variety of articles and books.

Thus began a historical search of materials published by women in nursing and sources from other disciplines on the interrelation between gender and nursing. From these sources, hundreds of articles and books were analyzed for possible relevance to this key area of concern. The organization and analysis of these sources confirmed the compellingly important influence of gender stratification and sex discrimination within the health occupations, in which about 70% of the workers are female. Discrimination, as documented in all social systems, adversely affects the individual nurse as well as her or his profession. Sexism is particularly important in understanding the development of the nursing profession, since it is almost totally female (97%).

Our primary focus has been to analyze the voices of nurses themselves, and of some non-nurses who have been concerned with gender issues in nursing. We have tried to stay as close to the words of the authors as possible, providing synthesis with other sources and critical analyses as appropriate. Our perspective is clearly directed toward women and their problems. Using sources only from English-speaking countries, we found that some of the writings are very sophisticated, and some, less so; thus, our syntheses and analyses are subject to both quality and quantity of published works. Since these are differentially distributed in varied cultures, the extent to which cross-national integration is possible also changes with the topics considered. For example, the interconnections between gender and expanded roles are more likely to be considered, even if only indirectly, in American sources. In comparison, British sources have been very concerned with the impact of men in nursing. Thus, the cross-cultural emphasis varies according to the sources available. Similarly, subcultural linkages among gender, race, and class are also limited to what is available in the literature. These linkages are infrequently made by many authors; thus, the interconnections among different forms of discrimination are still to be fully explored.

Ironically, in analyzing the published literature, it has been difficult to find writings from some historical periods that systematically express the interrelation between gender and nursing as a woman's profession. Nevertheless, we can establish and demonstrate a lineage of concern about women's roles, sex discrimination, health care, and nursing that extends over a century. There is a wide diversity in the writings of nurses themselves in their awareness of sex discrimination as a phenomenon to which all women are subjected. Thus, it is common to find in the earlier sources an underlying assumption that a gender-stratification system exists, for example, in economics and nursing, but no explication of that fact in the analyses presented. Also, it is common to find articles that do explicate facets of gender, such as in writings on nurses as mother surrogates, but, do not implicate *systematic* sexism within the body of the work. In contrast, some women, even in the earlier periods, were acutely aware of the gender-stratification system and clearly espoused feminist principles in their writings. Though we have chosen to focus on those sources that exhibit some understanding of the effects of sex discrimination and gender on the nursing profession, some nurses even now seem to be caught in the traditional subordination of women and exhibit little understanding of their own subjugation. The variations in *current* tactics and strategies for change still reflect the diversity of opinion on what a woman should be and what a woman's profession should be; thus, achieving political consensus in nursing has been extremely difficult.

Historically, there is a lack of a consistent theoretical position related to gender and a woman's profession; thus, it is difficult to analyze the historical materials from a coherent theoretical perspective. It was not until the 1980s that nurses themselves attempted to connect feminist theory to fundamental issues in nursing. Perhaps the best initial work comes from Peggy L. Chinn and Charlene Eldridge Wheeler (1985), who were among the first nurses to elaborate on four philosophic approaches in feminist theory for nurses. Liberal feminism, stemming from a civil libertarian emphasis on equal rights, stresses equal opportunity for women relative to men's. Marxist feminist theory originates in social structural thinking in which women and children are regarded as property in the social class divisions. Socialist feminist theory goes beyond traditional class analysis to focus on the integral relation between the private sphere of person, family, and reproduction and the public sphere of production and labor. Radical feminism arises from a woman-centered worldview and postulates that women's oppression is a fundamental universal experience. Chinn and Wheeler emphasize that feminism is not to be equated with lesbian ideology; rather, "it is committed to ending the isolation and divisiveness that exist among women in male-defined systems, advocating that women value themselves and other women" (p. 75).

What are the commonalities between feminist and nursing theory? Chinn and Wheeler propose that some concepts are essentially harmonious, such as the integral unity of human existence and environment, the interactive processes of caring and nurturing devalued by patriarchal systems, and reverence for life, for environment, and for individual uniqueness. Feminism adds the systematic analysis of oppression and power that, when applied to nursing, helps explain the devaluation of nursing, the low affiliation with others who are seen as "powerless" in professional associations, the frequent emulation of the powerful, as reflected in the medical model. But the analysis of power is not necessarily the enactment of power. It is a very common finding over the past three centuries that women who have written powerfully in behalf of women, or activists who have moved politically against discrimination, have taken the brunt of societal condemnation by men and even some women. In general, women can be activists as long as they agitate in behalf of others—children, sanitation, health, morality, and so on—but not for themselves. The most frequent accusation against activist women is that they are "unwomanly"; sometimes accusations of insanity and immorality have been directed toward women leaders. Perhaps the most distressing stereotypes have been "mannishness," common in the 19th century, and "queer" or lesbian, common in the 20th century. These stereotypes are intended to demean and trivialize feminists as well as weaken the unity among them. It is clear that feminism cannot be for only some women; it must be for all women of whatever race, creed, religion, or lifestyle. Without this unity, the masculist game of divide and conquer can be played out indefinitely.

Although ideal, it has not been possible to incorporate all of the feminist theories and research in this book; limitations on manuscript length have precluded this. Of the major feminist theoretical positions, however, the one that has been most consistently apparent in the sources analyzed on gender and nursing is liberal feminism, derived from the liberal or humanistic perspective, originating in the human rights tradition associated with the European, or more particularly, the British philosophical approach emerging in the 19th century. This was most eloquently expressed by John Stuart Mill (1869) in his book, *The Subjection of Women*, and in Harriet Taylor Mill's (1851) essay "Enfranchisement of Women." Thus, most of the sources assume a position based on an equality of rights. Exceptions to this trend can be found earlier, for example, in the work of Lavinia L. Dock (1907; 1909), who espoused in some of her thinking a more socialist-feminist position and sometimes even a radical-cultural feminism. These perspectives are best represented today by various writers who have been particularly concerned about the economic status of women as nurses, or who have been influenced by radical feminism, sometimes associated with feminist philosopher Mary

Daly (1980), and observed in the thinking and writing of some nurses (e.g., Ashley, 1976, 1980; Campbell, 1981).

Newer perspectives from critical theory, especially feminist deconstructionism, have not predominated in the research and writing about nurses and nursing, although some are evident in recent critiques of nursing education: Allen's (1986) analysis of familialism in nursing textbooks, Hagell's (1989) concern with nursing's overreliance on scientific knowledge and quantitative research to define its knowledge base, and Doering's (1992) feminist poststructuralist viewpoint on the development and maintenance of nursing-medicine power relations. Numerous theories specific to the fields of anthropology, psychology, and sociology clearly have influenced scholars writing about nursing; for example, feminist organizational theory, the role of women in complex organizations, psychological effects of war on nurses, and effects of employment on women and their children. Many of these theories, however, have not been used in a consistent manner to produce cumulative research-based bodies of knowledge.

Until relatively recently, research on gender and nursing has been somewhat limited. Few studies are available from the earlier periods, probably because nursing was yet to be established in university structures in which research was legitimized and expected. As more nurses have achieved advanced degrees, an increasing number of research studies on gender and nursing have appeared; and as more women's studies scholars attend to nursing, more analyses should be expected. Nevertheless, a large number of sources deal with personal expressions of dismay among nurses, and offer only short analyses of specific issues, often derived from the social sciences, and more recently, from feminist writers. These give us a sense of women's perceptions of nurses and nursing from a gender perspective over time.

It is apparent that a strong women's movement has directly affected the nursing profession. For example, at the turn of the century, when even nonfeminist women were organizing to achieve the vote and the rhetoric of feminism was widely heard, the movement to strengthen the nursing profession was significant. This same interrelation can be observed in the past two decades with the reemergence of feminism. For example, feminist issues such as pay equity are now widely espoused by nurses. Given this trend, however, it is clear that many nurses have followed the lead of women external to the profession, exhibiting a concern for gender issues somewhat later than their emergence among women external to nursing. Yet, a countervailing trend is also apparent: Nurses have retained their concern for feminist issues, such as working conditions for women and greater equity between male and female workers, even during periods of extreme gender conservatism. Although an overt feminist analysis is not often apparent in some of their writing, still such efforts could be classified as attempts to achieve greater autonomy and power—both important goals of feminism.

These trends represent only a few of those observable in the history of gender and nursing. All these trends influence the current situation in nursing and, unless gender issues are resolved through the historical analysis of their impact in previous decades, nurses will be unable to make forward progress because they will have little clarity on the essential, fundamental issues.

CREATING NEW PERSPECTIVES
FOR UNDERSTANDING NURSING'S HISTORY

From the enormous number of sources collected and analyzed to clarify the effects of gender stratification on nurses and the health-care system, it became clear that one volume alone could not do justice to fully explicating the complex relationship between the most fundamental social roles, defined by sex in gendered patterns, and the professional roles of nurses, whose lives, work, education, and practice represent in microcosm the realities of and restrictions on women in the general society. Thus, this book is the first of an interrelated set of texts that examine neglected areas in previous writing and research and provide a comprehensive perspective on gender and nursing. Drawing on sources from the United States, Great Britain, Canada, and, to a lesser extent, other predominantly English-speaking countries, the research on which these books is based interrelates historical sources to create new perspectives and to establish a basis for women's studies in nursing, a field, until recently, overlooked by most scholars.

The attitudes, beliefs, and behaviors that are directed toward women influence all segments of the practice and education of nurses. In this text, *Feminism and Nursing: A Historical Perspective on Power, Status, and Political Activism in the Nursing Profession*, the status of women is historically linked to the status of nursing and to nurses' awareness of feminist issues. The other texts are currently being edited and prepared for publication. *Sexism and Nursing: Historical Perspectives on the Struggle to Overcome Educational and Economic Inequities* focuses on the historical interrelation between nursing and the discriminatory patterns inherent in patriarchal educational and economic systems. Another text, *Nurses as Caregivers at Work and at Home: The Impact of Triple Duty, Inadequate Support, and Changing Gender Expectations on their Families and the Nursing Profession* analyzes major published sources, again historically organized, on the problems that nurses as women experience in juggling personal and professional roles in societies structured on male work patterns. *Nursing, Physician Control, and Medical Monopoly: A Historical Perspective on Gendered Inequality in Roles, Relationships, Rights, and Range of Practice* analyzes time-ordered resources that exemplify the writing of social scientists, nurses, and, to a lesser extent, physicians, on their gendered interrelationships from very early periods to the 1960s. A closely related and companion text is *Gender and the Nurse-Physician*

Game: The Impact of Changing Interrelationships on Autonomy and Range of Practice in Health Care. If possible, *Nursing, Physician Control, and Medical Monopoly* should be read first since it begins with earlier historical periods and provides more general analysis of gender and interprofessional relations. *Gender and the Nurse-Physician Game* begins with the latter 1960s and focuses on recent role changes involving nurses and their interactions with physicians. A special subset of nurse-physician relations, and the one most heavily contested, is related to childbirth, midwifery, and obstetrics. Thus, we have developed a preliminary anthology on midwives, nurses, and male control, focusing on the one area of health care women have been most reluctant to allow men to control. As such, obstetrics, midwifery, and nursing, considered historically, represent most clearly the conflictual relations between gender and professional authority. Another text, *Men in Nursing: Historical Perspectives on Prejudice and Privilege*, is devoted to the problems of male nurses, whose gender role is often perceived as incongruent with the professional nursing role. Although the history of men in nursing is actually quite lengthy, we are most concerned with writings produced in this century, and, more particularly, during the past three decades when publications on male nurses substantially increased.

As a result of our extensive bibliographic search, we have organized over 2,000 sources from which the books are produced. Some of these sources contain only peripheral information on gender and nursing and some are directly related. In addition, a bibliography on men in nursing provides a historically organized set of resources on this particular topic. Thus, a comprehensive repository of sources is available from the authors for scholars who are interested in broadening their perspectives on gender and nursing.

To understand the interplay between gender and professional subordination, we have attended to the voices of all nurses, *both* female and male. Nevertheless, female terminology is used to refer to members of the nursing profession since the emphasis is on the status of women in the general society in relation to women in nursing. Almost all writings of nurses refer to physicians as male; pictures in nursing journals invariably depict male physicians; until recently, even research does not usually distinguish between men and women physicians. In the not too distant past, when female physicians were studied, they were often dropped from analysis because of their small numbers. Ideally, a variegated analysis of the relations of male physicians and male nurses and of female physicians and female nurses should be compared with those of female physicians and male nurses and all these should be differentiated from the more common cross-gender interrelations of male physicians and female nurses. Given limited data, this is only partially possible at this time. Therefore, we follow the practice of nurses themselves, referring to physicians as male, except when there are differentiations made by specific researchers or authors. To the voices of nurses are added those of non-nurses, usually female, but sometimes male, social scientists or activists, who were concerned about nursing. The medical point of view on nursing is represented, but their history is widely known; thus, we have selected only the work pertaining to gender and nurses, paying particular attention to sources included by nurses in their own reference sources.

The complementary interconnections among the texts allow readers to obtain a comprehensive understanding of the processes of gender stratification and sex discrimination that influence nursing and health-care systems. Thus, it is possible to grasp the extent to which nurses have been aware of and have written about nursing issues from the perspective of their subjugation as women; to focus on nurses' conceptions of marriage and family roles as these influence the profession; to understand how societal institutions—economic, political, and educational—affect nursing and health care; to perceive the relationship between the "public" and "private" spheres of life; to connect these to interprofessional relations between men as physicians and women as nurses; to understand the search for autonomy in expanded roles in relation to gendered interactional patterns between professions; to see how women's biological functions in childbirth have been central to the gendered struggle for control; and to learn what happens to men who choose to enter nursing, a traditionally female field. For those who wish to do more investigation, the bibliographies provide a cross-disciplinary research orientation, drawing on research and analyses from the social sciences, nursing, and related fields.

The analysis and selection of sources used in the texts and bibliography should accomplish several objectives. First, they further clarify the gendered historical development of the profession so it can be reconsidered from a broader perspective and more accurately understood. Second, they significantly modify existing and traditional conceptions of the nursing profession. To use standard definitions of the nature of a profession without reference to the gender roles of the members of that profession is a continuing exercise in futility; thus, in the sociology of professions, scholars may be able to rectify the muddled state of affairs on the meaning of professional identity. A third objective is to provide nursing, medicine, and the social sciences with resources organized both historically and substantively as a foundation for further research. A fourth objective is to uncover and define new areas of knowledge, which may help refine existing concepts in nursing and provide directions for new research. A fifth objective is to influence curricular directions in nursing education by changing analyses of the nursing profession and its history, which as currently presented to students and understood by most nurse educators, are inadequately interconnected to gender, race, and class. A sixth goal is to provide women, both nurses and non-nurses, with a more accurate and precise understanding of gender and professional role identities and to establish these as a component of women's studies. A seventh objective is to provide men, both those in and out of nursing and medicine, with a clearer understanding of the historical and current discriminatory practices so they can be sensitive to change and help create different, more equal institutional and societal arrangements for women and men in the health-care system. Finally, from these new, more equal arrangements, consumers can hopefully obtain health care that is more holistic, less expensive, and more directly available to them in their homes and communities.

PURPOSE AND ORGANIZATION OF THE TEXT

In this text, cross-era, comparative sources are analyzed to better understand the relation between women's roles in society and the effect these have had on the nursing profession as it has evolved over time. Chapter 1 focuses on Florence Nightingale as the recognized founder of nursing. We examine her writings on and for women, particularly her philosophy of women's status, her feminist thinking, and her mystical perceptions of life and work. Included are others' perceptions of Nightingale's feminism and the changing images or moral iconography of her as a woman speaking about women and nursing in publications over the past century. In a sense, the debate on Nightingale as feminist or nonfeminist is a symbolic debate on nursing itself. In another sense, this issue revolves around her role as an early critic of family and of religion and in her creation of one woman's early system of "objective" spirituality.

Other voices from the past, other nursing leaders, have also spoken about women's roles and lives. In Chapter 2 we meet Clara Barton, Margaret Sanger, Lillian D. Wald, Adelaide Nutting, Lavinia Lloyd Dock, and, more recently, Wilma Scott Heide, all of whom wrote on women's lives and experiences. Those choosing a feminist path external to nursing often have their early work in nursing discredited or overlooked. Those doing their major work on feminism within nursing often remain unknown to both scholars and the general public.

Paralleling the emergence of the women's movement are the continuing series of men's wars, which impacted most heavily on women in nursing. In Chapter 3 we analyze nurses as healers in the military establishment over time. Devoted to healing and caring, nursing as a woman's profession has experienced both gains and losses as a result of male violence in the Crimean and Civil Wars and later in World War I, World War II, and the Korean, Vietnamese, and Iraq wars. Certainly, there was considerable debate among nurses about the First World War and much distress about subsequent wars. During the Second World War, women were urged into public work, but following the war, in the latter 1940s and throughout the 1950s, they were urged to return home. These contradictory directives were particularly problematic for nurses, who wrote during the war on nurses and the military, but subsequently wrote little on women. In general, the treatment of women and men nurses in the military has been discriminatory, causing substantial damage to individuals and forcing nurse leaders to struggle for decent treatment throughout this century.

In Chapter 4 we examine the feminist actions of those early nursing leaders who aligned themselves with non-nurse feminists in fighting for women's suffrage. The lively debate among nurses on suffrage during the first two decades of this century and subsequently on the "Lucretia Mott Amendment," or the Equal Rights Amendment, exemplifies the commitment of a few nurse leaders to women's equality, as well as illustrating the divisions in the ranks of professional nursing.

Chapter 5 makes it clear that, from the late 1950s through the 1960s, the sounds of transition could be detected in the few voices speaking about women's issues in nursing publications. They expressed their concerns about their status in the sense that every report or commission on nurses described a largely female group trying to sustain public professional roles during a time of severe conservatism about women's roles. In Chapter 6 we see how the turning point in the early 1970s gave rise to the much more decisive ring of feminism in nursing in the latter part of the decade. Thus, in Chapter 7, the dilemma of women leaders in nursing is analyzed. While power in nursing was being openly discussed, so was the fragmented diversity of nurses. Clearly, gender and professional role expectations were differently configured for women, both in and outside of nursing. The critical need for politically astute leaders and administrators was proclaimed with nurses presumably entering a confrontation-negotiation era. As we see in Chapter 8, this continued into the 1980s, although the conservative Reagan era had a significant effect in deflecting attention from feminist goals and activism.

Finally, Chapter 9 considers current relationships among gender, power, and leadership. Personal power gradually came to be associated with political action, which many nurses had previously seen as "unprofessional, unworthy, and unwomanly." Obviously, feminism had influenced nurses sufficiently that they begin to reject such assertions. Authors saw, in fact, the significant change in the profession as a newly found sense of women's competencies and worth associated with a determination to act; the newer thinking connected women's and nurses' rights with overt calls for action. Resocialization in consciousness-raising groups was connected to a call for cohesive, strong membership in political action to counteract male domination and authoritarianism. The struggles both in and outside nursing's body politic again called for assertive action. Nursing history was presented more frequently to gain a new perspective in the preparation of leaders. Organizational analyses of nursing, medicine, and hospital administration led to recommendations for different coalitions. By the 1980s women in nursing were writing on the politics of medical deception, challenging the trajectory of medical history. By the early 1990s an analysis of structured misogyny, detailing implications for the politics of care, had emerged.

Articles on barriers to women in top-level management and structural similarities between the corporate worlds of hospitals and business appeared simultaneously with those discussing nurses in feminist organizations, such as the National Organization for Women and others, considering new power strategies for women in management. Canadian and British nurses joined American nurses in analyzing power and legitimizing political action, connecting both to the provision of adequate patient care. American inbreeding and infighting among nurses in practical politics appears alongside British accounts of surgical sisters' successes and failures in retaining power in surgical theaters. Assertiveness training is advocated, and nurses are urged to speak out for their patients and the profession. More restrained but still useful analyses of gender and leadership are connected to nursing in some sociological work in women's studies. The need for women mentors for women (as detailed in earlier women's studies organizational analyses) is reconsidered in fine-tuned analyses of gender and sponsorship. Projections on power and gender are viewed from a futuristic perspective. Finally, recent successful efforts to wrest the control of home care and other areas of practice from physicians is documented, marking an increased sophistication in political actions by nurse leaders.

NURSING'S FEMINIST FUTURE

Contrary to popular opinion, many feminists argue that women's status has not substantially improved during the past decade. Indeed, Susan Faludi (1991) asserts that women have been convinced that their dissatisfaction and distress are caused by *too much* feminism; however, any minimal progress has actually been undermined. According to Faludi, virtually all outlets of popular culture have spread the backlash to women's rights. Promoting questionable studies on issues such as the "shortage" of men or the "epidemic" of infertility, the media has been joined by political actions that have reduced women's employment and reproductive rights. Indeed, the image of a "New Traditional Woman" covers up the actual losses in achieving equality. The rise of violence against women in films, television, homes, and jobs, and on the streets tells women that if they question their subordination beyond a certain level they will suffer the consequences. Indeed, Faludi claims that there is much left to be achieved and contends that feminism is *not* women's worst enemy but their only hope for real change.

Nursing professor Phyllis B. Kritek (1991) analyzes Faludi's work, praising it for its thorough documentation, but is appalled with the disturbing trends so obvious in Faludi's critique. Kritek agrees that there *is* a backlash and that women have lost ground over the past 10 years. As a female-dominant discipline, nursing reflects the status of that women in any culture; thus, Kritek wonders how the backlash of the 1980s has affected nurses. She urges nurses to return to Lavina Lloyd Dock, who a century ago perceived the intimate linkages among the status of women, women's health, nurses, and nursing. In environments not conducive to the collective hopes and visions of the future, Kritek warns that "the full development and worth of women is a troublesome and threatening agenda. . . . Sometimes the opposition will be substantial and deeply destructive" (p. 4).

Attorney Sondra Henry (1992), equally impressed with Faludi's work, felt compelled to interview her. As a Pulitzer Prize-winning journalist, Faludi's persuasive documentation (80 pages of footnotes) underpins her contention that women have become convinced that their dissatisfaction and stress come from too much independence and feminism rather than minimal economic and political progress. Faludi claims that society, not feminists, has downgraded women's work. The women's movement called attention to the systematic condescension and degradation of women's roles, for example, in the imbalances, status, and pay of nurses compared to physicians. Faludi states that describing the reality is not endorsing it: "The goals of feminism were, and remain, to add and honor in real ways the work that women do" (p. 40).

Faludi also notes that there was historically a conscious campaign to chase women out of the healing profession that was originally theirs. The situation for nurses today reflects that takeover. One wonders how so many nurses, conscious of the power differentials, can remain in the profession while being underpaid, overworked, and disrespected. Faludi claims that the key problem is the glorification of physicians in the medical structure, which must change if authority is to return to women. In mental health, women are now the majority of psychologists, competing effectively by being more affordable and offering less invasive, drastic, and more short-term solutions than higher-priced psychiatrists. Could not nurses use this as a model for entrepreneurial "medicine"? Faludi believes she could obtain more care from a nurse practitioner, who had her client's best interests at heart, than from medical care. Furthermore, shortages could force *organized* nurses to make strides in practice and policy.

Can nurses simultaneously sustain their own values while also changing inequities? Without real authority in decision making, Faludi warns that women's values cannot be fully expressed. Both efforts, then, must be undertaken simultaneously, and, if possible, in coalition with women physicians. But how can nurses change the stereotypes of them as self-sacrificing caretakers, intellectually inferior to physicians and unable to make informed clinical judgments? Faludi emphasizes that myths are perpetuated for a reason. If physicians continue to espouse publicly the handmaiden image of nurses, this will justify lower pay and diminished authority. Nurses must engage in publicity blitzes, law suits, and strikes, but they are discouraged from banding together on a massive scale and from recognizing their allied interests.

In the interview Henry pointed out that leaders of the backlash will often use the fear of change as a threat *before* the major changes can happen. Faludi agreed that there had been the veneer of change; thus, physicians pay lip service to nurses' contributions instead of acknowledging equal pay and authority. Henry said that despite changes, nurses are still patronized by physicians, who advise them to be happy so everyone can be happier. To this Faludi replied, "Nurses are not rocking the boat enough! No one was happy with the old arrangements. Fear kept our mouths closed. No one enjoys being devalued, looked upon as a glorified bed-pan changer" (p. 45). But when nurses challenge physicians, the medical profession has tried to import nurses from other countries or even created new categories of workers, such as registered care technologists. To this, Faludi said, "Backlash is felt more keenly when women challenge a profession that is seen as 'male'" (p. 45). Despite these more difficult problems for nurses, Faludi said the most significant gain in the past two decades was a change in women's own heads. Sexism was not even a word until the late 1960s. Women, even if not feminists, now say they expect equal treatment. Although women now have a different vision of themselves, only a small minority of men support real change; the majority in surveys still perceive the "ideal" woman as the one who puts family before work and defers to a man. Certainly men in power have not reshaped societal institutions to accommodate women's new vision. The enormous resurgence in women's anger is the most promising sign and this, with strength of numbers, can create change. The key tool in the backlash has been "to load down the word feminist with every epithet imaginable" (p. 134), forcing women to back off from the term but not the tenets of feminism. Women must get over the fear of public identification with feminism—to obtain the fruits of a political movement, women must participate in it.

If Faludi is correct, then this volume on nursing and feminism, and the other texts in process, may provide a real hope for substantial change in nursing and the health-care system, helping free women health-care workers to provide the care and cure people really need, and to reconceptualize health care in a more humane way, creating a model of human health and equality that is worthy of adoption throughout the world.

Chapter 1

"Awake, Ye Women, Awake!" Perspectives on Florence Nightingale

It is a peculiar characteristic of human groups that their founding members often take on symbolic meaning. This meaning becomes drawn and redrawn as the needs of the group change over time. In this sense, a moral iconography, a picture of the founder's image, is painted and repainted, according to the needs of each subsequent generation. Such is the fate of Florence Nightingale, revered for decades as the "lady with the lamp," with infinite compassion and dedication to the sick and suffering. As nursing became more complex and higher education for nurses more critical, the image of this moral icon altered so that Nightingale later came to be seen as an efficient administrator, and, most recently, an exceptional researcher and scholar. Over time, she has also been seen as a woman who at times disclaimed women, while simultaneously espousing the rights of women as nurses to a vocation of their own, administered and controlled by themselves.

In this chapter, we focus on Nightingale as a woman and on her views of women's position in society. To understand these, we consider her fundamental conceptions of life from which emerged her theoretical position that incorporated her ideas about women. Because of her voluminous writings, the scholars of Nightingale considered here present, over time, different perceptions of her. In this chapter, we ask several questions and consider possible answers. Was Nightingale a feminist or not? Did she approve of feminists and their goals? What capabilities did she think women had? Was she in favor of women's enfranchisement, and did she support the suffrage movement? Did she like women? Did she have close female friends to support her, or did she primarily rely on men? What were her thoughts on nursing versus medicine? Nurses' authority versus physicians' authority? Was she influenced by the thinking of certain philosophers, and in what ways? Were her actions motivated by mystical and spiritual experiences or traditional religious beliefs? How did her metaphysical views influence her attitudes and actions in nursing and in feminism? The answers to some of these questions become clearer as we consider various interpretations of Nightingale over time.

BETTER PAIN THAN PARALYSIS: FLORENCE NIGHTINGALE ON WOMEN

Florence Nightingale spoke on women in a work entitled *Cassandra*. Written in 1852 when she was 32 years old, the book was revised and privately printed in 1859 after her return from the Crimea. On the advice of Benjamin Jowett it was not published. Presumably, it would have interfered with Nightingale's development of nursing, since it expressed sympathy toward the plight of women in the Victorian era:

> Why have women passion, intellect, moral activity—these three—and a place in society where no one of the three can be exercised? Suffering, sad "female humanity"! What are these feelings which they are taught to consider as disgraceful, to deny to themselves? . . . What are the thoughts of these young girls while one is singing Schubert, another is reading the *Review*, and a third is busy embroidering? Is not one fancying herself the nurse of some new friend in sickness; another engaging in romantic dangers with him, such as call out the character and afford more food for sympathy than the monotonous events of domestic society; another undergoing unheard-of trials under the observation of someone whom she has chosen as the companion of her dream; another having a loving and loved companion in the life she is living, which many do not want to change? . . . And is not this all most natural, inevitable? . . . By mortifying vanity we do ourselves no good. It is the want of interest in our life which produces it; by filling up that want of interest in our life we can alone remedy it . . . . out of suffering may come the cure. Better have pain than paralysis! A hundred struggle and drown in the breakers. One discovers the new world. But rather, ten times rather, die in the surf, heralding the way to that new world than stand idly on the shore! . . . Passion, intellect, moral activity—these three have never been satisfied in a woman. In this cold and oppressive conventional atmosphere, they cannot be satisfied. To say more on this subject would be to enter into the whole history of society, of the present state of civilization. (Nightingale, 1859; cited in Strachey, 1928, pp. 396–398)

From Nightingale's essay, resurrected in the 1970s, we glimpse a woman who had a profound sense of the dilemma of female existence. Since *Cassandra* was privately distributed to only a few, Nightingale's passionate advocacy of a way to the "new world" was little known. In her most widely disseminated publication, *Notes on Nursing: What It Is, and What It Is Not* (1859), Nightingale did not engage in feminist analysis, but asserted the importance of educating women and affirmed an educated female approach to health matters: "It is often said by men, that it is unwise to teach women anything about these laws of health, because they will take to physicking" (p. 108). This "amateur [and] . . . reckless physicking" is, however, "what the really experienced and observing nurse does *not* do; she neither physics herself nor others" (pp. 108–109). Cultivating the health education of nurses, mothers, and governesses did away with "amateur physicking" and relieved physicians' work.

Nightingale espoused health education for all classes of women while recognizing that men held medical authority. In a society in which women were legally subordinate, it is difficult to see how she could have established the legitimacy of women's work without adroit manipulation of the prevailing system of beliefs. She admitted that some women misused drugs given by physicians and advised that "by far the safest plan is to send for 'the doctor'" because some "ladies who both gave and took physic, . . . would not take the pains to learn the names of the commonest medicines" (p. 109). Moreover, there were "excellent" women who, observing sickness in their neighbors, would obtain a prescription for themselves from a physician and then give it to their friends and neighbors. However, just as one is prepared to condemn Nightingale for elitist obedience to physicians and for denigration of women, these simplistic interpretations are modified by her subsequent recommendations:

Now, instead of giving medicine, of which you cannot possibly know the exact and proper application, nor all its consequences, would it not be better if you were to persuade and help your poorer neighbors to remove the dung-hill from before the door, to put in a window which opens, or an Arnott's ventilator, or to cleanse and lime-wash the cottages? Of these things the benefits are sure. The benefits of the inexperienced administration of medicines are by no means so sure. (p. 109)

Nightingale even went so far as to recommend homeopathy, since the principles were comparatively sound and would cause no harm. As a further example, she condemned the common error of taking "aperients" to achieve daily bowel movements, but then, *after giving her own opinion*, she deflected criticism by saying this was the physician's area of expertise and suggesting that women give no aperients without consulting a physician. She then made it unnecessary to do this by recommending that women regulate bowel movements by diet. Deficiencies of meat or vegetables could cause constipation, but "Home made brown bread will oftener cure it than anything else" (p. 109). Thus, Nightingale acknowledged medical authority but then withdrew the need for it since much of health care required no medical intervention. However, women themselves said "they cannot know anything of the laws of health, or what to do to preserve their children's health, because they can know nothing of 'Pathology,' or cannot 'dissect'" (p. 110). To Nightingale, this represented a confusion of ideas: "Pathology teaches the harm that disease has done. But it teaches nothing more. We know nothing of the principle of health, the positive of which pathology is the negative, except from observation and experience. It is often thought that medicine is the curative process. It is no such thing; medicine is the surgery of functions, as surgery proper is that of limbs and organs" (p. 110). To Nightingale, medicine did nothing more than assist nature by removing obstructions. In contrast, nursing places the patient in the best condition for nature's action. However, some women think "fresh air, and quiet and cleanliness extravagant, perhaps dangerous, luxuries . . . and medicine . . . the panacea" (p. 110). Medicine as a panacea, said Nightingale, is an illusion. Once again, she credited medical knowledge, but subordinated it to more general principles, ones that she urged women to act on.

Nightingale cautioned against the common idea among men and even women that a woman disappointed in love or incapable of other things could be turned into a good nurse. Popular writers, she said, invented ladies "fresh out of the drawing-room" who seek wounded lovers in war-hospitals, and finding them, abandon the sick-ward; these women were even extolled as "heroines" of nursing. Nightingale denied these stereotypes, claiming that the management of large wards and hospitals were matters of "sufficient importance and difficulty to require learning by experience and careful inquiry. . . . They do not come by inspiration to the lady disappointed in love, nor to the poor workhouse drudge hard up for a livelihood" (p. 111).

Nightingale concluded her *Notes on Nursing* by referring to nursing pioneer, Elizabeth Frye, and earnestly urged her sisters

To keep clear of both the jargons now current everywhere (for they are equally jargons); of the jargon, namely, about the "rights" of women, which urges women to do all that men do, including the medical and other professions, merely because men do it, and without regard to whether this is the best that women can do; and of the jargon which urges women to do nothing that men do, merely because they are women, and should be "recalled to a sense of their duty as women," and because "this is women's work," and "that is men's," and "these are things which women should not do," which is all assertion and nothing more. Surely woman should bring the best she has, *whatever* that is, to the work of God's world, without attending to either of these cries. For what are they, both of them, the one *just* as much as the other, but listening to the "what people will say," to opinion, to the "voices from without"? And as a wise man has said, no one has ever done anything great or useful by listening to the voices from without. You do not want the effect of your good things to be, "How wonderful for a woman!" Nor would you be deterred from good things, by hearing it said, "Yes, but she ought not to have done this, because it is not suitable for a woman." But you want to do the thing that is good, whether it is "suitable for a woman" or not. It does not make a thing good, that it is remarkable that a woman should have been able to do it. Neither does it make a thing bad, which would have been good had a man done it, that it has been done by a woman. Oh, leave these jargons, and go your way straight to God's work, in simplicity and singleness of heart. (pp. 111–112)

What is to be made of these assertions? On one level, Nightingale espoused a radical feminist critique: gender is not and should not be central to the identity and work of any person. Women and men are not to be defined by anything other than their individual efforts to do the best they can, to do the right thing for themselves and humanity. On another level, Nightingale seemed to deny the legitimacy of organized political action that would crack the sexist structures that restricted women to a limited sphere. Yet Nightingale herself was capable of very sophisticated political action that did, indeed, weaken the sexist conventions limiting women's roles and actions. What is the underlying structure of thought that produced these seeming contradictions? The answer: a mystical understanding of the fundamental identity, the essential *oneness* of all creation, which Nightingale combined with the duty to act on "the good," the essential quality of the universal essence as she understood this from her own mystical experience, the inner voice from which she directed her life.

It is a common misunderstanding that the mystic is a dreamer removed from life. The opposite is more often the case: a person in touch with a more fundamental reality feels called to act with compassion toward others whose lives can be rescued from darkness and misery. In this sense, Nightingale could not be attached to any "ism" because she understood that all "isms," even feminism and humanism, were only partial perceptions of the fundamental unity of humanity. Her theoretical base went beyond the language of civil libertarianism. Her followers, however, too often misconstrued her basic theoretical position, leading to a variety of conflicting interpretations of her philosophy and motivations. Nightingale, herself, was at times inconsistent in her expression of her mystical theoretical understanding. This also contributes to the confusion among her interpreters.

THE CHANGING MORAL ICONOGRAPHY
OF FLORENCE NIGHTINGALE

From the historical consideration of this influential woman, we find paradox: Nightingale, as the image of woman and nurse, and as a symbol of female strength, is used to simultaneously constrict and expand the strength of subsequent generations of women as nurses. A paradoxical, complicated imagery of Nightingale sustains over time, producing several themes in the iconography of this complex woman.

For example, Ray Strachey (1928) discussed the "prison house of home" and Florence Nightingale's relation to the earlier women's movement. On the ascendance to power of young Queen Victoria in 1837, Florence Nightingale, at 17, was a contemporary of outspoken feminists such as Harriet Martineau, Harriet Taylor, and John Stuart Mill, and literary figures like Charlotte Bronte, who was 21, and Marianne Evans (George Elliot), only 18. Joining in their revolt against women's cramped and guarded lives, Nightingale struggled "against the restrictions and limitations of young ladyhood [with] the same passionate force which enabled her in later life to carry out her magnificent achievements" (Strachey, 1928, p. 19). As Strachey noted, Nightingale, from her early life, believed herself to have a true vocation, a call from God. Saying little about her goals, she continued to move toward her mission in life, surprising and shocking everyone with her intention to become a nurse, which was considered worse than being a kitchen maid. Her opportunity came when the Crimean War broke out in the winter of 1853.

Strachey considered Nightingale to be a feminist of sorts, noting that Nightingale signed petitions and believed in women's suffrage, because "it is the first principle or axiom that every householder or taxpayer should have a voice" (p. 24). However, she frankly admitted that she did not expect much would be gained from enfranchisement. As Strachey stated, "even while she fought like a tiger for professional status for her nurses, she grew desperately impatient with the inefficiency and lack of mental power she so often met with among women; and did not hesitate to say so" (p. 24). In a letter to feminist Harriet Martineau, Nightingale declared: "I am brutally indifferent to the rights and wrongs of my sex" (p. 24).

It is clear that this complex woman fought successfully for the rights of women in the healing arts, struggled valiantly to make a vocation, a calling, for women in nursing; it is equally clear that she understood the severe constraints placed on females and yet she, at times, was a severe critic of women. Although fundamentally supportive, she was not active in, and even at times, was antagonistic to the feminist revolt of her period. It is this legacy of dedication to the profession, distress over the triviality and constraints on women's lives, expressing support for, but at times antipathy to, some of the proponents of organized feminism that has left a significant mark on the nursing profession.

There were other aspects of Nightingale's character that were not so well known, but had a significant impact on her life. Sir Edward Cook (1914) focused on the mystical, spiritual aspect of Nightingale: "'I do entirely and constantly believe that the *religious motive* is essential for the highest kind of nurse'" (p. 272). Cook stressed Nightingale's increasingly fixed purpose of caring for the sick, quoting from her diary: " 'The longer I live, the more I feel as if all my being was gradually drawing to one point, and if I could be permitted to return and accomplish that in another being, if I may not in this, I should need no other heaven' " (p. 19).

It is not easy to understand the enormous difficulties that stood in Nightingale's way, like the strenuous objections made on moral and social grounds that nursing work was unworthy of an educated woman. Cook also emphasized Nightingale's decision to remain unmarried: " 'I could not satisfy this nature by spending a life with him in making society and arranging domestic things. . . . To be nailed to a continuation and exaggeration of my present life, without hope of another, would be intolerable to me' " (p. 34). Cook noted that after meditating on what marriage means and deciding against it, Nightingale said, " 'I must strive after a better life for woman' " (p. 36).

Paradoxically, while striving for a better life for women and insisting on a woman's vocation as central to a woman's culture, Nightingale was not supportive of the move to make nursing a "profession." On the question of registration of nurses, a move toward professional autonomy in the view of many of her day, Nightingale wrote to the probationer nurses in the school she founded at St. Thomas' Hospital in London in 1888: "We hear a good deal now-a-days about Nursing being made a 'profession.' Rather, it is not the question for *me*: '*Am I* living up to my 'profession?' " (Nightingale, 1888; cited in *International Nursing Review*, 1971, p. 4). She continued: "Now, there is a danger in the air of becoming Parasites in Nursing (and also Midwifery)—of our being Nurses (and Midwives) by deputy—a danger now when there is so great an inclination to make School and College education, all sorts of Sciences and Arts, even Nursing and Midwifery—a profession, in the low, not the high sense of the word" (p. 5). It is clear that Nightingale wished to sustain the best from the culture of women by emphasizing nursing as a calling, believing that professionalization, by deputy, would denigrate nursing and eliminate the autonomy she strived to achieve. It is equally clear that her deep spirituality—not to be confused with an identification with organized religion—demanded a sense of "calling" to do the right thing, not the bureaucratic or even professionally "correct" thing.

In contrast to Cook's balanced, thorough, and mostly positive analysis of Nightingale, Lytton Strachey's (1918) *Eminent Victorians* mocked and debunked Nightingale and other prominent 19th-century figures. According to historian John Halperin (1980), the post–World War I generation was weary of the bungling and blundering of their wartime leaders and accepted too easily the inaccuracies, imagined details, and disinterest in political history that Strachey held in common with others of the Bloomsbury group, young intellectuals who rejected the Victorianism of their predecessors. However, Virginia Woolf, Bloomsbury feminist thinker, in her essay, "The Art of Biography," claimed that Strachey had succeeded in treating biography as a craft, but "failed when he treated it as an art" (p. 434). To her, biography imposes conditions based on fact that can be verified by others. The historian cannot, as Strachey had done, invent facts as an artist invents them, and then combine them with facts verifiable by others. As Halperin notes, Strachey's talk about history as art is "palaver" since he wrote history as "polemic" and focused "too much on personality and too little on the outside forces shaping personality" (p. 435). As a part of the negative destruction of the past, the First World War, nevertheless, forced a "shift in scale" and the young, postwar generation focused on their differences from their progenitors.

Lytton Strachey's view of Nightingale, despite its inaccuracies, has had a long-term, negative impact. Halperin claims that Strachey "used those aspects of her character he found repellent to illustrate characteristics of the age he abhorred" (p. 439). What Halperin does not say is that Strachey's attack was sexist and similar to those of other men who have trivialized women writers, activists, professionals, and leaders over several centuries (Spender, 1983). Strachey attacked Nightingale for her repression of erotic feelings, for her indifference to human relationships, and created "a sort of Amazon whose humanitarianism was based on a system rather than real feeling, whose sexual instinct became sublimated in good works" (p. 439). Halperin concludes that Strachey's distortions turned a 19th-century epic into a 20th-century mock-epic: "Florence Nightingale *was* a great woman; in Strachey's hands she appears less great than eccentric" (p. 440). His factual and sexist inaccuracies create a little girl who, he claimed, nursed her dolls; this she did not do. To Strachey, Nightingale was, as a woman, "demonic, a megalomaniac whose psychosis took the form of a desire to heal all of mankind" (p. 440).

To achieve this interpretation of "possession," Strachey claimed that Nightingale's hospital orderlies in the Crimea were miserable, convalescent soldiers, when, in fact, they were able-bodied noncommissioned officers. He stated that Nightingale appointed herself "purveyor of clothing," but she did not do this. He claimed her report on the Crimean War made her the "leading authority" on army administration; in fact, the document was privately published and little read (p. 440). According to one authority (Holroyd, 1980), Strachey reconfigurated Nightingale as " 'a female Dr. Jekyll and Mr. Hyde . . . a schizophrenic monster . . . a saintly crusader . . . at the next a satanic personality, resorting to sardonic grins, pantomime gestures and sudden fits of wild fury' " (p. 440). Halperin concludes that Strachey made Nightingale into "a symbol of the Victorian matriarchy that, he felt, emasculated men and bred neuroses—an embodiment of the woman who sublimates her sexual feelings in her pursuit of power over men" (p. 441). Presumably, her excessive demands for reform and action "murdered" Sidney Herbert and Arthur Clough; this claim is, according to Halperin, simply absurd. In both cases, the facts are fabricated to the extent that Strachey did not even name his prime ministers correctly for the periods involved! Strachey claimed that Nightingale lay for 50 years in a "dark stuffy room" with "hundreds of dignitaries" patiently waiting downstairs for an audience with her, but her biographers agree that her rooms were "painted white . . . always light and airy," and had large windows that faced south (p. 441).

Is it any wonder that nurses and women in general have had a difficult time in this century sorting out who their foremother really was? Yet nurses have, themselves, sometimes without in-depth knowledge, created different pictures of Nightingale according to their own needs.

When feminism was strong in the early 1900s, an editorial in the *American Journal of Nursing* (*AJN*) credited Nightingale with creating a new profession and reducing the death rate of the British army. Yet the chief reason for her "immortal distinction" went beyond these achievements to "her declared and reiterated explanation of *how* and how *only*, this was possible to her, and would alone be possible to her successors" (*AJN*, 1908, p. 333). Yet few people

pierced to the spring of that current which she set in motion . . . [and] ignore absolutely her basic principle. . . . The undivided control of nurses in all that relates to their teaching, training, and discipline must lie in the hands of women, themselves trained, and occupying positions of undisputed authority within the limits assigned to them. Medical orders for the patients do not lie within these limits; they are external to them. For physicians, or male secular authorities, to control the training of nurses, is, in her own words, "fatal to discipline." It is extraordinary that this first essential, viz., that women should be, in matters of discipline, under a woman, should need to be advocated at all. But so it is. (p. 333)

From the larger societal viewpoint, the brilliant essence of Nightingale's whole work lay in taking from men's hands "a power that did not logically or rightly belong to them, but which they had usurped, and seizing it firmly in her own, from whence she passed it on to her pupils and disciples. In this she was a glorious and successful revolutionary" (pp. 333–334).

When Nightingale's principles were accepted, nursing had made wonderful progress, but when ignored, conditions continued as bad as ever or declined: "This is not a petulant expression of revolt, though the lay nursing journals, will probably call it such. It is simply a plain statement of fact . . . easily verified . . . by inspect[ing] the hospitals of Southern Germany, Austria, Italy, and certain portions of France, where there has always been complete male control" (p. 334). Examples are given of physicians' efforts to deprive matrons of their rightful positions of authority in England and to disallow American nurses sufficient time for training, study, and rest. The preference for untrained attendants of former days was "openly declared by men whose genuine motive is a fear that nurses as a body are becoming too independent" (p. 335). Sham schools were flooding the market with half-trained women and untrained attendants; "male encroachment" into respectable schools was occurring, along with the denial of state registration of nurses. The *AJN* editor concluded: "If the women of our profession are timid they should remember that reaction is to be expected, but it should always be resisted, or it will drown progress and compel future generations to go through the whole painful struggle again" (p. 335). Clearly, the editor's knowledge of Nightingale was sufficient to support the accuracy of these assertions. Nightingale's most revolutionary act some 50 years previously was a seizure of power from men, returning nursing to women. There was no doubt in this editorial that Nightingale was a feminist leader.

But what of the future generations? Some 50 years later, in the conservative 1950s, British nurse tutor Evelyn C. Pearce (1954) considered the influence of Nightingale on nursing, saying that she had permanently stamped her own personality and ideals on the profession and that these had become the Spirit of Nursing. Gone was the image of a feminist Nightingale, who fought for and obtained power for women. Instead, Nightingale was depicted in childhood as seizing "every possible opportunity to tend the sick and care for tiny babies and old people" (p. 20). True selflessness was essential to Nightingale, said Pearce, and the source of her inspiration was nature, from which she "strove to understand the Meaning of Beauty" (p. 20) and its influence on life.

To Pearce, Nightingale was concerned with goodness, deeply examining her own conscience; introspective, often thinking of what could be done for others to the exclusion of herself; spiritual, needing close communion with God; mindful of the miseries of the world, desiring to relieve distress. She was a fragile, gentle lady, who became overnight a thoroughly efficient organizer; compassionate with patients, but ruthless against military red tape and indomitable in administration. The Lady with the Lamp, whose influence on suffering soldiers was almost unbelievable, she was also stoic and confident. Obliterating forever the vision of the intemperate and incompetent nurse, Nightingale was the "embodiment of the Sermon on the Mount" (p. 22). To Pearce, the Spirit of Nursing was strengthened by acts of devotion and sacrifice, which revived the Lady with the Lamp, whose true light was within her. Obviously, the question of feminism was, to Pearce, simply irrelevant to her portrayal of the Nightingale image.

It was not until ten years later that the first clear statement of the varied uses of Nightingale as a moral icon emerged. Elvi Whittaker and Virginia Olesen (1964) were two of the first contemporary nurse scholars to recognize and discuss the faces of Florence Nightingale as related to the functions of the heroine legend in the occupational subculture of nursing. They noted that Nightingale was still seen by some nurses as a symbol of the stereotyped "frail, delicate creature, dedicated and self-abnegating, moving alone, and at night, among rows of wounded and dying men" (p. 124), holding in her hand the symbol of strength, a lamp. However, a second picture painted of Nightingale depicted her as a fierce advocate for increasing the occupational status of nursing. Clearly, in the sacred imagery, the split between traditional and nontraditional gender roles for women is apparent and affects the perception of Nightingale.

Peculiarly, Nightingale was not the first recognized nurse, nor the founder of the first school of nursing, nor even the first "trained" nurse. Presumably, Nightingale's refusal to become deeply involved in the women's movement of the day made it possible for her to be used as an image of nursing, because it induced few cultural role strains that would negate the Victorian image of the self-sacrificing mother. From their research, Whittaker and Olesen noted that Nightingale was perceived by faculty and students in a traditional, hospital-based school of nursing as an indoctrinator and value-bearer, identified as "a nice young girl, dedicated and ambitious, working beyond the call of duty, a hard worker" (p. 128). However, in a university-based school of nursing she was seen as a widely educated woman, whose main contributions were the development of vital statistics, political power, and concerns related to administration. To the authors, nursing students, whether in hospital or university nursing programs, were given the idea that they could be nurses while still embracing all the female virtues of "femininity" as expressed in the traditional Nightingale image.

A decade later, offering still another interpretation, Jean Nelson (1976) claims it is "impossible not to smile at her stress on *intelligent* obedience to the doctor, . . . and the way in which she values thought in nurses above kindness and mere devotion to duty" (p. 40). Still, Nelson concludes, "Some of us imagine that we are sick of Florence Nightingale, when, in fact, we have never read nor heard from the lady's own pen; perhaps we are just tired of the image of her passed down to us" (p. 41). Thus, by the 1970s, the nonfeminist, traditional female image of Nightingale still prevailed. Though this image had gained ascendancy, it was no longer acceptable in the new feminist era, and Nelson advises nurses to go back and find out who Nightingale really was.

This is exactly what the Feminist Press did in 1979 when they published Nightingale's little known essay *Cassandra*, with an introduction by Myra Stark. Who, asks Stark, was Nightingale? The ministering angel, the haloed lady with the lamp, the ideal image of the tender, nurturing female? These sacred images, now attached to the profession she created, are not the full truth—the reality is quite different. To Stark, nursing, as Nightingale herself wrote, was not the most important function. Nightingale's accomplishments were more the result of "her concern with diet and dirt and drains, her understanding of sanitation and its relation to mortality, her ability to organize, to lead, to get things done" (p. 1). Her horror of the incompetence and criminal negligence of the Army Medical Corps and the War Office led to major reforms of the Army Medical Services, the living conditions of the British army, hospital construction and administration, sanitation, and even irrigation in India. Indeed, "she directed the purification of the Madras water system from her bedroom in South Street, London" (p. 2).

Stark recognizes that Nightingale encompassed in her lifetime many accomplishments, any one of which would have occupied the entire lifetime of one individual: the founding of the Nightingale School and Home for Nurses at St. Thomas' Hospital and the Training School for Midwives at King's College Hospital; the creation of a respectable, new profession for women when they had few alternatives for a decent livelihood; the founding of district and workhouse nursing; the expansion of public health services; the use of statistics to categorize diseases and to develop hospital accounting systems. Although Nightingale embodied the essence of Victorian femininity, to live for others, Stark says, "the real self-sacrifice for her . . . would have been to stay home, marry, and lead the life of a wealthy woman" (p. 3). She chose to become one of the "odd" women, the "redundant" women, an active doer in the world, not the inspirer and nurturer in the home. This, says Stark, she did despite the rigid sex segregation of the Victorian period; the total male economic power over wives; the complete control by men of wives' assets—property, children, and even women's bodies; the humiliating work of middle-income women; the grinding 12- to 14-hour work days of poor women; the barring of women from universities and professional employment.

As Stark points out, Nightingale did not rebel alone. Her friendships with women—Mary Clarke, Marianne Nicholson, and Hilary Bonham Carter—served as her support. With other women of her class, enforced idleness led her to fear for her sanity: " 'so many of my kind . . . have gone mad for want of something to do' " (p. 8). Nightingale had an intensely spiritual nature; God spoke to her, and called her to service on four occasions at key points in her life. To her, marriage made heroic service impossible: " 'Women don't consider themselves as human beings at all. There is absolutely no God, no country, no duty to them at all, except family' " (p. 9). Marriage of her highly trained nurses she saw as desertion: " 'Oh God, no more love. No more marriage, O God' " (p. 10).

Charitable philanthropy was an accepted woman's outlook, but, as Stark notes, Nightingale spoke contemptuously of women who dabbled in "poor peopling." To Stark, *Cassandra* was Nightingale's protest against the powerlessness of women: "their lack of control over their lives, their subordination to husband and family, their loss of any identity except through personal relationships" (p. 13). The boredom and triviality of women's lives, the waste of their energies and talents was, to Nightingale, a spiritual matter: "the waste of souls, against lives lived without any meaning or purpose" (p. 14). Stark points to Nightingale's choice of the mythological Cassandra, a prophetess cursed by Apollo, "doomed to see and speak the truth, but never to be believed" (p. 23).

Stark concludes that Nightingale would not, in modern terms, be perceived as a feminist; she did not give full support to suffrage and was critical and sometimes contemptuous of women's lives, probably caused in part by her struggle against her mother and sister, who tried to force her to conform to

Victorian feminine standards. Unfortunately, Stark relies on George Pickering's (1974) *Creative Malady*, in which Nightingale's invalidism following the Crimean War is seen as a psychoneurosis with a purpose—to isolate herself from her family. It is difficult to diagnose neuroses in any usual way in a woman who produced over 200 books, pamphlets, and reports and more than 12,000 letters. Nightingale simply goes beyond such superficial ideation and explanation.

Whether Nightingale was a feminist has remained a debatable issue. Muriel Skeet (1980), in her thematic conclusion to the republished *Notes on Nursing*, focuses on Nightingale's concern for the health care of women. For example, in 1871 Nightingale published her *Introductory Notes on Lying-in Institutions* in which her statistical evidence proved many obstetrical wards to be "pest-houses"; she emphasized the importance of isolation and extreme cleanliness, and furnished model rules, plans, and specifications for lying-in institutions. As Skeet notes, Nightingale urged the importance of training schools and pleaded for midwifery as a career for educated women. In a letter addressed to "Dear Sisters," she wrote: " 'There is a better thing for women to be than 'medical men' and that is to be medical women' " (p. 104). Nightingale was concerned about children's and women's health and their careers, but Skeet concludes that it is by no means certain that Nightingale would support today's women's liberation movement. Nevertheless, she did write in a letter to John Stuart Mill, in response to his invitation to join the National Society for Woman's Suffrage, founded in 1867, " 'that women should have the suffrage, I think that no one can be more deeply convinced than I. It is so important for a woman to be a person' " (p. 105). But realistically and accurately, she continued, " 'it will be years before you obtain the suffrage for women. And in the meantime there are evils which press much more hardly on women than the want of the suffrage' " (p. 105). However, as Skeet notes, Nightingale did join the Society a year later and allowed her name to be placed on the General Committee in 1871; seven years later she sent a written statement for publication.

In contrast to other researchers, Skeet, as a nurse, believes that Nightingale, who regretted not having had an opportunity for formal training, strongly supported women's education as essential to leadership. In nurses' education, Nightingale's mystical theory influenced her in her insistence on character training, on goodness. It is in this context that her statement, " 'To be a good nurse, one must be a good woman, or one is truly nothing but a tinkling bell' " (p. 109), must be placed. The more usual interpretation focuses on her need to differentiate nurses from the drunken, immoral "Sairey" Gamp of Dicken's imagination. While this is probably true, it is an insufficient explanation of Nightingale's understanding of and insistence on "goodness."

The debate on Nightingale's attitudes toward women continued in the 1980s. Nurse Florence T. Smith (1981) sees Nightingale as an early feminist, extolling her as a 20th-century woman in her ideas about nurses, their training, women's "place" and social class in nursing. Smith notes that Nightingale, classically educated by her father, became discontented with the passive woman's role in which " 'vacuity and boredom . . . are sugared over by false sentiment' " (p. 1021). Of women entering the workforce, Nightingale said, " 'I would say to all young ladies . . . called to any particular vocation, qualify yourselves for it as a man does for his work' " (p. 1021). According to Smith, the Crimean experience proved to Nightingale the need for education. After reducing the mortality rate in six months from 42% to 2%, Nightingale realized that some "gentlewomen" were not fit for demanding hospital work. " 'They flit about like angels without hands, and soothe souls while they leave bodies dirty and neglected' " (p. 1022). She scorned the prevailing conceptions of nursing, of the middle-aged woman "tamed" by having had a family: " 'No *man*, not even a doctor, ever gives any other definition of what a nurse should be than this—'devoted and obedient.' This definition would do just as well for a porter. It might even do for a horse' " (p. 1022). She stressed that nursing was the skilled servant of medicine, surgery, and hygiene, but not of physicians, surgeons, or health officers.

To Smith, Nightingale's concept of classlessness is illustrated in her acceptance of half of her students from lower income groups, subsidized by the Nightingale Fund, while the other half, from upper classes, paid tuition: " 'I have seen somewhere in print that nursing is a profession to be followed by the 'lower middle class.' . . . Why limit class at all? Or shall we say that God is only to be served in His sick by the 'lower middle class' " (p. 1023). Note once again that Nightingale's theoretical base derives from a mystical understanding of the unity of all life.

This point is not made by Smith, whose definition of Nightingale as feminist rests on what she was able to achieve for women in nursing and for their patients. Smith concludes that much of the philosophy of nursing—the vital role of public health nursing, the independence of nursing education from service, the administration of nursing education by nurses, the concern for accurate observations, good nutrition, therapeutic environments, preventive health care, nursing the patient, not the illness—are all derived from Nightingale. But are these signs of a *feminist* consciousness, or an enactment of values basic to a traditional women's culture? Peculiarly, the act of a woman wresting control of nursing from physicians, Lavinia Dock's major point, is not considered by Smith.

It is fascinating to see the differences in how women inside and outside nursing portray Nightingale. However, there is often one similarity: the exclusion of Nightingale's partially successful power play to wrest direct control of nursing from men. This fact is also missing in what is now a classic by Elaine Showalter (1981). In contrast to Smith, Showalter states that "Historians have often had to admit sadly that Florence Nightingale could not be counted among the great English feminists" (p. 395). Many concur with Ray Strachey that Nightingale had an " 'incomplete and easily exhausted sympathy with the organized Women's Movement'" (p. 395). In light of new developments in women's history, Showalter claims that new conclusions are possible. She concedes that Nightingale was relentlessly upper class in her reliance on money, privilege, and personal connections; that she was intellectually arrogant in her rejection of emotions and values of ordinary women; that she despised her mother and sister for fighting her efforts to gain independence and enter nursing. But, as Showalter notes, Nightingale seriously questioned the fundamental organization of family life, scoffed at the inflated virtues of motherhood and daughterhood, and criticized the sexism of the English church—institutions more formidable and resistant to change than Parliament. To Showalter, "The suppression of *Suggestions for Thought*, which included her best-known feminist essay, *Cassandra*, is one of the most unfortunate sagas of Victorian censorship of female anger, protest, and passion" (p. 396). Providing a missing link between Mary Wollstonecraft and Virginia Woolf, Nightingale's neglected work has both feminist and spiritual significance.

"A CALL FROM GOD TO BE A SAVIOR": NIGHTINGALE AS VISIONARY MYSTIC AND SPIRITUAL FEMINIST

According to Showalter, the genesis of Nightingale's "peculiar feminism" is found in a turbulent family life in which, as her mother put it, " 'We are ducks who have hatched a wild swan'" (p. 396). At age six, Nightingale considered herself a shameful anomaly, not like other people, unable to behave like others. William Nightingale educated both Florence and her sister, Parthenope, but by sixteen, Florence was her father's library companion and Parthenope was her mother's companion in the drawing room, where both lived an existence of social ambition, intellectual laziness, and infantile emotionalism—the expected and stereotyped mode of life for Victorian ladies. To Showalter, Nightingale, gifted but thwarted, translated her intellectual and vocational drives into the acceptable language of religion, experiencing the first of four revelations before her seventeenth birthday, when she claimed that God spoke to her, calling her to His service. In this, Showalter sees the feminist yearning for freedom translated into religious language more acceptable for women; however, as she notes, Donald R. Allen (1975), in a psychohistorical interpretation, explains the voices as related to extremely intense emotional and psychological stress, characterized by self-doubt, dissatisfaction, depression, and a sense of failure. Peter T. Cominos (1972) sees female religious ecstasy as an outlet for repressed sexuality. An alternative explanation from research on mysticism is very simply that Nightingale experienced an alternate reality (a common experience over the centuries for many women and men of great genius), but clothed it in the terminology of the day. From this perspective, Nightingale the mystic is exactly what she said she was: a person inspired by the experience of another reality from which she drew the spiritual direction and its applied manifestation in her life.

For the next fifteen years, following her calling, Nightingale unhappily carried out her family and social duties, while her attempts at autonomy were sabotaged by her mother and sister. After refusing marriage and finding her efforts to receive serious training as a nurse blocked, she became deeply depressed. During this time, however, she wrote the ambitious three-volume work *Suggestions for Thought to Seekers After Religious Truth* (1860), which would "justify the laws of God" to working men and women. She attempted in the first volume to create "a new philosophic religion that would combat atheism" (p. 399). In the second volume, the new system of thought was based on her empirical research in religious psychology derived from her practical deductions on her own experience with altered reality or God. The third volume concerned divine law and moral right. *Cassandra* was a memoir related to volume 2 and originally conceived as a problem novel about women. According to Showalter, from Nightingale's private writing during this time, she concluded that she must go forward in her nursing career, but when her family was informed, a violent scene with her mother and sister caused Florence to faint. Nevertheless, she studied at the Kaiserswerth Hospital, subsequently considered joining a Catholic religious order, and began work in two Catholic hospitals run by nursing orders. Nightingale's sister retaliated by having a complete nervous breakdown; Parthenope was advised to break relations with her sister. Florence, who felt she was being devoured, was now allowed to leave home so that her sister, " 'the Devouree might recover health and balance which had been lost in the process of devouring' " (p. 400).

From this circumstance, Florence derived a permanent annual allowance from her father and later took a nursing superintendent's position. In 1852 she experienced her second revelation, " 'a call from God to be a savior' " (p. 400). In 1854 she left with 38 nurses for Scutari in the Crimea. Even after she became a heroine, her mother and sister continued their demands. This "lifelong contest," according to Showalter, scarred Nightingale and made it impossible for her to adopt a "model of feminist consciousness" that today is "based on the premise that full reconciliation with one's own mother and sisters is fundamental to personal and political authenticity" (p. 401). Nightingale believed that children should be brought up in well-managed child-care centers or "creches," and felt that she had " 'expended more motherly feeling and action in a week than my mother has expended for me in thirty-seven years' " (p. 402).

Showalter seems to accept Allen's argument that by choosing nursing, " 'with all of its outer-directed and masochistic implications,' " Nightingale could " 'absorb her fury, satisfy her drive for power,' " and presumably " 'placate her extremely strong superego' " by aiding others in God's name (p. 402). This peculiar interpretation of nursing as masochistic and outer-ordered becomes even more problematic when connected to subordinated power and the superego. How would nursing, presumably outer-directed and masochistic, allow Nightingale's strong ego to be fulfilled in a drive for power? The contradictions in such an analysis are obvious, as is the stereotyping of nursing on which they depend.

Showalter's interpretation of Nightingale allows us to understand her conflicting feelings as derived from her mother's obstructions, but at the same time reduces Nightingale's greatness as understandable only in the narrow terms of the old Freudian paradigm of id, ego, and superego. To explain Nightingale's greatness in such terms is to demean the altruism, the brilliance, the spirituality, and the genius of this exceptional woman. To understand Nightingale's theory of a rational mysticism, one has to deal with Showalter's assertion that Nightingale rejected an androgynous Jesus; in fact, Nightingale stated that the next Christ might be female. It is far more likely that Nightingale saw mystically the centrality, not of a strong, masculine God, but of a spiritual force of which the Christ spirit was only a manifestation. And it is equally likely that her command to be a savior was derived from the essence of the alternative reality, the joyous unity described by so many mystics before and since Nightingale.

From this perspective, the choice of nursing was not a form of masochism, nor a fulfillment of a drive for worldly power, but a genuinely altruistic endeavor. It follows, is consistent and logical, that Nightingale's rebellion against the sexist restrictions on women would be a necessity; thus, her feminism would also flow naturally from the unity, the equality of all things in "God" or the universal matrix of meaning in which no thing or person, male or female, is subordinated. One must grasp the essence of the experience of alternate reality to understand Nightingale's feminism, because her basic theory derives from her inner voices, certainly clothed in conventional God imagery, and not from external political thought systems.

If, as Showalter claims, the emergence of Victorian interests in sisterhoods, Anglican or Catholic, is also the first sign of incipient feminism, then Nightingale's interest in finding a way to express herself in a women's religious community would have offered one of the few traditionally acceptable paths for her rebellion. But it is inaccurate to interpret Nightingale's sophisticated differentiation between spirituality and religiosity in the simple terms of mother rejection. Showalter quotes Nightingale as saying that the Church of England was an "idle mother," offering only homilies, giving neither work to do nor education for it (p. 405). To equate Nightingale's rejection of Mother Church with her rejection of her own mother is to deny Nightingale's assertion that she would have given her head, heart, and hand, but the Church would not have them because it did not know what to do with them. Obviously, the Church of England would not know what to do with a rebellious and questioning daughter, particularly one who was a visionary mystic and whose understanding of spirituality extended beyond the homilies of organized, patriarchal religion. In this sense, such an organization *is* like a mother; both parent and church become moral only when the children or members are allowed intellectual and spiritual inquiry.

Nightingale viewed the Roman Catholic Church as " 'an over-busy mother' " (p. 405), who imprisons, reads letters, penetrates thoughts, and regulates every hour. While it is true that female mother images are used, it is likely that Florence the mystic is reflecting on the fate of mystics such as St. Joan when she concludes that the Church " 'burnt us if we had been thinking wrong' " (p. 405). Commonly, not mothers, but the Church, referred to as female or Mother Church by everyone, burns its children. Surely, Nightingale could and did make this distinction in her thoughts. She obviously knew what could happen to rebellious women and to female mystics.

Showalter concludes it was inconceivable for Nightingale, who struggled to escape from a family ruled by mother and sister, to have lived in a sisterhood with her unresolved ambiguities of feeling toward women. It is highly probable that after her battle to be free, "she could not submit to the will of others" (p. 405). While this is probably true, it is equally true that in the usual mystical experience the " 'thought of God' " did not, as Nightingale said, involve people acting like dead bodies " 'surrendering up the whole being to the superior' " (p. 405).

While affirming Nightingale's powerful individualistic feminism, Showalter states that Nightingale's experiences with religious sisterhood were disastrous, that she was unable to trust other women, that she engaged in her writing in feverish outbursts against some women, that she turned to men to present and carry out her plans, that she submitted her *Suggestions for Thought* to male rather than female intellectuals. Benjamin Jowett was unlikely to sympathize with Nightingale's "originality of religious thought, pungent forthrightness of expression, and explicit angry feminism" (p. 407). And, indeed, he modified, subdued, reorganized, and eliminated her anger, asking her to soften her antagonisms and fondly advising her against publication.

Given her mystical experience, it would probably have been difficult for her to find anyone, male or female, who also had such experiences, or who would publicly admit to having them. Certainly, spiritual feminists would have been no more likely to have shared experiences of alternate realities with her or the public. Nightingale's critique of both Roman Catholic and Anglican doctrine made her, according to Showalter, "a heretic . . . by any conventional religious standards" (p. 408). Indeed, from the mystical viewpoint, religions too often exclude the spiritual in which the full development of strengths and abilities requires the freedom for all, regardless of gender, to achieve their best. In short, the mystical theoretical position embraces a fundamental, even absolute, equality in the essential unity of all being.

Nightingale, as spiritual feminist, evoked a God who gives freedom, not self-denial, to do the best, to learn the right, then to do what we like, to have all of one's abilities brought to light, so as to achieve harmony and contentment in human existence. To achieve this absolute equality of opportunity to be all one can be, marriage and family roles would have to change; Nightingale envisioned a commune with "'all ages and both sexes really living and working for each other'" (p. 409).

To Showalter, the image of the prophetess Cassandra, doomed to predict and express truth without being heard, emerged from Nightingale's understanding that "women must be shocked into an awareness of their own anger and frustration . . . must risk pain in order to grow" (p. 410). Nightingale said, "'out of nothing comes nothing. But out of suffering may come the cure. . . . Awake, ye women, all ye that sleep, awake'" (pp. 410-411). Clearly, a radical feminism is coupled with a mystical sense of reality. In one sense, Nightingale demanded that women awake from their slumber of servitude; in another, she used the time-honored mystical metaphor of sleep for those who are unaware of another more fundamental state of reality. For example, Plato used the analogy of the viewer of shadows on the cave wall who mistakes these for reality, never going to the cave door to see the light that is the true source of the shadows. Similarly, Nightingale, as mystical feminist, cried to women to awaken both to the true reality in themselves as human and an alternate reality of being. Perhaps then, as Nightingale said, the next messiah *would* be a female savior who understood other levels of consciousness, of meaning. But to complain, to have the "'continual gnawing feeling of the miseries and wrongs of the world'" (p. 411) and not act, creates unheeded altruism that turns into hatred.

According to Showalter, Nightingale believed in women's emancipation, not women's rights. It would probably be more accurate to say that Nightingale was impatient with women who complained, but did not act on injustices, as she herself had done in creating modern nursing, sanitation reform, and a dozen other major innovations. To Showalter, Nightingale never became a feminist leader in her own time, but presents an image of women "who demand freedom from women's culture as much as from women's sphere" (p. 412). Alternatively, one could look to Nightingale as the progenitor of modern feminist spirituality and an activist who tried to create alternatives for compassion in nursing consistent with her understanding of a deeper reality; and who, in Dock's terms, wrested control of nursing from men and placed it in the hands of women.

THE NATURAL LAWS OF UNIFIED BEING

To better understand the theoretical basis of Nightingale's thinking, Nancy Boyd (1982) takes a closer look at Nightingale's *Suggestions for Thought*, which presumably bases its theology on a combination of early church saints and 19th-century rationalists. Clearly, Nightingale was attempting to integrate opposing perspectives in a rational mysticism, and, as Boyd notes, her theoretical position gave her the basis of both her choice of social causes and her methods of procedure: First, Nightingale reflected on God's plan in creation; second, she analyzed evidence of natural laws; third, she chose issues of social importance; and, fourth, she focused on nursing, health, hospital, sanitary, and poor law reforms to help " 'man create mankind' " (p. 197).

Nightingale's notes on the spirituality of mystics are not widely known. As previously mentioned, her three-volume set was privately printed but not published. Boyd is critical of Nightingale's thought because her overall theological argument presumably lacks cohesion, although it does contain some insights that are original and important. Nevertheless, it is clear that Nightingale was not enamored of popular religion, neither Anglicanism nor Roman Catholicism, or of predominant philosophies, neither liberalism nor scientific positivism. Nightingale believed religion focused on denominational affiliations in which expressed beliefs were largely devoid of spirituality as applied to daily life. Twilight belief, or darkness of unbelief, replaced the search for spiritual truth. She deplored a monster God, who would forever torture people in purgatory, who would create beings whose existence came about through no will of their own and whose fate would be, for many, everlasting misery. Similarly, Nightingale deplored atonement to a God, the wrathful Father, who must receive bloody sacrifice. To her, forgiveness is freely given, not based on quid pro quo.

Philosophy also provided inadequate alternatives. Liberalism provided no religion to replace those torn down; gave no sympathy or insight into God and the highest ways of humanity. Liberalism made " 'a great show of enquiry and of power; but there is nothing behind, nothing within, nothing with the principle of life in it; it is all temporary, negative, unreal' " (p. 203). The overt atheism of positivists was simply "disgusting" to Nightingale. Boyd wondered why Nightingale could not see the affinity of their ideas to her own. Was it, Boyd asks, her childhood faith or her dedication to the "God" of the mystics? It is surprising to find this questioned.

If God spoke to Nightingale, she clearly existed in more than one reality and understood the mystical reality. Thus, she did not deny, but used empiricism, love of science, faith in logic, as expressions of the order inherent in the natural laws of unified being. According to Boyd, Nightingale "stubbornly maintained against all comers" (p. 203), but more aptly put, she consistently affirmed her empirical knowledge of other states of reality in her belief that there is a "necessary connection between empirical fact and rational truth . . . [which] originates and derives its universality from God" (p. 203). It should not be surprising that Nightingale attempted to create empirical theology, referring not to supernatural miracle but to universal lawful action. To Nightingale, positivists claimed that everything is lawful, but disclaimed any ability to apprehend a Lawgiver. As a mystical theoretician, Nightingale responded that this is " 'not only not true but is absolutely absurd—the fact being that we have *no one* more *intimately* present to (everyone of) us or more constantly present than God'" (p. 204).

Nightingale asserted that there is increasing evidence of lawful order, of a perfect Being, and that we are continuously approaching to perfection. This, she claimed, was no less a metaphysical assertion than the positivists' formula of the metaphysical. "'Metaphysical is,'" she said, "'*What I think*'" (p. 205). Obviously, Nightingale had gone beyond a two-dimensional or even three-dimensional world and attempted to convey the experience of other dimensions to a flat-world people, who could not believe other dimensions existed because they had not engaged in the empirical search of inner being, which was needed to find them. To the multidimensional Nightingale, "'mankind marched towards a vision of perfected humanity'" whereas positivist Auguste Comte's "religion" of "Collective Humanity" was redeemed by no vision (p. 205). Humankind in its sorry state could not be worshiped; it was, she said, "'a collection of 'me's.' Is this what I am to reverence . . . to work for?'" (p. 205). If one life was a disappointed fragment, said Nightingale, then the mass of unfinished lives, without ultimate meaning or purpose, remained a collection of aborted existence.

Boyd states that Nightingale was prepared for systematically investigating the nature of God because, previously, she had set up rigorous systems of evaluation for nursing. This comment might be seen by some as demeaning the intensity of Nightingale's inner struggle to comprehend the universality of all things. Clearly, Nightingale preceded by more than a century current feminist critiques of both science and religion and attempted to find a way out of the traditional patriarchal cosmology. She affirmed omnipotence as power without contradictions; spirit as "'living thought, feeling, purpose, residing in a conscious being'"; love as the "'feeling which seeks . . . the greatest degree and best kind of well-being'" for others; wisdom as the thought by which love is accomplished (p. 206).

Evidence for the existence of a general law, or of the expression of God's thoughts, she discovered in patterns of predictability, the laws of science, and mathematical symmetry—in the natural world from which God cannot be separated. To her, evil was illusory and suffering was only a means toward spiritual perfection. John Stuart Mill objected to Nightingale's view of evil, claiming the species may be ruled by unchanging laws, but these do not necessarily protect the individual: "the suffering of the innocent still stands" (p. 208). Nevertheless, Nightingale saw "no contradiction between the knowledge that the ultimate solution to pauperism lies in social and economic law and the impulse to help the individual pauper" (p. 208). If people are hungry, feed them instead of simply accumulating more knowledge or dismissing hunger as God's will.

Boyd notes that Nightingale's belief in the link between the specific and universal was provided by God; this idea formed the basis for her accumulation of massive numbers of specific facts from which she abstracted generalizations; she used the individual fact as an illustration of a general law. When Nightingale meticulously amassed facts on mortality rates, she then was able to generalize that death was preventable when the rates changed markedly after she introduced sanitary reform. To Nightingale, the laws she uncovered provided an organization that led to power. Similarly, Nightingale's analysis of the relation between architecture and mortality rates proceeded from studying floor plans of individual hospitals in which she found that death rates in maternity wards attached to general hospitals were four times higher than in those housed in separate buildings. From such facts, Nightingale generalized; she found both orderly reason and spiritual significance in the lawful order she uncovered. Nightingale accumulated facts from whatever fields of inquiry were available, extending eventually to include sociology, botany, and economics in her work on sanitary reform in India.

To Nightingale, reforms, for example, of education, poverty, and crime, required the reformer to discover the social cause and the means to alter it. "Mankind," through such acts, creates "mankind"—this is the work, said Nightingale, which God called people to do, to play an extraordinary role in creation: " 'There will be no heaven for me nor for any one else, unless we make it' " (p. 215). Nightingale believed that prayer, a sincere wish to do right, and good intentions were insufficient. "To preach to a man to do right and then 'send him back to the pigsty where he cannot but do wrong is nonsense' " (p. 215). Instead, Nightingale demanded that the pigsty be improved. Many "saviors" were needed—people who learn by the consequences of human errors and "save" others from them.

According to Boyd, Nightingale renounced the joys of ordinary human companionship and chose the solitary route of a savior. True to her mystical understanding, Nightingale rejected the Resurrection and the uniqueness of Christ as the only son of God. To her, there were many saviors, self-giving, and this itself was the key to spirituality—a life of service in accord with one's own nature. In contrast, Nightingale's contemporaries had, according to her, no time left in their schedules for inspiration, for that intercourse so necessary to the mystical contemplative understanding of another reality. This, she observed, was even typical of women, who had no type of such intercourse, no model to follow out of the morass of family obligation that monopolized all their time in lives squandered. To expect daughters to give up their own lives for their parents is, said Nightingale, perversion; daughters have " 'the right to expect that their powers shall be exercised, their lives made worth having, opportunity given them for developing all their faculties' " (p. 219). Michelangelo and Beethoven did not work at odd moments to achieve their goals. People fritter away their power and, "Lacking a larger arena, the imperative to service turns inward" (p. 219). To Nightingale, denial of a serious calling would inevitably lead to spiritual death or madness.

Nightingale believed that mothers were especially captive to the family and home; when overly defined in their maternal roles, they give "undue importance" to children from whom they may receive little sympathy; this, in turn, leads a woman to consider herself a failure, adding guilt to loneliness. Marriage and courtship, too often spent on trivial social expectations, place inequitable requirements on women: "Behind *his* destiny woman must annihilate herself, must be only his complement. A woman dedicates herself to the vocation of her husband; she fills up and performs the subordinate parts in it, in nine cases out of ten. . . . The fact is that woman has so seldom any vocation of her own, that it does not much signify; she has none to renounce. A man gains everything by marriage; he gains a 'helpmate' but a woman does not" (p. 221). As Boyd stresses, this feminist critique is part of Nightingale's theological writing in which she portrays a society that has lost its sense of purpose. A society that encouraged all people to know spiritual laws and enact these would be equally liberating for men and women; but it is to women, Boyd says, that Nightingale directed her message. The core, the heart of Nightingale's feminism was " 'first to infuse the mystical religion into the forms of others' especially among women, and secondly to give them an organization for their activity in which they could be trained to be 'Handmaids of the Lord' " (p. 221). With a conviction of a calling to a life of purpose, women would, according to Nightingale, have the strength to rid themselves of the restrictions of home and family since they, as God's ministers, were equal to and independent of men. Marriage would then occur only as a union of those who shared a true purpose for humankind and God.

To Boyd, Nightingale disappointed feminists in their fight for the vote since "She was concerned with the rule of Almighty God, not with that of a majority opinion that generally paid little attention to the will of God" (p. 222). More accurately stated, it is not the rule of God, but the union with universal being, another level of reality. Boyd claims that Nightingale consciously sought out "the classics of the mystic tradition, borrowing books from Georgiana Moore, copying out fragments on bits of paper for her own guidance and support" (p. 223). She hoped to incorporate the thinking of such women mystics as St. Angela of Foligno, Jane Frances de Chantal, and St. Teresa of Avila, and of gentle men such as St. Francis of Assisi into a volume, *Notes from Devotional Authors of the Middle Ages, Collected, Chosen and Freely Translated by Florence Nightingale.*

The women Nightingale turned to, such as her Aunt Hannah Nicholson, saw an opposition between love of God and love of self; thus, Florence's impetuous spirit, her need to "confront the whole of reality, unswerving honesty, even intellectual abilities" (p. 224)—these gifts came to be seen as sins. According to Boyd, the experience of light and an inner voice, like that of Joan of Arc, brought further ambivalence to Nightingale. Perhaps it would be more accurate to say that Nightingale was purposely blocked by sexist limitations imposed on her, complicated by the very real difficulty of differentiating between her own ego needs and her experience of a different reality. The dark night of the soul is not uncommon to mystical life. A period of severe questioning and uncertainty for Nightingale would have been compounded by her honesty. It is genuinely difficult to know at times whether the inner voice represents one's own wishful thinking or another, more fundamental essence. Of nursing, compassionate work itself, Nightingale said, " 'This is life. Now I know what it is to live and love life' " (p. 226).

In middle age, Nightingale expressed mixed feelings, but continued to regard mysticism as her true vocation; spiritual religion, no matter how imperfectly she lived it, was and always would be enough. Where, she asked, will I find God? The answer? In myself. How to do this? By placing the self in a state for union. When more was known about this state, mysticism would not be a "series of extraordinary emotional events punctuating the long stretches of time when the ordinary and the rational seem to have the upper hand, but a permanent state" (p. 227). To Nightingale, " 'The 'mystical' state is the essence of common sense if it be real; that is, if God be a reality' " (p. 227).

As noted earlier, experience of alternate reality often leads, in the Western tradition, to greater action in the world; thus, mystics such as St. Catherine of Siena, politician, and St. Catherine of Genoa, medical missionary, and St. Teresa of Avila, organizer and administrator, were Nightingale's female models. Boyd claims that Nightingale was within the tradition of church martyrs, but she believed that each person is called to be a savior; in this, she is simply espousing the unity of all, commonly experienced in altered realities. It is probably incorrect to place Nightingale within any traditional church lineage. Her work went beyond those earlier female mystics who were tied to orders; for example, her effort to unify rationality and mysticism, her rejection of formal religion, and her feminist rejection of constricting family roles and stunted development of women. It is not odd, as Boyd thinks, that Nightingale questioned her union in another reality; to the contrary, outside of any conventional religious congregation or order, she needed confirmation that her ego in this reality was not dishonestly replacing the inner sense that went beyond. She established her own criteria: " 'the feeling, approved by the sense of justice, conscience or whatever other faculties we perceive' " (p. 229) combined with evidence from reason. Note the insistence on the integration of emotion and intellect, a recent trend in feminist thinking on women's epistemology (Belenky, 1988).

It is precisely because Nightingale went beyond previous mystics in her lonely quest and because she affirmed equality for women as a necessary condition for a full life that she is important. She accepted self-denial, not self-contempt, although she said that " 'It is much easier for some of us to hate our lives than to love them' " (p. 229). Asceticism, as Nightingale said, is erroneous; to remove worldly enjoyment is a mistake: " 'It should be our enjoyment to do the world's work' " (p. 229). That she fell short of living constantly in the state of grace, the other reality, is not, as Boyd suggests, an indication that she did not love her life, but rather an expression, common to mystics, that she was not able to bring her two realities together in a consistent and harmonious manner. How any woman, fighting against all the sexist restrictions of her age, succeeded as well as she did remains the miracle to be explained. She sounds particularly modern when she says, " 'All is tendency, growth . . . each present mode of being is part of a development from a past without beginning, towards a future without end' " (p. 233). Nightingale shared with her close friend, Hilary Bonham Carter, the sense of the invisible world as she experienced it in nursing: "How one feels that the more real presence in the room is the invisible presence which hovers around the death-bed and that we are only ghosts, who have put on form for a moment, and shall put it off, almost before we have time to wind up our watch" (p. 233).

Without doubt, Boyd gives us the most perceptive modern analysis of Nightingale. Her work has been referred to at length in order to establish the theoretical basis of Nightingale's thought. It is clear that Nightingale's feminism was imbedded in a broader view and that her nursing innovations flowed from both her feminist and mystical understandings of the nature of reality, though little has been written about her in nursing from these perspectives.

In 1986, Marylouise Welch did try to place Nightingale's thinking in the context of the philosophical writings of other intellectuals of the Victorian era—all men (John Stuart Mill, Auguste Comte, Henry Thomas Buckle, and Benjamin Jowett). Welch is particularly interested in the concept of the person in Nightingale's work, but she misses entirely the feminist and the mystical, the two components that distinguished Nightingale's work from those of her male contemporaries. The concept of universal laws existed a priori for Mill, who said such laws were confirmable and could be empirically substantiated. Buckle and Jowett agreed with Nightingale that the general concept of universal laws provided order and predictability to life. Comte thought that natural law passed from theological to metaphysical to positivist, the latter dealing with the world as it is and studying human nature in terms of laws.

To Comte, the person moved away from a belief in God, theism being only a transitory state. On the existence of God and free will, Mill, a self-described rational skeptic, believed in a first cause for laws, but not that this was a God. Only Jowett would agree with Nightingale that universal laws derived from an originator. Welch notes that *Suggestions for Thought* contained Nightingale's philosophy, but *Notes on Nursing* applied her philosophy in which she asked, for example, as a general principle whether all disease was not more or less a reparative process and asserted that the laws of the body were still to be learned.

If natural laws existed a priori, what of free will? Mill's law of necessity allowed for self-improvement. But Nightingale saw natural laws as successive; a person could learn these and, thus, determine the development of his or her life by making free choices, but only through knowledge. Welch does not deal with the mystical in the successive stages, nor does she differentiate, as Nightingale did, the female's choices, given societally imposed restraints.

How does one acquire knowledge? To Mill, it was through the experience and observation of phenomena; thus, empirical methods were needed and to these Nightingale subscribed, criticizing Comte for his positivist belief that repeated facts, never contradicted, could be accepted as true. As Welch points out, Nightingale, as an empiricist, changed this idea to "never contradicted in *human* experience," which for the moment might be true, until some new or different phenomena called for a revision of accepted fact. Thus, she emphasized learning from experience and observation. By studying groups of people, patterns, tendencies, and probabilities would become evident; thus, Nightingale used statistics, as Buckle also recommended, in approaching natural laws. Welch provides no evidence on Nightingale's observations on women, once again losing a distinctive contribution different from those of most male thinkers of her day.

According to Welch, Nightingale did not subscribe to dualism, the reduction of elements, for example, to body and soul or good and evil. Given her mystical experience, she could only stress holism; on the social level, the person working toward the discovery of knowledge and truth created a better society, and on the individual level she wrote to Jowett, "'it is absurd to consider man either as a body to be improved or as a soul to be improved separately'" (cited in Welch, 1986, p. 9). Although influenced by some of the men thinkers of the day, Nightingale, says Welch, had her own ideas.

Still another attempt to place Nightingale in the context of male philosophical thought is that of Virginia E. Slater (1994), who believes Nightingale was most strongly influenced by Plato, Descartes, Rousseau, and Stewart. Nightingale as a young girl and woman would have learned much about these philosophers during the many hours spent with her father studying philosophy, language, mathematics, astronomy, and other sciences. To Slater, Nightingale was not ahead of her time, but very much a woman of her time, presumably reflecting the prevailing philosophies of the day. No one would deny that even the greatest thinkers reflect the prevailing thought, but one could certainly question whether Nightingale reflected male thinking in, for example, *Cassandra* or in some of her writings for nurses. Certainly, Plato's metaphysical belief in ideal form and his espousal of gender equality, at least for educated and enlightened men and women, would have been very attractive to Nightingale, both as mystic and feminist.

A 19th-century more democratic variant of Plato's approach was represented by Dugald Stewart, who spoke of "enlightened conductors," those elite members of society (primarily men, but a few women, too), who would diffuse knowledge and lead people, through education, to the highest intellectual and moral status of which they were capable. There is no doubt that Nightingale believed in educating all women and accepting all classes into the nursing profession. She also emphasized, as did Stewart, that the "practical rules" learned from experience should be written down for the benefit of future generations. Unlike Slater, Boyd interprets Nightingale's approach as motivated by her spiritual mission and, thus, the elite, the "enlightened conductors," would be those who had achieved not only worldly knowledge, but an apprehension of other realities. Furthermore, from her feminist writing, it is clear that she felt that women en masse and certainly all nurses were to be educated, and from these women would emerge leaders whose calling was most evident.

The influences that Descartes and Rousseau had on Nightingale are more difficult to assert, though Slater believes these philosophers also affected her. However, it is difficult to see how Nightingale the mystic could have subscribed to Descartes' premise of the separation of mind and body. To him, all material things were "machines," except humans, to whom God gave souls. Those humans who did not have minds, however, did not have souls, and, thus, remained machines. The debate over whether women had minds and souls was a longstanding one; many saw them as machines, put on earth only for man's purpose and pleasure. Certainly, Nightingale did not subscribe to this aspect of Descartes' philosophy, nor is it clear that she accepted the separate nature of mind and body, as Slater states. Her belief in unified being, in the connectedness of all, denied a philosophy of dualism or separation. When Nightingale wrote of caring for the "flesh and the spirit," did she really see these as *unconnected* parts of a whole, as Slater postulates? Or did she rather see the necessity of caring for *both* or all parts of a human being to achieve harmony and wholeness? Given Nightingale's fundamental mysticism and her philosophy of nursing care, her approach is most probably holistic. Welch (1986) also takes this position, as noted earlier.

Rousseau thought little of women, believing them to be created for men's uses and purposes. Consequently, women should not receive the same education as men; rather, their education should be "relative to man," learning to please and nurture men and making life "agreeable" to them. It is difficult to imagine Nightingale accepting this philosophy, especially in view of her writings on women's roles in home and family. Yet Slater believes Rousseau's influence on Nightingale is demonstrated by her understanding and compassionate care of the soldiers in the Crimea, and by her ability to work with men such as Herbert in carrying out her reforms.

If one is to accept the premise that Nightingale was significantly influenced by any philosophic theorist, it most probably would have been Stewart. But even this conclusion can only be made with hesitation. As Welch points out, Nightingale was a critical analyst of the philosophic thinking that prevailed during her era and found fault with many premises and assumptions advanced by the philosophers she studied. In contrast to Slater, Welch believes that while Nightingale may have been somewhat influenced by these thinkers, she was essentially a woman with her own ideas, often forced to act on these ideas against the tide of prevailing popular values and notions.

FLORENCE NIGHTINGALE AND WOMEN'S ENFRANCHISEMENT

Central to any conclusions one might make on the influence certain male philosophers had on Nightingale is the issue of her feminism. If indeed she was a feminist, her basis for thought and action would be distinctly different from the antifeminist male philosophers. Evelyn L. Pugh (1982) focuses specifically on the issue of Nightingale's feminism and the debate between her and John Stuart Mill on women's rights. Their exchange of letters between 1860 and 1867 never became public, remaining unknown until the correspondence was published (receiving little attention) in 1935 in the journal, *Hospitals*. As noted by Stark, Nightingale initially refused to sign a women's suffrage petition in 1866 to the House of Commons and delayed becoming a member of the National Society for Women's Suffrage. The actual correspondence between Nightingale and Mill received little notice, but Pugh claims that, in retrospect, the letters illustrate the dichotomy between Nightingale, the pragmatic reformer, and Mill, the feminist theoretician: "Within that context it becomes more understandable why Miss Nightingale, despite her enormously influential practical work in elevating the status of women, failed to become allied with Mill in the initial stages of the women's emancipation movement" (p. 119). Nevertheless, Mill, in his *Subjection of Women* (1869), was "perhaps more indebted to her for reinforcing the validity of some of his own preconceptions than has been previously realized" (p. 119). Nightingale sent her *Suggestions for Thought to Seekers After Religious Truth* to Mill for review. As noted earlier, this three-volume, 829-page work included *Cassandra*. Clearly, women's issues were imbedded in Nightingale's more general spiritual concerns. But Mill focused on and took issue with her *Notes on Nursing: What It Is, and What It Is Not*, specifically over her advice to avoid "jargons." Mill was concerned since the volume was "immensely popular, 15,000 copies of the first edition selling within a month of publication" (p. 121). (By 1946 the book had been reprinted at least 50 times.)

Nightingale retained the "offensive" jargon section, and Mill wrote that she had given the prestige of her name to those who denigrate proponents of women's rights, the very people who contend that women or men cannot find out what they can do without being allowed to try. Essentially, Mill claimed that Nightingale had given support to the "'gross injustice to women that men should pass sentence in the matter beforehand, by peremptorily excluding them from anything'" (p. 121). To this she replied that Mill had misunderstood her; Mill responded that her implication may be that women should not be excluded from trying any mode of existence open to men, which was the contention of women's rights advocates, one that could not be condemned as mere jargon. Nightingale replied that she accepted his interpretation, but protested that jargon was an appropriate word since she knew more about women than he did. Mill, she said, had never been "a 'scatting' female . . . among a world of 'scatting' females (and some very odd ones too)" (p. 122).

Pugh believes that Nightingale's personal experience with many women of different creeds and nationalities led to disappointment. In letters to women friends she claimed that men had helped her most, her doctrines having taken no hold on women; that she had not found a woman whose opinions had altered her life; that women lacked the sympathy that men had given her; that she was willing to pay five hundred pounds a year to obtain a woman secretary, but could not find one. She was, according to Pugh, highly annoyed with the talk and writing about women when, after opening a new field for women, there were more employment opportunities than applicants. Nightingale claimed she received hundreds of requests for nurses that remained unfilled, and she recommended that the writers on women's rights "each train ten women for a demand already in existence" (p. 123). Clearly, her frustration with the lack of progress in nursing colored her perceptions of feminists; nevertheless, she retained her friendship with feminist Harriet Martineau, who published newspaper articles suggested by Nightingale and a book on the maltreatment of soldiers based on Nightingale's reports.

Nightingale's *Notes on Nursing* contained scattered negative comments on women who dispensed unauthorized medicines, who were unobservant and unable to follow directives, and whose dress was unsuited for anything useful: "fashionable crinoline and starched petticoats . . . rustled and disturbed patients . . . [were] a fire hazard . . . [and] an affront to decency" (p. 124). Pugh, however, notes that the "jargon" on women did not include Mills, to whose work she heartily subscribed and deferred. Pugh pointedly asks, Would Nightingale's reaction have been so laudatory if she had known that Mill's work was more that of Harriet Taylor, his wife, than his own? In fact, as Pugh states, Nightingale identified the "jargonists" as the contingent of American women doctors led by Elizabeth Blackwell, about whom British feminists had written at some length. Indeed, Nightingale herself was given credit by one male physician as the person who had provided the basis for women doctors since nurses were neither unfeminine nor indelicate; in fact, nursing exposed women to far more repulsive and painful duties than those required for medical examining and prescribing. Nightingale acknowledged Blackwell as a friend; nevertheless, she saw medical women as potentially "third-rate men," who would probably fail to do any good. In this context, it is important to point out that Nightingale was unimpressed with the entire medical profession and, as Pugh notes, demanded that women doctors should reform medicine, not merely earn a living from it.

Pugh rightly states that Nightingale wrote in *Cassandra* one of the "most moving and profoundly feminist statements in existence . . . a scathing indictment of a society which reduced women to spiritually and mentally impoverished creatures . . . a devastating picture" (p. 127). Mill complimented her on " 'an appeal of an unusually telling kind on a subject which it is very difficult to induce people to open their eyes to'" (p. 128). According to Pugh, Mill's book (*The Subjection of Women*) reflected Nightingale's writing in "similarities . . . too striking to be ignored" (p. 128). For example, Mill's explanations of the causes of women's intellectual differences and attainment, of time as sex-related, of the trivialities of conventional idleness and nervous susceptibility and attendant ills, closely parallel Nightingale's. Pugh claims that for several pages in his book, "Mill was, in effect, describing Miss Nightingale's life during her 'Cassandra' phase" (p. 130). Furthermore, both regarded family as an instrument of tyranny, the culprit in continuing the subordination of women. If Mill's thought is, in part, derived from Nightingale, who, one might ask, is the pragmatist and who the theoretician?

By 1867 Mill resumed his correspondence with Nightingale, asking for her support for suffrage, and she again responded. But Pugh points out that Nightingale asserted "proudly that she could not have had more administrative influence" (p. 131) than if she had been a member of Parliament. Working behind the scenes had been a more effective method for her, to which Mill replied with a lengthy lecture on the fundamental principles of political liberty, arguing that women's enfranchisement was more readily obtained than other reform. Nightingale did not agree with the efficacy of the franchise, believing Mill would be disappointed with the results of giving women the vote. Would starving wives and daughters of workhouse paupers be helped, she asked? Will giving women the vote remove even the least of these evils? Pugh concludes: "She retained her skepticism about the franchise while simultaneously admitting that without representation there could be no freedom. . . . Women's rights, in the political sense, remained low on her list of priorities" (pp. 133–134).

Pugh believes that Nightingale, who had broken through sexist barriers and provided an example for other women, could not perceive that her own situation as a wealthy woman was unique in relation to the masses of women. The irony is that a "woman of genius, demonic energy, iron will, and a profoundly manipulative spirit" stated in an 1881 letter to nurses that they should have "'quietness, gentleness, patience, endurance, forbearance'"—all characteristics of the ideal Victorian woman (pp. 134–135). Her *Cassandra* never was published in her time, and was only brought to light by Ray Strachey in 1928 in a watered-down version in which the most angry and feminist assertions were missing, clearly showing the censorship urged by Benjamin Jowett. As Mill said, women often had ideas that were lost to the world or credited to men. Ironically, Nightingale recognized that Mill in his book had "'quoted' her 'stuff'" and should not have done it (p. 136).

Essentially, Pugh portrays Nightingale as suffering from the Queen Bee syndrome: I made it by myself, so why can't you? Additionally, Pugh explains the contradictions in Nightingale's statements by developmental phases: the Cassandra phase, an earlier phenomenon, followed by increasing conservatism arising from "little understanding of the legal basis of society and the democratic process" (p. 137). Presumably, Nightingale relied on the prestige and personal contacts traditionally used by the English upper classes: "As a practical matter, which she undoubtedly realized, she could only have such influence if she did not insist it was done as a matter of political principle" (p. 138). To Pugh, Nightingale chopped the branches off the tree of sexism but Mill attacked the trunk. This interpretation is open to question. In his book, Mill relied on Harriet, his wife, and "borrowed" from Nightingale. Whose branches and whose trunk are we talking about? Further, if Nightingale was intensely critiquing religions and philosophies in a fundamental way, who was the deeper thinker? The cosmologist or the political analyst? The civil libertarian or the woman who attacked the most basic belief systems of society?

POLITICAL ACTIVIST OR RECLUSE?

Little of Pugh's analysis and none of Boyd's appear in most of the literature written by nurses about Nightingale in the 1980s. However, nurse Irene Sabelberg Palmer (1983a) focuses on some of the political implications of Nightingale's work. To her, "Nightingale placed nursing, clearly and unequivocally, under medical and administrative authority" (p. 229). Palmer states that Nightingale clearly recognized the power of physicians and tried to avoid inciting their hostility. Nightingale probably had few choices open to her in the decisions she made, claims Palmer, pointing to the absence of a reputable, disciplined, and knowledgeable group of women, since they were yet to be produced. Nevertheless, Palmer believes that female subservience to male power sustained a century of male resistance to women who, nevertheless, led the way to hospital reform and decreased mortality. Men took the credit for these advances while leaving the work to women. Another reason for the choices Nightingale made was the need to change the social perception of the nurse as a degraded woman who did not merit authority. Nightingale's solution was to provide a system of education under the direction of female nursing leaders, who were indirectly controlled by men in hospitals in order to obtain the necessary approbation. Since Nightingale was a patrician who distinguished between ladies and women en masse, she believed authority could be extended to the matron, but not to nurses as a group. Nightingale herself was a power-oriented activist and a politically shrewd woman; thus, a new version of the icon is painted as Palmer quotes the founder: "Let us take care not to be left behind . . . and don't let us be like the chorus at the play which cries, 'Forward, Forward,' every two minutes; and never stirs a step" (p. 233).

Palmer (1983b) attempts to disentangle the myth from the reality of Nightingale, noting that she has "not escaped unscathed from speculation . . . mystery and rumor [about] her health, sexuality, personality, work and philosophy" (p. 40). In 1855 Nightingale succumbed to "Crimean Fever," probably undiagnosed typhus or typhoid fever. Problems with sciatica were compounded by episodes of dysentery and cardiac irregularities. Palmer speculates that Nightingale's immobility was also related to spinal problems since it is known that she wore corrective shoes. Inactivity combined with menopause could also have created osteoporosis. The magnitude of her physical difficulties was probably associated with the "psychical and physical trauma she experienced during the war" (p. 40), leading to irreversible debilitation associated with preexisting conditions, such as the "weak chest" noted in her childhood and youth.

The emotional turmoil of witnessing 2,000 deaths in the Crimea during the winter of 1854–55; the frustration of available, but inaccessible, supplies and clothing to prevent starvation and neglect; the problems with nurses and the blocking and thwarting by officialdom—all these, Palmer states, combined with life-threatening illness, led to severe physical debilitation. Indeed, recent analyses of Nightingale's physical condition and health problems include the suggestions that Nightingale may have suffered from post-traumatic stress disorder (Brook, 1990), supporting Palmer's thesis, or possibly from systemic lupus erythematosus (Veith, 1990). Brook's and Veith's interesting ideas, along with those of other current scholars on Nightingale, are presented in the fine anthology by Bullough, Bullough, and Stanton (1990), a culmination of papers presented at a 1989 conference on "Florence Nightingale and her Era."

Crediting Palmer with being the first investigator to trace Nightingale's invalidism to physical causes, Veith observes that Palmer deals only minimally with Nightingale's symptoms of sciatica, spinal troubles, and postmenopausal osteoporosis, giving more attention to discounting rumors about venereal disease and morphine addiction as causes of Nightingale's invalidism. According to Veith, Nightingale was diagnosed as having at least four illnesses in her lifetime: Crimean fever (probably either typhus or typhoid fever), sciatica, rheumatism, and dilatation of the heart. All of these had the potential for crippling side effects and a pattern of excessive bed rest. In the absence of an adequate health and illness history, Veith hypothesizes that Nightingale's ailments became chronic and tormented her throughout her life. In addition, Veith agrees with Woodham-Smith that from 1842 to 1852 Nightingale had severe episodes of mental illness, but whether, as in her terms, she was simply going mad for want of something to do, is not clear. Like Stark, Veith relies on Pickering's psychoanalytic interpretation, which is clearly open to question. Indeed, Nightingale's lengthy illness in 1844 could be explained, even by Pickering, in physical terms since it is possible that she visited cottages where people were sick with scarlet fever; possibly she contracted the disease, thus, accounting for her later cardiac problems. In 1853, while in Paris studying various hospitals, she contracted "measles," but at age 32 measles is rare and since she reported having them previously, Veith considers alternative explanations, such as systemic lupus erythematosus (SLE), particularly since many of her symptoms and complaints were consistent with such a diagnosis, one that was unavailable to physicians and nurses in Nightingale's time. Whether using opium or morphine for persistent pain might have led to some addiction is left open by Veith, although Nightingale herself complained that opium hardly improved the vivacity or serenity of her intellect.

Two themes dominate the literature on women and disease in the 1800s: woman as an invalid by nature, at the mercy of her biology; and woman as a victim, subject to biased and sexist perceptions and treatments by men physicians, whose actions sustained the patriarchal status quo. Alternatively, the theme of inadequate medical knowledge could lead to a third interpretation: woman as chronically ill, improperly attended by physicians whose ignorance made it impossible to deal with women's illnesses. Certainly, it was common to diagnose neurasthenia and to administer opium to women, causing addiction. Subsequently, both the diagnosis and the treatment have been rejected. Certainly, Nightingale was subject to the medical conceptions of women of her time, but whether she was influenced, as Veith contends, by these ideas is open to question. Veith compares Nightingale's correspondence to that of an American woman, Ann Phillips, who also voluntarily shut herself off from the world, claiming to grow sicker everyday, but living to her 90s, as did Nightingale. Since both women wrote melancholic letters describing their ailments, Veith sees this as evidence of the influence of the prevailing Victorian conceptions of women. There is one clear difference: Nightingale remained active intellectually, engineering multiple and major reforms, both facts admitted by Veith, while Phillips accomplished little. Thus, the comparison is inadequate.

Whatever the truth, Palmer sees Nightingale's rage and resentment turned inward, and a return to earlier patterns of withdrawal. How her seclusion could be considered withdrawal, when, without adequate time for recuperation, Nightingale produced voluminous writings, reports, and recommendations, seems a problematic interpretation. It should be remembered that women in public were anathema. Surely, Nightingale, being a shrewd politician, could wisely assess her best tactics and strategies. And surely she was well aware that privacy was necessary to produce the tremendous amount of work needed to effect reform. Indeed, Palmer notes that Nightingale, during her first two years back in England, did leave her home frequently, collecting data all over London. Later, after developing cardiac problems, she worked at her country home and took carriages into London; in later life, she also took carriage rides in London.

Palmer asserts that the invalid image of Nightingale should be dismissed in favor of the active intellectual, encouraging and engineering multiple reforms. Some scholars have claimed that after 1868 Nightingale wrote nothing new. But Palmer states that Nightingale engaged in intensive correspondence with nurses and wrote her finest paper on nursing in 1893: "Such allegations discount her letters of advice to her nurses, or her delineation of nursing's parameters and responsibilities . . . [and] deny the importance of Nightingale's effect upon nursing, hospital construction and management, and district nursing as well as denying the social significance of the profession" (p. 40). Furthermore, the idea that Nightingale had succumbed by about 1866 to using morphine regularly for unremitting pain is not supported by her written work on nursing, which gives no evidence of confusion, euphoria, or fantasy.

Palmer also deals with the rumors ascribing Nightingale's death to venereal disease, an assertion discounted by her health certificate, which specified old age and heart failure, and by the fact that she certainly would have experienced nervous system paralysis and become demented in 20 years if untreated. Could Nightingale have produced her voluminous writings over 35 years if so affected, asks Palmer? She concludes that Nightingale's upbringing and religious convictions would not argue for sexuality outside of marriage. But given Nightingale's views on marriage and the family, this assertion must remain speculative.

In contrast to some authors who state Nightingale did not like women, Palmer notes that at least one biographer claimed that Nightingale had unresolved homosexual tendencies because of the nature of her female friendships: her depressions when her governess died, when her Aunt Mai married, and when Marianne Nicholson rejected Florence's friendship when she refused to marry Marianne's brother. To this, Palmer counters that Nightingale expressed anger and resentment toward women as unsympathetic, interrupting and delaying her work, abandoning her, refusing to take up her causes, rejecting useful work and nursing.

What evidence is there for alleging Nightingale's same-sex preference? Some writers have used Nightingale's letter to her friend Mary Clarke-Mohl in 1861, in which she complained of her disappointment with women: "And my experience of women is almost as large as Europe. And it is so intimate, too. I have lived and slept in the same bed with English countesses and Prussian *bauerinnen*, with a closeness of intimacy no one ever had before" (p. 41). Palmer believes Nightingale had a bent to exaggeration and that it is improper to take this sentence out of context, particularly in view of alternate definitions of "intimacy" in Victorian life. Using as proof the sustained friendships that Nightingale had with many men and their wives over her lifetime, Palmer argues for Nightingale's heterosexuality. However, a stereotyped view of homosexuals as incapable, unwilling, or unable to maintain friendships with men cannot be used as valid evidence. None of Nightingale's relations with Milnes, Herbert, Sutherland, Galton, or Jowett were apparently sexually based; how then do they provide evidence for or against heterosexuality? One may perceive the nature of female homosexuality as excluding any sexual experience of men but research suggests otherwise. There is also the implication that male friendships are excluded, but again, the research evidence on lesbians does not support this assumption. Palmer is probably more accurate when she concludes that Nightingale had many protracted friendships with *both* women and men that were sustained over many years, serving business, pleasure, and social functions.

In contrast to other scholars discussed previously, Palmer focuses our attention on Nightingale's friendships with women and her support of women in nursing. This is in contrast to some of the interpretations of scholars external to nursing, who are more likely to minimize Nightingale's positive relations with women and maximize her work with men. Whether Nightingale had sexually intimate relations with other women will probably never be known since the evidence is insufficient; certainly the "mature adult," regardless of sexual orientation, is quite capable of long-term, deep, and sustained friendships with both sexes.

Palmer rejects the excessive attention given to Nightingale's personality, concluding that she was dedicated to her work and could be both compassionate and tyrannical. More important, Palmer claims there is too little attention given to Nightingale's intellect, to her concepts of the nature of the universe, to her philosophy, although these are restated within the more traditional definition of religion, rather than the "positivist mysticism" as delineated by Boyd. Palmer notes that Nightingale's intellect was appreciated by Queen Victoria and by others, including two of the "feminine" (presumably feminist) writers of the day. She believes that Nightingale understood the Victorian mores about her gender; thus, she shunned publicity, worked behind the scenes, and enlisted support to obtain a broader base for her reforms. Focusing on Nightingale's tactics and strategies for effecting change, Palmer concludes: "My respect for this tremendous woman . . . who emerged as one of the world's greatest social reformers, grows daily" (p. 42).

MEDIA PORTRAYALS OF THE SACRED ICON

Over the past two decades, the centrality of imagery to the public's conception of nursing has increased in importance to nursing researchers. Central to this development is the thoughtful reconsideration of the Nightingale imagery by nursing historians Beatrice J. Kalisch and Philip A. Kalisch (1983a, 1983b), who analyze Nightingale as a "Heroine out of Focus," first, as portrayed in popular biographies and stage productions, and second, in film, radio, and television dramatizations. Since Nightingale's death in 1910, her legend is primarily derived from a series of specific images of her from only a short, 21-month mission in the Crimea (1854–1856). These depict a "slender, graceful lady walking through miles of darkened wards full of wounded soldiers . . . easing pain by her gentle manner, transforming morbid, filthy barracks into a clean hospital" (1983a, p. 181). To the Kalisches, the combination of legend and biography creates a peculiar problem for scholars since much of Nightingale's work, even in nursing, is excluded from media productions, which serve to reinforce the public's traditional perceptions of what is important about nursing.

The Kalisches found 10 separate dramatizations of Nightingale's life between 1915 and 1965, making her "the most dramatized woman in history" (p. 182). Media productions have been based primarily on three biographies: *The Life of Florence Nightingale* (Cook, 1913–1914), *Eminent Victorians* (Strachey, 1918), and *Florence Nightingale: 1820–1910* (Woodham-Smith, 1951). The Kalisches claim that none of these sources is properly documented, and that "Nightingale's life and career cry out for professional evaluation" (p. 182). Although all agree on her importance, the vastness and complexity of Nightingale's work are so great that biographers have focused more on her motives and behaviors. "Most troublesome of all have been attempts to explain Nightingale-the-woman in the masculine world of politics and war" (p. 182). Concern with personality, rather than accomplishments, and with "feminine identity" obscures Nightingale's historical significance: "nursing reform, military organization, hospital and barracks construction, workhouse reform, sanitary and military reform in India, all facets of public sanitation, and the articulation of a new religious ethos—to name the most prominent" (pp. 182–183).

Cook, overwhelmed with Nightingale, was additionally constrained as her official biographer to exclude information embarrassing to her family and friends; thus, he acknowledged but softened the difficulties that Florence had with her mother and sister, and continually reminded readers that "harsh remarks found in private notes and intimate correspondence had no counterpart in Nightingale's conversation" (p. 183). According to the Kalisches, Cook's Nightingale was a woman who combined an intense feeling with a profound intellectual grasp, yet he never sentimentalized her. For example, " 'She was at once Positive and Mystic' " (p. 183), and did not fit into easy categories. The Kalisches point out that everyone has plundered Cook, whose work was the source for a 1915 film, an obscure piece in 1922 by Edith Gittings-Reid, and a radio drama in 1950.

The Kalisches discovered that Lytton Strachey's imbalanced, unscholarly, and sexist interpretation of Nightingale unfortunately has had the widest impact. Evidently, Strachey's view of demonic possession was more interesting than the previous angelic legend to subsequent producers of media presentations. In feminist thinking, particularly Mary Daly's (1980), the sexist technique is reversal: in Nightingale's case, the "angel" becomes the "devil," turning upside down the woman's reality, focusing on the dark side of her personality, even claiming, as noted earlier, that she had driven her friend, Sidney Herbert, to his death. To the Kalisches, Strachey took the most dramatic episodes of Nightingale's life and simplified her complexity into the single-sided, fierce crusader, a view dominant in William Dieterle's 1936 film, *The White Angel*, and Reginald Berkeley's 1929 stage play, *The Lady With a Lamp*.

Cecil Woodham-Smith's *Florence Nightingale* (1951) influenced the television play "The Holy Terror" in 1965. The Kalisches claim that Woodham-Smith's work is flawed—transposing Nightingale's quotations to alter the original meaning and ignoring "documentary evidence . . . that contradicted her conclusions" (p. 184); using written notes and letters as though they were the "spoken word"; characterizing Nightingale's mother and sister as totally negative while disregarding her concern for them, focusing instead on her "disgust and antipathy." As noted earlier, Allen's psychohistory, to the extent it relied on Woodham-Smith, is, thus, also heavily flawed.

Woodham-Smith's view of Nightingale as having the "'hard coldness of steel,'" as the Kalisches observe, is a distortion. The biographer referred to Nightingale as *both* emotionally unmoved and yet dreaming of Milnes, who proposed marriage to her. Furthermore, Woodham-Smith, as noted indirectly by Palmer, quoted Nightingale's "effusive language—the language of Victorian friendship—yet never informed her reader whether or not she was implying an improper or excessive intimacy between Florence and her female friends" (p. 185). Rephrased, did Nightingale quietly engage in sexually intimate relations with other women, which in much current feminist thought is considered neither improper nor excessive? Or did she simply use the "effusive" loving terminology of the day? Translated, did she love women, but not act on her love sexually? The feminist debate over the interpretation of Victorian friendships began in the 1970s and continues; it remains unresolved. Certainly, the importance of this issue to Nightingale's life is central since so many writers have assumed that she was negative about women and feminism. If indeed she was "effusive" in her affection toward her women friends and consistently supported her nurses, the understanding of her feminism would have to change.

The Kalisches note that Edith Gittings-Reid's 1922 play focused on the "often humorous gap between legend and reality . . . [but] the entire play distorts the audience's appreciation of Florence's extremely difficult labor" (p. 185), failing to demonstrate the opposition she experienced to her reforms. On the other hand, Gittings-Reid's Nightingale deflates rhetoric, emphasizing the practical nature of her efforts, that she managed people well, used charm, wit, and enthusiasm to sway others, deferred to medical authority, and insisted on control of her own nurses in the Crimea to prove by controlled experiment the value of organized and disciplined women.

In contrast, Reginald Berkeley's play in 1929 relied on Strachey, but exceeded even him in "acidity and bitterness," portraying a Nightingale whose yearning for love and domestic happiness was unfulfilled, leading her to submerge herself in work for relief. As the Kalisches note: "Florence's relationships with men in the Berkeley play all suffer from ambivalence, as if the playwright could not understand a woman dealing with men without romantic or sexual tensions, yet was determined to so present his heroine. He did this by turning Florence Nightingale into an insensitive and sharp-tongued shrew who bullies the men around her" (p. 186). Again, there is the reversal of historic fact: a lovable, or at least likeable woman, becomes unlikable and unacceptable. As the Kalisches state, the emphasis on her suitor "does not allow Florence's refusal of this marriage proposal to be indicative of a mature, fully decided mind" (p. 187). The playwright invented unrealistic, unhistorical barracks scenes. Finally the husband-to-be dies, saving Nightingale from leaving her work in nursing. Similarly, Nightingale's friendship with Sidney Herbert is overridden by an invented "long-simmering conflict" with Elizabeth Herbert in which both women "square off" against each other, making Nightingale appear condescending, demanding, and resentful of "Liz," who, in turn, appears vicious, petty, intellectually inadequate, and jealous, and finally, years later, tells Florence that her "prolonged old age and gradual debilitation" is Florence's deserved "purgatory" (p. 187). This cruelly sexist inversion of Nightingale is historical fantasy. The impact on nurses is obvious when Berkeley pits one nurse, who believes Nightingale is a saint, against a younger nurse, who replies that saints are "'sinners who've gone soft'" (p. 187) and states she does not believe in making idols.

The Kalisches (1983b) also analyze media images of Nightingale in film, radio, and television dramatizations, which do not "mirror" reality but create an impression of it—"the result of both conscious design . . . and unconscious integration and reproduction of cultural paradigms" (p. 270). The patriarchal paradigm consistently emerges, influencing the public view not only of Nightingale but of the profession she represents in the popular imagination. Three feature films of Nightingale appeared. The first, *Florence Nightingale*, was shown in 1915 and consisted of a series of silent scenes; ironically, this early work represents the only dramatic effort to review Nightingale's entire life. Now lost to modern viewers, the Kalisches believe the film may have been used to motivate women to serve in the British Red Cross.

The White Angel (1936), drawn from Strachey's work, depicts a father who supports his daughter to free herself from her mother's social world; but, claim the Kalisches, William Nightingale actually withdrew from the domestic difficulties in his home into a world of books and other interests. The film concludes with Nightingale reciting her oath and pledge, which was actually written by another woman many years later. The Kalisches conclude that the film fails to recognize that Nightingale's life work began *after* she returned from the Crimea and that she faced enormous opposition. Instead, the sexist stereotypes of womanly virtues—goodness, gentleness, nurturance—appear, but none of the energy, labor, and vision required to reform military hospital services. Still, the film is a "loving, reverential view of the founder of the nursing profession. [It] remains an important component of the regeneration of the Nightingale legend . . . and . . . the extent to which one dedicated person can make a difference in human history" (p. 272).

In 1952 a British version, *The Lady With a Lamp*, filmed on location by Harold and Anna Neagle Wilcox, relied on Berkeley's play, but excluded the inaccurate romance between Nightingale and Henry Tremayne, as well as the nonfactual "battle" between Nightingale and Elizabeth Herbert. Instead, the film focused on Nightingale's nursing care and supervision of nursing activities; nevertheless, she remains "intensely feminine throughout her life . . . yet . . . keeping a firm . . . control over her own emotions" (p. 273). The Kalisches conclude that this is the "best dramatization" produced, but reviewers claimed that portraying Nightingale as " 'a lady in the best sense of the word' was 'outdated' " (p. 274).

In contrast, radio and television plays have remained "superficial and unoriginal," with Nightingale cast as a "romantic and tragic heroine, disappointed in love" (p. 274). In 1941, for example, a radio production starring Helen Hayes portrays Nightingale's voice as gentle and determined. A later version in 1948 produced a less sympathetic Nightingale whose suitor again takes prominence. In this version, Florence, speaking with "feminine distress," appeals to a lieutenant for help. Nightingale is dismayed to find her injured suitor on her own ward, but refuses to send him home, because he should not be given "special favors." She cries when she learns later of his death, and, again, cries in an audience with Queen Victoria and Prince Albert. These sexist and inaccurate interpretations lead the Kalisches to say, "Florence's persona . . . emphasizes a certain feminine weakness and inconstancy, as if Florence could not be loved if she appeared strong and able to control her emotions" (p. 274).

A 1950 radio production featuring Irene Dunne emphasized Nightingale as a nurse, but excluded all her other concerns and projects. Again, Nightingale is used by the media to recruit women to alleviate the severe nursing shortage and to assist the Red Cross. Once again, Nightingale is portrayed as "intensely womanly and gentle . . . a nurturing, comforting presence whose idea of nursing means cleanliness, prayer, offers of encouragement, and assistance to doctors in surgery" (p. 275). The conflicts that characterized Nightingale's life in reform work were again mostly ignored.

In 1965 the first full television dramatization, "The Holy Terror," by James Lee, appeared. In this version Nightingale is portrayed as "a driven fanatic," probably derived from Woodham-Smith's work in which Nightingale "stages" ill health to keep her family away. The portrayal is of a woman who is "a chilling human being who lacked any warmth and feeling for others, despite the surface wit and sense of fun" (p. 275). Revealing little gentleness of spirit or manner, Nightingale is the Joan of Arc, the woman of divine calling, allowing no one and nothing to hinder her work. In this production, Nightingale unhistorically behaves outrageously at the ambassador's residence, exposing her bald head (supposedly the result of fever, but, in fact, it was only a short haircut), and describing the "gory details" of barracks conditions. In Lee's version, Julie Harris as Nightingale becomes paralytic to blackmail her family. Furthermore, she hounds and bullies friends. The Kalisches comment: "How unfortunate that this last production, seen by millions of American viewers, should have presented this exaggerated portrayal of Nightingale" (p. 276). A recent television production (1989), starring Jaclyn Smith, attempts perhaps to dispel Lee's earlier interpretation. But again, Nightingale, as in previous productions, is depicted in her Crimean, ministering angel role, gentle and quiet, with only minimal attention given to her fight to obtain adequate supplies and care for the soldiers.

What is the impact of these images on nursing? The Kalisches conclude that all productions show the "enormous value of [Nightingale's] efforts to establish nursing as an honorable and worthy profession for women . . . associated with bravery, nobility, and selfless dedication" (p. 276). But what constitutes a nurse, other than cleanliness and submission to strict discipline, remains vague. What constitutes a feminist or a brilliant reformer also remains unclear. As the Kalisches point out, there are no other nurses in any dramatizations that rival Nightingale; they "appear in a sympathetic light only because of their unfailing loyalty to Nightingale, who . . . remains the exceptional, atypical nursing figure . . . [other nurses] remain pure, discrete, loyal, and dedicated to the welfare of others" (p. 277). It seems that a woman who is not defined by her relationship to a man must be redefined. A strong and attractive woman, who chooses of her own will to reject marriage for a career of humanitarian service, pays, for example, in Berkeley's play, a heavy price, becoming frustrated and bitter, turning against others. Indeed, in Lee's work, "he not only defeminizes her, he dehumanizes her entirely" (p. 277).

The Kalisches recognize that the emphasis on self-sacrifice, discipline, and obedience in the earlier Nightingale iconography no longer appeals to nurses. They affirm Nightingale's life as a field for discovering the scientific and creative forces that shaped modern nursing. To them, Nightingale is still a strong role model for nurses and the general female population, which should not be "shelved" as out-of-date. Obviously, the extent to which Nightingale herself supported women, not only in nursing, is critical to her importance to women in general.

Except for Jaclyn Smith's 1989 traditional portrayal, Nightingale has not been presented in the media in the past two decades. More recent analyses of Nightingale by nurse scholars have provided the profession with a more thorough, well-balanced portrait of its founder, but these interpretations have not been systematically shared with the public. People outside the nursing profession continue to embrace the legendary, traditional image of Nightingale, presented by uninformed biographers and dramatists. This leads, of course, to a continuing controversy over who Nightingale really was.

AN UNFINISHED PORTRAIT:
THE NIGHTINGALE CONTROVERSY CONTINUES

Inaccurate, nonfactual written biographies of Nightingale's life have made as negative an impact on her image as have pictorial presentations. The Kalisches are very alert to the sexist denigration of women leaders, clearly sustained by F. B. Smith's (1982) "highly pretentious 'biography' . . . a polished exercise in character assassination with highly sexist overtones" (Kalisch & Kalisch, 1983b, p. 278). An alternative explanation, of course, is that the fundamental purpose of Smith's book *is* the sexist destruction of a strong female figure. Since it shows no awareness of the constricted opportunities for power available to Victorian women, nor the constrained female sex roles in the 19th century—factors certainly well established in historical research—Smith's work is clearly sexist, not only in overtones, but in fundamental purpose. As the Kalisches observe, the qualities of leadership praiseworthy in men became highly negative when applied to Nightingale, who is portrayed as a " 'boastful, lying, cheating, and egotistic' woman" (p. 278). As with other authors, Smith remained ignorant of research in the history of women, of nursing, and of medicine to achieve his sexist biography, one containing many errors of fact, which the Kalisches claim constitutes "the ultimate insult" to Nightingale, one that should cause nursing leaders to demand a "more equitable modern account" (p. 278).

Smith's book seems to have been largely ignored by American nurses. According to Evelyn R. Benson (1991), "a search of the literature did not reveal a single review of this book in American nursing journals" (p. 6). Although it was considered in the *American Historical Review* and in several Australian and British nursing journals, it remained in limbo in the United States. Benson's tardy review notes Smith's vituperative language, sarcasm, and skepticism and his intent to destroy forever the image of the ministering angel, the lady with the lamp. "With one blistering comment after another the author calls Miss Nightingale a master manipulator, a fraud, a titillating fabulist . . . secretive and deceitful . . . he trivializes her deeds, and disparages her motives" (p. 6). Strangely, says Benson, the author's tirades are often concluded by "begrudging admissions of her noteworthy accomplishments and positive qualities" (p. 6). Nightingale was presumably inept and insensitive, but had superb intelligence, a beautiful floating walk, and a voice peculiarly soft with clear intonation. Benson notes still more incongruities: an attack on Nightingale's religious beliefs, but praise for saving the nurses in the Crimea from getting caught up in petty religious rivalries.

Smith attacks not only Nightingale but other Victorian women as well. Benson states there is "a disturbing bias that permeates his writing . . . [and] language that can only be regarded as misogynistic" (p. 6) when he refers to Victorian women as females who adopted bizarre, unpopular causes and remained unmarried by choice. Again, Benson notes the inconsistency when

Smith credits Nightingale for justified interference in the reforms in India, radical reform of the Poor Law for the sick, and her positive impact on soldiers through the reform of the military. Surprisingly, Benson recommends Smith's book as an "important item" on a bibliography and of "value" to historians of women and nursing. Still, the complete absence of any American review, until Benson's, has served a useful purpose: to ignore any misogynist books that engage in character assassination may be the best way to silence such authors.

The changing iconography of Nightingale has influenced not only women, but young girls as well, as is clear in Martha Vicinus' (1990) excellent paper on biographies of Nightingale written for girls. Studying popular biographies of heroines from the 1870s to the 1950s, Vicinus found a focus from 1870 to 1900 on religious faith and channeling innate inclinations; from 1900 to 1920 on progress and overcoming the constraints of society in the later period of the first wave of feminism; in the 1950s, the focus had shifted to choosing between heterosexual love and personal ambitions. Indeed, Vicinus concludes that the biographies in the earlier periods gave girls *more* freedom and scope for public work than those in the mid-1900s.

Using Nightingale as a case study, Vicinus found that over some 80 years the presentation of this one woman included or excluded very different materials. In the Victorian period, self-sacrifice, a key feminine virtue, was stressed in Nightingale's rejection of her wealthy way of life. That she "loathed these activities was ignored" (p. 94). Her enormous labors to reform the army and public health were suppressed and her efforts to create a respectable female occupation were emphasized; thus, her political actions were denied and stereotyped womanly characteristics were stressed. But even her propensity to "nurse" was pictured as developing under the auspices of caring males, of her minister, teachers, or relatives, who, says Vicinus, were described as introducing girls to the outside world and giving moral approval and help in developing their skills. Even though the men guided, the girl herself followed her "natural" inclinations to nurse or teach or study.

The heroine had to overcome opposition without a contentious spirit or disobedient action, but Nightingale's difficult relations with her mother and sister violated these norms, so biographers focused on her relationship with her father, leaving family love inviolate. Vicinus notes that even public opposition was characterized as an abstraction—unbelief, ignorance, worldliness, or bureaucratic muddle; specific persons were not blamed, although some did change their minds. Thus, in Nightingale's biographies, the inefficiency of unnamed "authorities" or "officials" caused military chaos, but her indomitable will, not her specific methods and actual behaviors, caused changes. Her daily work was also elided. Thus, the sacred icon, the Lady with the Lamp, hid "the complexities of achieving social change" (p. 97). The reader could then allow imagination to create a different, wider life: "A shadowy Nightingale could be invested with desirable characteristics more easily than one encumbered with complex motivations" (p. 97). Although womanly obedience was the message, independent action was the possibility.

In the 20th-century biographies, interesting alterations occurred, although the theme of overcoming personal difficulties and social opprobrium to bring public progress was sustained. According to Vicinus, details of Nightingale's home life, sometimes called the "gilded cage," began to appear, but a major change was the emphasis on her wealthy background, so her self-sacrifice, no longer fashionable, became redefined as the loss of material goods. Opposition was still abstract; actual unnamed but real people were still absent, but society was caricatured, for example, as moralistic spinsterish women, who were horrified with a woman going to the battlefield. It is important to note that Vicinus found that spiritual strivings were replaced by material issues.

The suffragists, however, "saw Nightingale as a great leader whose true accomplishments had been obscured" (p. 99). In one feminist pamphlet in 1913 she was redefined as a controversial figure, a strong, capable, "brainy" woman with force and bold authority: "The most popular heroine in history had to pay the price that is exacted of all pioneers. Bitter venomous attacks, misrepresentation, irredeemably vulgar slanders, signalled her departure for the Crimea. Before her name became for all time a name to conjure with, it was the butt for coarse wit and ridicule of the day" (p. 99). To feminists who wanted wider leadership opportunities for women, Nightingale as an administrator, sanitarian, and strong-minded and firm-handed genius was the model, not one of the gentle, caring female, the Lady With the Lamp.

Subsequently, Strachey's and even Cook's biographies, says Vicinus, diminished Nightingale's reputation and her name was less frequent in biographies of famous women for girls. However, in the 1950s she appeared suitably psychologized into a typical idealistic adolescent, who was a real problem to her parents. The focus on the temptations of material wealth and family quarrels undermined the perceptions of duty, individual initiative, and responsibility. Indeed, a male lover was given credit for influencing Nightingale's interest in the poor: "romance, rather than the early childhood inclination, became the impetus for doing public good" (pp. 100–101). Adding sexual interest shifted the plot, says Vicinus, from the self and the public world to a triangle of self, romance, and public duty. With the growth of the "feminine mystique," romance, the nuclear family, and subordination to men were reflected in stories for girls: "When the biographies focused upon the heroine's struggle to choose between romance and public duty, they became stories of a failed romantic heroine, rather than a successful public figure" (p. 103). The heroine's identity became defined by desire: "Once romance was admitted, a woman could not be portrayed as a whole person if she had rejected a suitor" (p. 103). Thus, seeking affirmation outside the home, girls found that they could never escape their sexual identity—"a lesson many feminists have been fighting their whole adult lives" (p. 103). In contrast, the Victorian biographers of Nightingale were not invested with sexual conflicts and widened the definition of the possible. Vicinus concludes that "Familiar feminine characteristics in unfamiliar places were a potent appeal for social change. Is it too far fetched to speculate that formulaic biographies for girls may have engendered powerful fantasies that empowered the first feminist movement?" (pp. 103–104). To this the only response is, no—it is not far-fetched and is quite possible.

CONTRADICTORY POSITIONS ON NIGHTINGALE

Renewed interest in Nightingale is evident in the 1983 reprint of Cecil Woodham-Smith's 1951 biography. In 1984 Charlene Eldridge Wheeler published an essay in response to the republication of the biography. Although out of print for some years, the biography is still widely cited in nursing articles, and Wheeler, in contrast to the Kalisches, considers the biography balanced in viewpoint, "presenting a picture of a multitalented woman who defies easy classification," and about whom it is "difficult to distinguish myth from malice, fact from fantasy, and bias from realism" (p. 75). To Wheeler, both the "lady with the lamp" and the "neurotic, ambitious woman" images serve to "diminish her . . . [and] deemphasize . . . her contributions to health care" (p. 75). In fact, claims Wheeler, the terms used in current literature are "so disparate it is difficult to know if they all refer to the same individual": Was Nightingale an "'obstructive reactionary . . . passionate humanist . . . early feminist . . . radical genius . . . [or] benevolent despot?'" (p. 75).

Snapshot images, frozen caricatures, too often show Nightingale as an eccentric with a few good ideas, but easy to discount and dismiss; this, says Wheeler, has an insidious, dangerous influence on perceptions of the nursing heritage, which, in turn, can also be discounted and dismissed. To Wheeler, Woodham-Smith provides overwhelming evidence that Nightingale was both a passionate humanist and creative genius, who "created a paradigm shift in nursing and health care" (p. 76). But whether Nightingale was an early feminist is still open to interpretation. Wheeler selects the oft-cited paragraph from Nightingale's correspondence with Mill, in which she affirms her support of women, but interprets this as bringing "to the issue of women's rights and suffrage the same global analysis she used in issues of health care" (p. 76). According to Wheeler, Nightingale disagreed with method, rather than content, and, although she might not have been a feminist, because she did not actively work in the women's movement and aligned herself with powerful men to achieve her goals, still her commitment and accomplishments "contributed greatly to the cause of women" (p. 76).

In contrast to writers external to nursing, Wheeler focuses on Nightingale's revolutionary accomplishments in nursing, including a scheme to pipe hot water to every hospital floor, a windlass installation, a lift to deliver patients' food, and bells for each patient with valves that opened and remained open in the corridor for nurses to see. Wheeler perceives Nightingale as a woman who knew every student and corresponded with many of them for years. Given Nightingale's concern for these women, Wheeler has difficulty with Woodham-Smith's view of Nightingale as tyrant and benevolent despot. Further, Nightingale's concern for her close friend, Hilary Bonham Carter, is selected by Wheeler as a fact that reinforces Nightingale's concern for other women. Wheeler rejects the label "obstructive reactionary," for example, in Nightingale's fight against other women over nurse registration. Such a label obscures the context of the controversy.

According to Wheeler, various authors have arrived at flatly contradictory positions regarding Nightingale. For example, Irene Palmer (1983a) concludes that Nightingale saw nursing functioning under medical and administrative authority. In contrast, Kelly (1976) maintains that Nightingale placed " 'nursing service responsible to a nurse administrator, not other administrators or physicians' " (p. 78). This issue, an important one from a feminist perspective, continues to plague nursing to this day. Clearly, as Wheeler notes, at least some physicians did not like Nightingale's system, or the idea of " 'an independent female hierarchy' " with its main objective of being " 'independent of all males . . . considered as the natural enemies of the organization' "(p. 78).

Wheeler believes that Woodham-Smith's biography clarifies the issue of female subservience, since it emphasizes Nightingale's belief that accurate assessment depends on educated women. According to Wheeler, this assertion contests Palmer's belief that Nightingale devalued the intellectual component of nurses and focused on them as trained servants. This, says Wheeler, is inaccurate, since Nightingale stated that nurses were " 'not to act as lifts, water-carriers, beasts of burden, or steam engines . . . [these] can be had at vastly less cost than that of educated human beings' " (p. 79). To Wheeler, Nightingale consistently supported the ideal of education for women—a major feminist goal. Although Wheeler appreciates Woodham-Smith's work, she concludes that the picture of Nightingale is still far from complete, with many questions unanswered and information missing.

Whether Nightingale was feminist or not is important to both nurses and non-nurses since this issue relates to multiple problems in nursing, not the least of which are education, obedience, and, more generally, politics and power. Lynda Nauright (1984) focuses on this issue, claiming that the picture of the "self-sacrificing do-gooder tiptoeing around soldiers" is replaced by the image of a "courageous, independent, fiercely liberated woman" (p. 5). Interestingly, Nauright uses Nightingale's injunction against "jargons" as evidence for her independence and determination. These characteristics are also obvious in Nightingale's meditation on marriage as " 'an initiation into the meaning of the inexorable word Never . . . which brings in reality the end of our lives and the chill of death with it' " (p. 6).

Nauright focuses on Nightingale's need to create a better life for women, which she did by establishing nursing as a suitable profession for women. The author rejects the poet Longfellow's image of the "lady with a lamp" as an exaggeration of only one aspect of Nightingale's life. According to Nauright, Nightingale was adept in working with powerful men, but she could not be called a feminist or radical: "Her service to women was that of example and leadership. She opened doors for women that had been closed . . . established precedents for women's achievement in nursing, hospital administration, medical statistics, public health, and politics" (p. 8). The new pride in this version of the sacred icon is expressed in Nauright's conclusion that Nightingale was "compassionate, tender, and devout . . . brilliant, creative, and powerful . . . politically astute, a genius at statistics, and mischievously clever . . . [she] defied her family and social custom . . . exerted leadership in the fields of sanitation and medical statistics . . . influenced the military power structures of Great Britain, France, and the United States. And she was a nurse" (p. 8).

As noted previously, little has been written about Nightingale by women studies scholars outside of nursing. Some recent portrayals present still another image, one not usually portrayed to students in the profession or to nursing practitioners. Feminist scholar Dale Spender (1983) says the following:

> Florence Nightingale gives every indication that she understands why the two sexes are required to behave in the manner that they do, and why it is that women's loss is men's gain. If it was this aspect of the woman question that she had in mind when she stated that she didn't expect much from the vote, her assessment was completely justified and her conventional portrayal as anti-feminist is then cast in a very different light. The changes that she sought (and which to some extent she managed to procure for herself—as did Harriet Martineau) were so radical that there was little likelihood that the vote would have been much assistance in bringing them about. (p. 402)

THE BONDS OF WOMANHOOD AND FEMALE FRIENDSHIP: NIGHTINGALE'S RELATIONSHIPS WITH OTHER WOMEN

According to Lois A. Monteiro (1984), if Florence Nightingale is compared to Elizabeth Blackwell, considered to be the first woman physician in the United States, there emerge two different versions of women directed by their separate visions. Differing from Pugh, Monteiro analyzes the correspondence between the two women as friends and colleagues. Meeting in London in 1850, they parted with tears in 1851—Nightingale to face hostility from male physicians in the Crimea and Blackwell to face similar antagonism in the New York Infirmary for Women and Children in the United States.

In 1857, on her return to England, Blackwell wanted Nightingale to join her in opening a hospital for women under the control of women physicians and staffed by female nurses. But Nightingale saw "only failure for a small, weakly financed women's hospital" (Monteiro, 1984, p. 524). Blackwell's ulterior motive was to establish a medical college for women at the hospital. Nightingale felt that this would alienate the men in power and jeopardize her plan to start a nurses' college in connection with a large London hospital. Monteiro sees a fundamental difference between the two women, expressed by Nightingale: " 'on different roads, (although to the same object). You to educate a few highly cultivated ones—I to diffuse as much knowledge as possible' " (p. 525). Nightingale went further in other correspondence: " 'I wish to see as few Doctors, either male or female as possible, for, mark you, the women have made no improvement—they have only tried to be 'men,' and they have only succeeded in being third rate men' " (p. 526).

Monteiro sees the two women as representing two different viewpoints in feminist thought: an equal rights orientation from Blackwell and a women's cultural point of view from Nightingale. To Monteiro, Nightingale represents one theoretical position in 19th-century feminism. Thus, the icon is now not merely repainted, but dipped in the different wash of feminist historical analysis, which places all women within the context of her story.

Monteiro's (1990) continued research on Nightingale and the women with whom she corresponded provides the clearest picture of Nightingale's attitudes and interactions with other women. As noted previously, feminist Harriet Martineau was important in Nightingale's life, but Monteiro considers her more a professional peer than a close friend. Although admitting that Martineau, too, like four other women friends, worked to help Nightingale, Monteiro focuses on Mary Clarke-Mohl (Clarkey), Hilary Bonham Carter (Hilly), Elizabeth Herbert (Liz), and Selina Bracebridge (Sigma), who all called Nightingale "Flo." Mohl was married but led an independent life; Bonham Carter was a single woman dominated by family obligations; Bracebridge was a married woman, who lived in her husband's shadow; and Herbert was also similarly situated until her husband (Sidney Herbert) died, after which she emerged as an author. The evidence is that these women shared a culture of womanhood, accepting male/female separation in their lives.

To Monteiro, Mohl (1793–1883) was the central figure, well acquainted with all the other women and most "modern" and most like Nightingale in personality. She was 45 years old, 27 years older than Nightingale when they met in Paris, where Mohl introduced her to her intellectual circle. Monteiro observes that Mohl took Nightingale seriously. And Nightingale wrote to Mohl about being fed up with inaction, with domestic lists and ornamental instruments of culinary accomplishments, asking if all the china, linen, and glass were necessary to make people progressive. She doubted it was good to invent wants in order to supply employment.

Hilary Bonham Carter, a cousin of Nightingale and a friend of Mohl, wrote to her about Florence's visit to Kaiserswerth, asking her to keep it a secret.

Mohl replied that Florence should be free to do her own "foolishness," even "wickedness," and if she wanted to go to some "wicked" place, she would keep the information "snug" from the folks in England. When Nightingale obtained her first nursing position through another woman friend and wrote of problems with the Governing Committee, Mohl replied, " 'Trample on the committee and ride the Fashionable Asses roughshod round Grovesnor Square' " (cited in Monteiro, 1990, p. 45). In 1856 she wrote of Florence as a great artist with a strong, creative individuality, who only after bursting out like a thunderbolt was able to do anything worthwhile: " 'What folly and cruelty to have made her for years give up her individuality under pretence that she must live for other people' " (cited in Monteiro, 1990, p. 45). After the Crimean period, until Mohl's death in 1883, they were, according to Monteiro, more relaxed, talking of kittens and cats, mutual friends, and Nightingale's responsibility at 55 for her mother, who had lost her mental faculties. Nightingale wrote: "from slavery to power . . . from power to slavery again. . . . It is the only time for 22 years that my work has not been the first reason for deciding where I should live; and how I should live. Here it is the last. It is the caricature of a life" (cited in Monteiro, 1990, p. 46).

Hilary Bonham Carter (1821–1865) was Florence's childhood friend and a year younger. Following her father's death, Hilary at 17 was the eldest daughter and her mother relied on her to help with a large family. After visiting Mohl in Paris, the two women worked together to find ways to help Florence visit hospitals. Mohl urged Hilary to live and study art in Paris, but Hilary left, feeling she was a failure in oil painting although she was competent in drawing. Nightingale, said Monteiro, confided in Hilary that everything seemed unreal, like a dream, in the social life she was living. Increasingly, Hilary, stopping her art lessons, took on more family work and Mary described her as someone who had been boned, as meat is, giving up all for others, losing all power of enjoyment, all because she was single and at everyone's beck and call, without a soul of her own.

In 1860 Hilary moved in to care for an ailing Florence, who felt ambivalent, thinking Hilary should be pursuing her own work and encouraging her to do the woodcuts for illustrations in one publication. Nightingale finally told her cousin to leave, that it was not right to absorb Hilary's life in letter writing and housekeeping. She confided to Mary, however, that "cutting off Hilary was like cutting off a limb" (p. 49). Mary questioned Florence's decision, but Florence stuck with it, inviting Hilary for visits. Subsequently, Hilary died of cancer after a year of illness. Florence wrote to Mary that there was not a single person who did not think that Hilary's family had engaged in her slow murder, thinking her worth nothing better than to be sacrificed to the "fetichism of family." Such a sad life was not uncommon, notes Monteiro, for unmarried oldest daughters in the 19th century.

When she was 25, Elizabeth Herbert (1822–1911) met Nightingale in 1847 in Rome through Selina Bracebridge, and in 1851 Florence stayed with Liz for six weeks before she had her second child. It was Liz, not her husband Sidney, who, as a Harley Street Committee member, fought to get Florence her first job. Monteiro notes that, when Nightingale decided to go to the Crimea, it was to Liz she wrote, asking her to negotiate her release from her Harley Street position and to gauge Sidney's reaction to the plan. (He had already sent a letter asking her to take charge.) On her return from the Crimea, when she was working closely with Sidney, Florence and Liz wrote to each other frequently, concerned over Sidney's health. On his death, Liz asked Florence to carry on the work and to keep Sidney's memory alive. Liz's own work included setting up lodging houses for farm workers, helping emigrating families and, later, writing.

Selina Bracebridge (1799–1874), about 20 years older than Nightingale, was, according to Monteiro, a mother surrogate for Florence and an ally in Nightingale's struggle against her own mother and sister. Both Charles and Selina Bracebridge were, in Florence's terms, more than an earthly father and mother to her. Nicknamed "Sigma" because of her love of Greece, Selina, too, was on the Harley Street Committee and she and Liz later interviewed the nurses to be sent to the Crimea. Selina went with Florence to the Crimea, but returned earlier.

Monteiro is very clear that the five women, including Harriet Martineau (1802–1876), were good friends not just to Florence, but to each other, forming a support system, a cross-linked group. A political journalist, Harriet's interaction was greatest following the Crimean War and through the years of parliamentary reform. Well-educated and widely traveled, Martineau was a columnist for the *Daily News* and, as noted previously, received confidential reports from Florence to help with her reforms by communicating Nightingale's knowledge to the public and thus, putting pressure on politicians.

Monteiro's research makes it very clear that this group of women ranged in their degree of conventionality—but some were clearly role-breakers and all supported Nightingale in her work, helping her achieve her goals. The picture of Nightingale from her personal correspondence is different from the "totally self-sufficient, independent woman" (p. 57) often portrayed; she also "accepted help from other women and recognized her indebtedness to them . . . [and] experienced the bonds of womanhood and of female friendship. . . . The private Hilary, Harriet, Selina, Mary and Liz were essential to the public Florence" (pp. 57–58).

To Monteiro, homosocial bonding, not homosexuality, was the issue. In Natalie N. Riegler's (1990) paper on Lytton Strachey's biography of Nightingale, this issue is again mentioned, although the main thrust of Riegler's article is on the inadequacy of Strachey's character sketch, his use of letters taken out of context, and his inaccuracies. He even credits Nightingale with quoting in 1861 a poem by Robert Browning that was not published until 1864!

Essentially, Riegler is in agreement with the Kalisches, but she also questions whether Strachey's bisexual relationships influenced his interpretation of Nightingale's relations with other women. Previously, Cook had claimed that a cousin and another man, both unnamed by him, were attractive to Nightingale, but he said she would never have considered marrying her cousin (Henry Nicholson). But Woodham-Smith claimed that Nightingale formed a relationship with Henry because it brought her closer to his sister, Marianne, for whom she had been seized by the "most serious" of all passions. Riegel concludes that Nightingale's relationships with her women friends were not homoerotic and were typical of 19th-century women. However, blaming Strachey's presumed sexual proclivities does not resolve the issue, which will probably remain unresolved. In contrast, Monteiro's work helps settle the question of whether Nightingale valued female friends, who formed a support network for her. Clearly she did. Thus, the accusations against her as biased against or hostile to women cannot stand and this lends support to the interpretation of her writing in *Cassandra* as clearly sympathetic to women's plight or as feminist in orientation.

Is there evidence that Nightingale also shared her work on spirituality, not only with men, but with women, too? Again, the answer is yes. JoAnn G. Widerquist (1990) also rejects F. B. Smith's caricature of Nightingale, providing research on her relationship with Mother Mary Clare Moore of the Sisters of Mercy, whom Nightingale trusted and loved, sharing her spiritual life in a mutually sustaining friendship. Georgiana Moore, leader of four nuns from Bermondsey, accompanied Nightingale on the ship to the Crimea and they continued their relationship on their return.

Widerquist asks, How in a time of "sectarianism, religious prejudice, and distrust could these two women of different faiths and national origin find so much common spiritual ground?" (p. 290). Nightingale was not religious in any orthodox sense; indeed, her beliefs were eclectic, heterodox, and essentially spiritual; she trusted that the perfectibility of people would lead to harmony, a happiness equaling perfection. The practical and rational and the mystical sides did not, according to Widerquist, mesh neatly and Nightingale's drive, not to dominate, as F. B. Smith said, but to achieve perfection led her to demand the same from others, who could not often meet the level Nightingale expected of herself. Mother Moore was an outlet for Nightingale's spiritual struggle. Their correspondence began in 1855 and continued to 1868, stopping perhaps because of failing health and heavy responsibilities. Moore died in 1874.

When Moore left Scutari because of ill health, Nightingale wrote that this departure was a severe blow to her. She recognized that Moore was superior to her in administration and spiritual matters and asked forgiveness for any pains inflicted. On Nightingale's return, she appeared alone and unannounced at the Bermondsey Convent, clearly demonstrating this contact to be one of her primary concerns after reaching England. That Moore had experienced the mystical state of another reality is clear when she wrote " 'our faith is the same' " (p. 298). The two women shared not only the thoughts of mystical writers, but the mystical experience itself. Books exchanged as gifts and loans included biographies of St. Catherine of Genoa, St. Therese, St. Catherine of Sienna, St. Frances De Sales, St. Francis Xavier, and St. John of the Cross. Of the latter, Nightingale wrote that she feared she had not entered even into the first "Obscure Night," even though it seemed so applicable to her. Clearly, she was struggling to integrate her altered reality with the practice of it in daily life.

Nightingale credited Moore with living fully in the other reality in her daily life and said she was never in full possession of that feeling. It was not simply longing for God's presence, but living in both that other reality and in the practical reality simultaneously. She saw that St. Teresa's strength and that of other mystics came not from " 'their doctrine of a God . . . but in their absolute purity of intention—their absolute linking of themselves in the idea of service' " (p. 302). Nightingale's longing for a deep spiritual life, says Widerquist, was apparent in all her letters, and she despaired over her want of "calmness" in her work. In 1889, writing to Jowett, Nightingale said that her two thoughts from God were "First to infuse the mystical religion into the forms of others (always thinking they [nurses] would shew it forth much better than I . . .). . . . Secondly to give them an organization for their activity in which they could be trained to be the 'handmaids of the Lord' " (p. 302). Widerquist believes that "The relationship of mystical life and service in nursing history needs further study by nursing scholars" (p. 302). How these interconnect with feminism, work in behalf of women to ultimately improve the whole of humanity, needs further analysis.

Widerquist rejects Smith's characterization of Nightingale's need for power, concluding instead that she needed perfection and mutuality, a fellow feeling in her relationships, which was often lacking, but not with Moore: "There was mutuality between these two women" (p. 304). Nightingale wrote in a spiritual essay, "What Is Friendship?" that there must be " 'A third in all these 'twos' to make them real or 'ideal' friends. And that third must be God' " (p. 304). Here again God was the experience of another reality and Moore and Nightingale must have shared this. Widerquist compares Nightingale's assertion with that of Irene Claremont de Castillejo (1973) who, a century later, said that " 'For there . . . to be a meeting . . . a third, a something else, is always present' " (p. 304). It may be called love, or the Holy Spirit, or according to Jung, the Self, but if this Other is present a meeting between persons cannot fail.

To Elizabeth Gaskell, noted 19th-century novelist, Nightingale's difficulty in loving individuals might be a gift if taken in conjunction with " 'her intense love for the race: her utter unselfishness in serving and ministering . . . but she is really so extraordinary a creature that impressions may be erroneous' " (p. 305). Moore shared with Nightingale the struggle to integrate the practical work of life with a vision of another reality. Widerquist's excellent work draws attention to Nightingale's drive, not for worldly power, but for the spiritual ideal of perfecting herself and humanity, though she does not connect Nightingale's feminist rejection of the shackles on women that impeded them from achieving this goal. Nevertheless, it is obvious that her rejection of women's roles and of organized religion allowed Nightingale herself to move toward a union of different realities. It is in this sense that women nurses as "handmaids of the Lord" should be understood, not in the conventional sense of sectarian religions.

In contrast to her friendship with Moore, Nightingale was not accepting of Mother Mary Francis Bridgeman, who headed the second contingent of nurses sent to the Crimea. According to Mary P. Tarbox (1990), Nightingale rejected, for example, the efforts of at least one Irish nurse to convert and rebaptize soldiers before their deaths. Bridgeman, the "personification of Irish Catholicism," in her memoirs said her major contention with Nightingale was over the unity of the church, which was not upheld since the Irish nurses and their chaplains were not allowed sufficient freedom. Furthermore, she objected to Nightingale trying to unify nuns from various motherhouses and thought it was a mistake to place the nuns under a secular supervisor, particularly if that person was a Protestant. Finally, she objected to the inadequate material provisions for human needs, an objection with which Nightingale, from a different perspective, would have agreed. Although Nightingale is conceived as the "embodiment of English Protestantism" in Sister Mary Gilgannon's (1962) doctoral dissertation, it is clear that Nightingale wanted to go beyond sectarian divisions, unifying nurses from all backgrounds. Clearly, she could do this with Moore, who shared the "same religion," the mystical reality of the ultimate, but not with Bridgeman, who seemed intent on maintaining sectarian religious divisions and purposes. Thus, Nightingale did not embody Protestantism; rather she was ecumenical in her approach.

THE NIGHTINGALE MYTH CONTINUES

Despite such scholarly efforts to understand Nightingale in her full complexity, Monteiro (1991) reports that the old Nightingale myth continues, as illustrated in the birthday memorial service for her at Westminster Abbey on May 8, 1990, the 170th anniversary of her birth on May 12, 1820. Organized by the Florence Nightingale Memorial Committee, the commemoration also honored all nurses who died in the service of Great Britain and whose names were on the Nurses Roll of Honor kept in Westminster Abbey. Attended by nurses and students, representatives of the Red Cross, and the military, the service was conducted by the dean of Westminster, Michael Mayne, and included a reading from Proverbs by a man and a reading from the Beatitudes by another man, followed by a procession of nurses bearing the Nurses Roll of Honor. After Dean Mayne's short prayer, there followed the hymn, "Dear Lord and Father of Mankind Forgive Our Foolish Ways"—a somewhat peculiar choice for a woman who felt the next savior could be a woman!

The first words from a woman were heard in the sermon by Sister Frances Dominica, who focused on faith in the midst of illness and death, and this was followed by "Hail the Resurrection Thou," again an interesting choice for a woman who questioned the existence of a judging God. Following this, a Procession to the High Altar, led by a female chief nursing officer and 20 students, "continued the Nightingale myth, the themes of service and the 'lady of the lamp'" (Monteiro, 1991, p. 5). The handing of the lamp from a sister to her staff nurse signified the passing on of the tradition of nursing; but the lamp was then handed to Dean Mayne who placed it on the high altar. Again, a somewhat ironic location for the spirit of a woman who questioned the rituals of organized religion. A prayer said in unison remembered Nightingale's sacred calling to serve the sick and injured that was passed on to nurses, who received this calling with "gladness and humility." Dean Mayne then prayed for the Lamp to shed light to praise the Father in Heaven, and gave thanks for Nightingale's vision, courage, and compassion that brought light to human suffering and sorrow.

What was a nurse historian's reaction to this commemorative service? To Monteiro, the themes emphasized service to others; loss of life in military duty; the meek and the poor from the Beatitudes; the lamp as a symbol received with humility; and the hierarchy in nursing. "The memorial service did not recognize the other dimensions of Nightingale's life and career that are being studied by current scholars, Nightingale as a social reformer and sanitarian, whose actions did not fit well into the mold of tradition and humility" (p. 6). Monteiro concludes: "The myth was what Nightingale expressed a wish to avoid, even though she did want the recognition she believed her work deserved. By emphasizing only the myth we continue to do a disservice to the broader, more complex woman, and as a memorial to Nightingale the service did not do justice to that true woman" (p. 6).

Are American nurses doing a better job of dealing with the complexity of Nightingale? In 1993, Judith Calhoun considered the history of the Nightingale pledge chanted by generations of nurses at their graduation ceremonies. Ironically, "Nightingale, in fact, knew nothing of the pledge until she was sent a copy after its completion" (p. 130). The pledge was created in 1893, but its origin was unknown, said the editor of the 1911 *American Journal of Nursing* (1911a). Responding to this statement, Lystra Eggert Gretter (1911b) said the pledge was prepared by the Farrand Training School Committee, composed of three nurses and a male reverend, associated with the Harper Hospital, Detroit, in 1893. This committee named the pledge after Nightingale, as a token of esteem for her, even though it closely paralleled the second paragraph of the Hippocratic Oath. Pledging the nurse to pass her life in purity and to loyally aid the physician in his work, these additions had become antiquated; "the pledge now epitomizes the nurse as subservient within the nurse-physician relationship, a role disdained by most professional nurses of today" (p. 130).

As Calhoun notes, the Nightingale Pledge remained unchanged until 1935, when the concept of service to the community and human welfare was added. The idea of loyalty to physicians remained intact; thus, Nightingale received credit for a pledge she never created and one that fostered dependence and obedience to physicians. Calhoun notes that the roles of women and nurses were ambiguous during the earlier women's movement, leaving nurses particularly vulnerable to moral and ethical conflicts regarding loyalty and duty based on a woman's responsibility to care. The solution was to create a role for women that compromised, using Susan Reverby's (1987a) terms, between total deference and outright defiance. Thus, "sacrifice, service, obedience to the physician, and ethical orientation were evident in the Nightingale Pledge" (p. 132). Nevertheless, Calhoun believes that the pledge is a commitment that survived the passage of time as threads are still woven into today's formal guidelines, although the sentence on loyalty to physicians has been changed. Calhoun concludes that the antiquated promises of the Nightingale Pledge are "outmoded and no longer viable" (p. 135). Ironically, to nurses who do not know the history of the pledge, Nightingale herself might be seen as outmoded when, in fact, she neither created the pledge nor necessarily condoned it. Thus, the American continuation of the moral iconography may involve a rejection of Nightingale for something she did not write.

From the publication of these more recent research studies, the complexity and character of Nightingale, so central to the public image of nursing, are better understood. Nightingale has been the primary icon and symbol of the nursing profession and what a nurse should be; her actions, motivations, and theoretical positions have been, over time, interpreted in a variety of ways, giving rise to different moral imperatives for nurses as societal values changed. Of one thing we can be certain: Nightingale's mystical view of women, humanity, and life itself must be understood if her feminism is to be placed in proper perspective. Less than this creates a caricature of this complex woman. She was the precursor of a different cosmological understanding and a practitioner of what she wanted for women, a life free of the sexist constraints of family. She fought for a legitimate occupation for women, led by women, in a world of lawful rationality infused with mystical meaning of another more fundamental reality.

Chapter 2

Nursing Leaders as Activists and Feminists

While feminist perspectives on and analyses of Florence Nightingale were more noticeable after the 1960s, nurse scholars also discovered that several of America's early nursing leaders had engaged in feminist activities, had fought for women's equal rights, and had campaigned against many social injustices of their period. As feminist scholars uncovered more and more of women's history and their social activism, nurses began to rediscover their nursing foremothers, often noting with surprise early nurses' activism, and, indeed, sometimes learning for the first time that certain well-known women were also nurses.

In this chapter, the feminist and sociopolitical activism of several major American nurse-feminist leaders from the mid-1800s on are presented and analyzed. Nurses such as Clara Barton, Sojourner Truth, Margaret Sanger, Lavinia Dock, Elizabeth Carnegie, and Wilma Scott Heide, for example, expressed their feminism and social consciousness in different ways and with varying intensity. In considering the nurse scholars who wrote about these women, we seek answers to many questions: How did the feminist activities of these women differ? Did they publicly express their support for women's rights and social injustices, or did they work "behind the scenes," manipulating men in power to achieve their goals? Was their activism expressed within nursing, or were some of these women forced to accomplish their work outside of nursing? Did they have any female networks or support systems to help them achieve their goals? And, most important, has the early legacy of nursing's social activism been lost to a narrow focus on intraprofessional concerns?

"AMERICAN WOMEN, HOW PROUD I AM OF YOU":
CLARA BARTON

Beyond Nightingale, the only woman whose name alone symbolizes nursing to the general public is Clara Barton, but even she cannot approach the worldwide icon of a nurse as represented by Nightingale. From a strictly political, feminist point of view, Barton, of the two women, probably deserves the greater recognition for her work on behalf of women. Like Nightingale, whose self-censorship of her most important feminist book may have allowed her to accomplish more with men in power, because she was not identified as a feminist, Barton, too, probably had to tone down her affiliation with feminism at times. Unlike Nightingale, however, Barton, over time, expressed her feminist thought and feelings much more openly. In societies controlled by men, the open espousal of women's rights can be the political death knell for women reformers and activists, who, nevertheless, need the support of other women to create social change. In Barton's case, her efforts to found American military nursing, and, subsequently, the International Red Cross, might have been hampered by her open identification with the women's movement. Nevertheless, Barton took a strong public stand on feminism; Nightingale, who faced similar problems, resolved them by engaging in manipulation of upper-class men in power and by subsuming her feminist thought in positivist mysticism.

In Elizabeth Brown Pryor's book, *Clara Barton: Professional Angel* (1987), the paradoxical juxtaposition of the two words in the subtitle represents the dilemma of a woman who represented the best in female culture while working with the professional tradition from male culture. Somehow "professional angel" demeans both or at least draws a picture of the irony and difficulty in bridging gendered worlds. Barton, who painfully and slowly overcame a scanty education and had difficulties in earning an income, was a natural candidate for feminism. According to Pryor, Barton's wartime work contributed even more significantly to her dedicated feminism. Barton believed that women had shown their sincere wish to contribute to society and proved to be "a political force in every soldiers' aid society and abolitionist rally" (p. 151). In a lecture never delivered, Barton wrote that woman had proved that she could be earnest, have character and firm purpose, and was competent in many crises. In poetic form, Barton said in "Women Who Went to the Field" that their work was marked by hindrance, pain, effort, and cost, yet through these came knowledge, which is power, " 'to accomplish the purpose our spirits have met' " (p. 151).

As Pryor points out, reactionary—and one might add, sexist—male observers delighted, as one said, in watching Barton, a "feminine" woman, speak in public, because she had not forsaken her "womanhood," earning her right to speak from " 'charitable ministrations . . . appropriate to her sex' " (p. 150). She did not engage in a "masculine crusade" against imaginary or greatly exaggerated abuses. But in Barton's own words, she declared her entire, earnest, heartfelt sympathy and cooperation to the thousands struggling for " 'the early and complete enfranchisement of my sex, and the admission of women of whatever race to all the rights and privileges . . . which as an intelligent human being belongs to her' " (p. 150).

Barton, on meeting feminist leaders Elizabeth Cady Stanton and Susan B. Anthony in 1867, began, according to Pryor, a long and productive relationship with them, particularly with Anthony, with whom she sustained a mutually supportive friendship. Clara spoke at women's conventions, attended rallies, and bestowed her reputation to the movement by simply sitting on the stage. In turn, Anthony advertised Barton's lectures in the publication, *The Revolution*, and in this way helped Clara obtain a livelihood from her lectures. She was subsequently supported by feminists in her struggle to organize the Red Cross. Barton also used her strong bond with veterans: " '*Soldiers! I have worked for you*—and I ask of you, now, one and all, that you consider the wants of my people. . . . God only knows women were your friends in time of peril—and you should be hers now' " (p. 151). On one occasion, Barton was publicly advertised as a speaker who was not a strong-minded woman; that is, she was not like Susan B. Anthony and her "clique," a class of women to which Barton did not belong. Barton gave her speech, but then read the offensive paragraph to the audience, claiming it not only misrepresented her as a woman, but maligned her friend, Anthony, abusing the " 'highest and bravest work ever done in this land for either you or me' " (p. 152). She continued:

> You glorify the women who made their way to the front to reach you in your misery, and nurse you back to life. You called us angels. Who opened the way for women to go and made it possible? Who but that detested "clique" who through the years of opposition, obloquy, toil and pain had openly claimed that women had rights, should have the privilege to exercise them. The right to her own property, her own children, her own home, her just individual claim before the law, to her freedom of action, to her personal liberty. Upon this, other women claimed the right and took the courage, if only to go to an army camp, and drag wounded men out of a trench, and try to save them for their families and their country. . . . No one has stood so unhelped, unprotected, so maligned as Susan B. Anthony, no one deserves so well; and soldiers, I would have the first monument that is ever erected to any woman in this country reared to her. . . . Boys, three cheers for Susan B. Anthony! (p. 152)

Barton later wrote that after this speech, applause caused the very windows to shake in their casements.

Women who try to protect other women are particularly at high political risk. As Pryor notes, Barton worked for the women's movement for forty years, but toiled for advancement in all areas, fearing that overemphasis on securing the vote for women would retard changes on other issues. It is, of course, wrongly assumed that Stanton, Anthony, and Matilda Joselyn Gage focused their efforts only on suffrage, a fact recognized by Barton. Thus, her refusal to allow her name to be put forth as an officer, or in one case as vice president, of the National Woman Suffrage Association had to be motivated by her political need to accomplish nursing and health goals, which may have been threatened. Additionally, Barton's nursing experiences in the Civil War made her recognize men's burdens and also led her in the fight over the proposed 15th Amendment to support Black men's right to vote, even if it did not include women's right to vote. She sided with the "Negroes," whose wrongs in slavery she perceived as greater than the sufferings of women in general. Furthermore, she could not believe that "the Negro, whom women had helped for so many years, would shut this door in their face" (p. 153). Barton herself had worked in Washington, DC, to bolster the spirits of the freed men and women.

Later in her life, suffering visual problems, she was taken to Europe by friends. Despite bandaged eyes, she wrote most of her letters—many on feminist issues—to female friends, penning them in the dark as if playing "blindman's bluff." When able to see, Barton was shocked, according to Pryor, with sights of European women being beaten as a matter of course and harnessed to carts like dogs, working in the fields all day, dragging tools back home while the men walked at leisure. Seeing one woman repeatedly attacked and insulted by a group of soldiers, Barton perceived "woman's plight with new eyes" (p. 172), feeling an even stronger bond with feminists.

In London, she was offended by her exclusion from an international prison conference, but while seated in the visitors' gallery, noted that the women were very disorganized. More significant, "Though living only a few blocks apart, she avoided visiting Florence Nightingale, who also declined a meeting with the American heroine whose work had been so like her own" (p. 173). Pryor believes that though "Remarkably similar in personality and aspiration, neither could brook a competitor" (p. 173). Just what caused the meeting to be avoided probably requires more analysis, but it is clear that Barton was annoyed with being called the Florence Nightingale of America; no one ever referred to Nightingale as the Clara Barton of Great Britain. The well-deserved accolades Barton received were never sufficient to bring her fully into the sacred iconography even of American nurses. Nor has she yet received her just reward for her feminist work from current feminist scholars.

On her return to the United States, Barton, in close proximity to feminist leaders in New York City and Rochester, reestablished her ties and spoke at conventions, wrote endorsements, and donated money to the feminist cause. In one letter, Anthony hoped that Barton would now "'do as much for women's emancipation as you did for the slaves & the soldiers,'" calling on her to "'organize, systematize, vitalize & marshall its forces . . . and come to

the help of the weary & worn in the service of woman'" (p. 198). Despite her heavy duties with prisons and the Red Cross, Barton accepted many invitations, contributed letters and articles to several feminist publications, subscribed to *The Woman's Journal*, attended suffrage conventions, and publicly endorsed the feminists' work. Even in her 1879 Decoration Day salute to the nation's soldiers, she said, "'American women: how proud I am of you; how proud I have always been since those days to have been a woman'" (p. 198). She declared that Abraham Lincoln said that without women's help the rebellion could not have been put down nor the country saved; "'Since that time I have counted all women citizens'" (p. 198).

Politically astute, Barton, to obtain support for the Red Cross, refused formal leadership roles with the suffragists, "sensitive to the dangers of having that organization indelibly connected with the women's rights movement" (p. 199), a cause unpopular with politicians on whom she had to depend for support. Feminist Lucy Stone questioned Barton's commitment to the suffrage cause, and to this she replied: "'I did not suppose that to be a matter of doubt. If on the occasion to which you so kindly invite me, there shall be in your assemblage one woman who doubts this, say to her for me, . . . Sister you do not know me'" (p. 199).

As a woman straddling reforms in both men's and women's cultures, Barton's position was difficult: ill health, pressures of Red Cross business, misunderstandings with feminist leaders—all these were intermixed with her anxiety that the Red Cross would be seen as just another organization of "interested women" trying to do what good they could. Unable to devote full time to feminism, she was again criticized, but Clara responded that she had "'shown a great deal of reticence in not telling the movement's leaders how to run their organization'" (p. 252), and even questioned the value of universal suffrage over "discriminative" suffrage. Later, at the request of Alice Stone Blackwell, editor of *Woman's Journal*, Barton sent dispatches, supposedly from the Dakota Territory, claiming that the time was ripe for a suffrage vote there. Barton was in Texas when the feminists discovered that Barton had never been to the Dakotas and, fearing their legitimacy would be attacked, they questioned whether her reports from Texas were equally flawed. Barton, writing to Anthony, who had criticized her in public, expressed pain at the implications for her sincerity and for her loss of the "'loving confidence of a friend unshaken by suspicion'" (p. 253).

Several years later, Barton again appeared at suffrage conventions, claiming that her place was not at the podium because she had "'not toiled as you have toiled'" (p. 253). Pryor believes that Barton would have sacrificed the vote for fair employment standards and for education for women and girls. She advised young women to "'put by your embroideries and your laundry . . . and commence your studies'" (p. 253). However, it is clear that many feminists supported not only suffrage, but very broad societal changes; thus, it is not

possible, as Pryor does, to delineate sharply between Barton and other women leaders on these issues.

There was considerable variation among feminist leaders in the 19th century. For example, Barton's approval of the Woman's Christian Temperance Union would not have received support from feminist Matilda Joselyn Gage since, in *Women, Church, and State* (1896), she had indicted the Christian church as historically central to women's oppression. According to Pryor, Barton approved of the WCTU women, of their competence, organization, and skilled debate, which to her were superior to many men's meetings, which frequently "degenerated into evenings of drinking and carousing" (p. 254). Barton saw women coming of age, breaking out of historical restrictions: " 'There have been great women in all ages, but never an epoch when *all* women were so great. . . . Women begin to *dare* to do, aye, dare *be*' " (p. 254).

By the late 1880s Barton renewed her work on suffrage at meetings of the major organizations. She spoke at several suffrage rallies in 1888, emphasizing women's intellectual and moral equality with men, ridiculing the need to beg for a right fundamental to all human beings. After one speech, Barton said, a dazed, bewildered feeling came over her when she was urged to ask for a privilege for women. She asked, " 'Of whom should I ask this privilege? Who possessed the right to confer it?' " (p. 254).

Barton was sorely pressed to deal with both her speaking engagements and Red Cross activities. In 1888, when a yellow fever epidemic broke out in Florida, she was overwhelmed with hundreds of applications from nurses. Concerned that those chosen for service be immune from the disease, she allowed the New Orleans Red Cross to select only those nurses who had already been exposed to yellow fever. According to Pryor, a group of thirty nurses, White and Black, female and male, left New Orleans for Jacksonville without Barton, who was not immune. She delegated her power and duties to Colonel F. R. Southmayd, secretary of the New Orleans Red Cross, who found, on his arrival in Jacksonville, several groups competing for the nurses' services. Unfortunately, the nurses were chosen only because of their immunity to yellow fever, and several of them behaved inappropriately, even scandalously. Southmayd attempted to organize the deteriorating situation, but succeeded only in offending the army and local physicians. Clearly, Barton's Red Cross activities, her development of nursing, and her feminist commitments demanded time beyond that available to mere mortals. Eventually, frictions and infighting within the Red Cross caused her power to be eroded. She attributed this partly to her being a woman, since few would dare to challenge directly her authority if she had been a man. Forced to rely on men in high government positions, she stated: "Mine has not been the kind of work usually given to women to perform, and no man *can* quite comprehend the situation. No man is ever called to do a man's work with only a woman's power and surroundings. How can he comprehend it?" (p. 346).

Barton, as Red Cross president, began to feel at a disadvantage with the highly educated and confident, brash new women who "ignored her work and took her small successes for granted" (p. 346). She resented and found ironic that "her removal from the Red Cross would come at the hands of her own sex, for whom she had worked for forty years" (p. 346). Feminist leaders saw this as a personal attack; Anthony sent many affectionate letters, and, according to Pryor, other leaders singled out Clara for praise, included her in conventions and rallies, and sought her out for her valued opinions. She received a standing ovation when she delivered a speech on the Red Cross at the 1902 Women's Suffrage Convention. At the 1904 convention, she was given a "teary-eyed tribute" from Susan B. Anthony, who called Barton to the stage and with her arms around Clara, spoke of her long work for women, starting with the first suffrage meeting in Washington in 1869. In Barton's own words, " 'there were only us left now to stand together at this last meeting tonight . . . we both realized that we should never stand together again before a Washington audience' " (p. 347). Barton had lived to see conferences of women eagerly attended and widely accepted by women who debated, presided over meetings, and ran their own organizations. In contrast, Pryor notes, "In her girlhood she had been barred from speaking out on school reform in her home town because of her sex, and as a lecturer she had faced audiences that were as curious to see a female speaker as they were to hear her words" (p. 347).

Ironically, Barton lost control of the Red Cross and subsequently avoided her feminist friends, lest some harm might result by others observing their friendly relations. According to Pryor, she gave only two interviews in the last few years of her life, both to young women reporters. Two groups could still persuade Barton to appear publicly, the Grand Army of the Republic, her "boys" from the Civil War, and feminists, for whom she appeared as a pioneer. In 1905, at the New England Woman Suffrage Association meeting, she was lauded along with Susan B. Anthony and Julia Ward Howe as " 'all that was left of the Old Guard' " (p. 367). In Baltimore in 1906 Anthony was too weak to speak on stage, so Barton and Howe spoke, with Clara giving the opening remarks and a tribute to Anthony, charging the younger women to take courage from the "hardships of their predecessors and to work on through disappointment or ridicule" (p. 367). She was the last survivor of her generation, writing tributes to Howe and Anthony upon their deaths. To her, women " 'unwritten, unrewarded, and almost unrecognized' " (p. 368) were the glory of the nation. Her bitterness over women's roles in forcing her removal from the Red Cross remained, and when hearing of the 1911 London suffrage parade, she said that she regretted " 'that the course of women toward me personally has been so hard, as to take the sweet from the triumph I should so much enjoy' " (p. 368).

In contrast to Nightingale, Barton directly engaged in feminist activities, establishing nursing and the Red Cross while standing firmly and publicly in behalf of all women. Her theoretical base was rooted in the tradition of civil libertarianism in contrast to the empiricist, spiritual basis of Nightingale's feminist belief system. It is the civil libertarian tradition that has most influenced subsequent nurses, who, with little access to *Suggestions for Thought*, probably retained traditional affiliations. Certainly those in religious orders remained more traditional. Since the history of women nurses in such orders has not been fully integrated into the more secular histories of nursing, it is difficult to interconnect the feminist ideologies of secular nurses and nursing sisters. Indeed, even recent research continues the separate analyses of these groups of women, but does show extensive efforts by women religious to improve the social conditions for women, children, and the poor.

THE CROSS AND THE DOVE:
MOTHER MARY FRANCIS CLARE

In 1989 Ursula Stepsis and Dolores Liptak edited *Pioneer Healers: The History of Women Religious in American Health Care*. Although this collection of short biographical accounts does not consistently integrate gender and social issues with those of nursing, one woman, Mother Mary Francis Clare, profiled by Terri Pollard, stands out as a strong proponent of women, the poor, and the disenfranchised. Margaret Anna Cusack was born in 1829 to an aristocratic family of English origins at Coolak, County Dublin. According to Pollard, her physician father influenced Margaret in caring for the needy, but her father's career was halted by cholera and Margaret, with her mother and brother, returned to her grandmother in Exeter, England, where she received the benefits of both wealth and education. Cusack became keenly aware of great social inequities: increasingly interested in social reform, she sought justice and peace, which meant to her relief from pain and suffering in a just social structure.

In 1853 she joined the Anglican Sisterhood, but after five years came to believe that petty matters took priority over the relief of human deprivations. Leaving the order, she said, " 'I do not believe in offering the Gospel of small talk to starving people' " (p. 212). In 1858 she converted to Roman Catholicism, taking her new name as a member of the Order of the Poor Clare nuns. In 1861 she was a founding member of a new convent in Kenmare, Ireland, where, as a gifted writer, she deluged newspapers with letters in which she "openly demanded equality for all, especially women" (p. 213). Equal pay for equal work, opportunities for equal education, and property rights—these and other reformist demands spread her influence in both Europe and the United States, where she was known as the Nun of Kenmare.

The Irish famine of 1879 forced her to appeal for help from supporters, and with the $20,000 she raised—a large sum at the time—she fed both starving

Catholics and Protestants. Instead of praise, Mother Clare received censure from local authorities, who viewed her as a "mere woman" interfering in politics and a menace to the patriarchal social structure; even her life was threatened. The archbishop of Kenmare closed her Famine Relief Fund and refused to see her, an action emulated by her sister nuns, leaving her alone in her room with a heart condition. Mother Clare wrote: "'As long as your Christianity is merely theoretical, they are well pleased with you, but once they find you are practical in carrying it out, they part company from you angrily'" (p. 213). Eventually, she left to establish a convent in County Mayo, where she proposed and then raised funds for an industrial school for women with a day care center for children. Again, she encountered disapproval from the local clergy, who did not want a nonconformist, a people's liberator, a woman, and a nun to change the rule of the Poor Clare Order to include social work. The men confronted her bitterly, issuing an edict that prohibited further contact with her sister nuns.

To the clergy's relief, Mother Clare left Ireland in 1883, leaving behind "the living testimony of the many thousands of people she had helped and loved" (p. 214). Fortunately, a group of like-minded sisters followed her to England, where they founded the St. Joseph Sisters of Peace. She and Sister Evangelista Gaffney went to Rome to seek papal dispensation for the new order. There she met with Pope Leo XIII, who, according to Pollard, commented favorably on Mother Clare's books on history, social issues, and church causes. He encouraged her to continue to write and assumed the complaints about her were unsubstantiated. Settling the new community in Nottingham, where the nuns were welcomed by the clergy, the women brought relief to the squalor associated with the Industrial Revolution, nursing the sick, visiting the poor, opening new schools for children, and teaching adults in the evenings. Other women joined them and their work spread to other towns.

Subsequently, Mother Clare sailed to New York, where she presented letters of support from the pope and her former bishop to Archbishop Corrigan of New York. He would not and did not see her for the next three years. She moved to New Jersey, where she received a warmer welcome, and began another community. There she proposed the idea of institutions for training the blind, only to meet with repeated refusals, all influenced by Corrigan, who even banned her from buying property in New York. Three years after her arrival in the United States, Mother Clare decided to leave, but only after publishing a book, without Church approval, striking out against Archbishop Corrigan, who had expelled a liberal priest, "'who loved the poor exceedingly . . . what matter? Obedience has been maintained, discipline has been supported'" (p. 216). Before her departure, she finally had a meeting with Corrigan, in which he inaccurately accused her of fund-raising in his diocese, said nothing of her book, and told her he never wanted to see her again.

Sadly, Mother Clare left her Catholic sisters, returned to Protestantism and the Anglican Church, and continued to write and lecture in England. Pollard notes that after Mother Clare's departure, Bishop Bagshawe, the original sponsor of the order, proclaimed himself its spiritual guide, and later the motherhouse was transferred from Nottingham to New Jersey: "The bright blue habit with its cross and dove insignia eventually gave way to the plain black habit, and . . . Mother Francis Mary Clare quietly faded into the past" (p. 216). Knowing of her pain, Sister Evangelista Gaffney, Mother Clare's close friend, moved the community and sisters to Newark. It was not until 1961, when the Second Vatican Council urged religious orders "'to return to the original spirit of the institutes, and to study their "founders" spirit and special aims'" (p. 216) that Mother Clare's memory was restored by a new generation of sisters who recognized the seeds of liberty and equality for women planted by their founder. Nevertheless, as Nightingale recognized, religious organizations provide inadequate theoretical bases for free women since the theologies are historically too often antithetical to full female liberation.

"RED EMMA": RADICAL ACTIVIST

Equally committed to social justice for all, but in sharp theoretical contrast to Mother Clare, is Emma Goldman (1869–1940), a radical activist who began her nursing career in prison. According to Vern L. Bullough (1983–84), Goldman, a Lithuanian Jewish immigrant, settled in Rochester, New York, worked in a clothing factory, and, after a brief marriage, left her husband and moved to New York City. Passionately dedicated to anarchist theory, she divorced her husband and took a number of lovers, one of whom was jailed for the attempted assassination of a steel magnate. "Red Emma" spent years lecturing, calling on her listeners to rebel against societal restrictions. These activities led to a trial at which she was convicted for inciting a riot. Ironically, this experience started her nursing career. At Blackwell Island prison in New York, she was assigned to the penitentiary hospital and trained there as a practical nurse. Goldman's account of the hospital was a severe indictment: patients with various diseases, such as tuberculosis and pneumonia, and those following major operations, were all treated in the same room. Goldman said that the patients' groans were nerve-racking, but despite long and strenuous hours, "'I loved my job . . . [and] I was gradually given charge of the hospital ward'" (p. 4). On her release from prison, she went to Europe, where she studied at the Allgemeines Krankenhaus in Vienna, receiving both nursing and midwifery certificates. While in Vienna, she also studied with Sigmund Freud.

Returning to New York, Goldman practiced midwifery, but, as Bullough notes, "Her anger mounted at the number of unwanted pregnancies she saw" (p. 4). Unable to perform requested abortions, she joined the movement to disseminate contraceptives, becoming acquainted with European leaders, often socialist, who promoted birth control. When her socialist lover, Alexander Berkman, was released from jail in 1906, she joined him in touring the country, working intermittently as a private duty nurse to support them. Speaking against the draft and other issues, they were deported in 1917 to the Soviet Union, where Goldman, according to Bullough, became disillusioned with communism. She later moved to England, where she continued her work with women, contraception, and her thinking on anarchist theory. Banned from the United States, she traveled to Canada where her family could visit her more easily.

It was in the prison hospital that Goldman had been " 'brought close to the depths and complexities of the human soul; here I found ugliness and beauty, meanness and generosity' " (p. 4). She even claimed that New York State could have rendered her no greater service than to send her to the penitentiary. Peculiarly, Bullough concludes, "Her trouble as a nurse was that she became upset at the way the poor and helpless were treated" (p. 4). Wanting to nurse all of humanity, she spent more time at the barricades than in nursing. One could revise this conclusion and ask what would have happened had *more* nurses become upset with the way the poor and helpless were treated and took to the barricades as Goldman did?

THE REVOLT OF WOMAN AGAINST SEX SERVITUDE: MARGARET SANGER

Another nurse who took to the barricades for women was Margaret Sanger (1879–1966), who has lately been reconsidered by several feminist historians, usually with little attention to her early training and work in nursing. In 1986, however, Mary-Ann Ruffing-Rahal published an article on Sanger as both nurse and feminist in order to reexamine the feminist legacy related to the current controversy over women's rights to control their own bodies. An early inductee into the American Nurses Association Hall of Fame, along with Lillian Wald, Lavinia L. Dock, Annie Goodrich, and Adelaide Nutting, Sanger, the sixth of eleven children, was influenced by her father's socialist perspective, which emphasized contributing to society. According to Ruffing-Rahal, Sanger's early life in Corning, New York, could not have been easy as a child of the town radical, who was an outspoken advocate of suffrage and emancipation, even though "he relegated all household work to his wife" (p. 246). Irish Catholic immigrants in "large, unruly households" were a sharp contrast to the smaller families in "orderly homes," leading Sanger to associate " 'poverty, toil, unemployment, drunkenness, cruelty, fighting, [and] jails' " with large families (p. 246). At age 48, her mother died of tuberculosis, a condition not helped by 18 pregnancies. Sanger herself contracted the disease. After her mother died, Sanger was accepted as a nursing probationer at White Plains Hospital.

In New York, Sanger became deeply involved in radical social movements, later credited by her to her early work in nursing, but she eventually focused her attention on birth control. Although biographers have downplayed Sanger's nursing career, she, in her own autobiography, does not. During her years in New York City, nurses were in great demand since few people wanted to go to hospitals to be "practiced" upon. Sanger (1971) noted that this attitude was vehemently held by women toward childbirth: "A woman's own bedroom, no matter how inconveniently arranged, was the usual place for her lying-in" (p. 86).

Sanger was often summoned to homes where families welcomed her advice and followed it. More and more, she worked with women from New York's Lower East Side, where she "hated the wretchedness and hopelessness of the poor" (p. 86). She began to expand her outlook, seeing the woman's unique background and her potentialities as an individual. Patients welcomed nurses with fruit, jellies, and gefilte fish, and Sanger noted, "It was infinitely pathetic to me that they, so poor themselves, should bring me food" (p. 87). The women would sit down for a "nice talk," frequently asking for birth control measures, some self-protection since they could not rely on their husbands. The worst circumstances were for women from the "submerged, untouched classes." No sun penetrated the apartments; garbage and refuse were profuse; fetid odors permeated airless rooms; derelicts were "boarders" and people slept six to a room; little girls were violated and abused—these conditions were associated with pregnancy, "a chronic condition." The doomed women implored Sanger to reveal the "secret" rich people had. The women stood in groups outside the office of a five-dollar abortionist, and Sanger heard repeated tales of women who had gone to the hospital, never to return, or who had simply committed suicide. Destitution linked with excessive childbearing caused a "Waste of life . . . utterly senseless" (p. 89).

Sanger cared for one woman, with an induced abortion and consequent septicemia, who recovered and asked how to prevent another pregnancy that would now surely kill her. The doctor advised her husband to sleep on the roof. The woman turned in absolute despair to Sanger, saying the doctor was a man so he could not understand and pleaded for a woman's help. Sanger could not help and weeks later returned to find the patient pregnant and in a coma from which she never recovered.

Sanger walked for hours that night in the hushed streets, seeing images of women in travail, bringing forth babies, naked, hungry, wrapped in newspapers; children, "pinched, pale, wrinkled faces, old in concentrated wretchedness . . . white coffins, black coffins . . . interminably passing in never-ending succession" (p. 92). She went to bed, knowing she was through with palliatives, that she would try to "change the destiny of mothers whose miseries were vast as the sky" (p. 92).

After marrying William Sanger in 1902, she bore three children and lived in Westchester County for several years. When the family eventually returned to New York City, both she and her husband became active in the Socialist Party, associating with trade unionists, socialists, and anarchists. However, none of these groups seemed to regard the issues of domestic freedom for women or gender inequities as pertinent to the need for social change. Sanger was, in her own words, "'enough of a Feminist to resent the fact that woman and her requirements were not being taken into account in reconstructing this new world about which all were talking. They were failing to consider the quality of life itself'" (p. 247).

Sanger began speaking to groups of women for whom she published a series, "What Every Mother Should Know," in *The Call*, a socialist newspaper, followed by "What Every Girl Should Know." One article was not printed because certain venereal diseases were named. Supporting striking textile workers, she evacuated 119 of their children, found shelter for them, and screened them for communicable disease. Later, in Washington, DC, she provided testimony in support of the strikers. On her return to New York City, she resumed her nursing career, providing home delivery and baby care through referrals from her sister, a staff nurse at Mt. Sinai Hospital. Later, she worked with visiting nurses from the Henry Street Settlement.

Sanger's anger, dismay, and agitation about the plight of the poor, particularly women, her usual cases, were shared by other nurses, who in textbooks of the day questioned whether public health nurses were happy and, if not, advised other work because the poverty and misery of so many might prove to be too depressing. Sanger herself found no satisfaction, hating the wretchedness and hopelessness of the poor. Her concern changed from her early hospital attitude: "I could see that much was wrong with them which did not appear in the physiological or medical diagnosis. A woman in childbirth was not merely a woman in childbirth. My expanded outlook included a view of her background, her potentialities as a human being, the kind of children she was bearing, and what was going to happen to them" (p. 247). Thus, she left nursing because she "'could not go back merely to keeping people alive'" (p. 248).

Sanger subsequently traveled to Europe, where she found greater acceptance of birth control. Returning to New York, she helped found the National Birth Control League and initiated a magazine, *The Woman Rebel*, in which she announced that contraceptive information would be published for women in the next issue. The Post Office, giving no reason, pronounced the issue "unmailable," but Sanger, aware that providing information on contraceptive techniques was illegal, also knew that general discussion of the issue was not. She goaded officials to action "by publishing an article on assassination (prohibited under the same law as birth control!) . . . [and] was charged with nine counts of violating the Federal Statutes" (p. 248). Arranging for her children's care, she published *Family Limitation*, which gave explicit information and illustrations about contraception, and then fled to Europe to avoid certain prosecution.

After studying Dutch contraceptive clinics, Sanger returned to New York in 1915, and in 1916 the government dropped its charges against her. Defying political, legal, and medical authorities, Sanger opened the first birth control clinic in the United States, directly violating the law that allowed only physicians to give contraceptive information solely for the purpose of preventing disease. Her clinic was closed down and she was arrested. The court recommended leniency if Sanger would promise not to violate the law again; she accepted this, but only until she could appeal the verdict. Consequently, she was sentenced to 30 days in the workhouse. After her release, she quickly published *The Birth Control Review* and continued to send out issues of *Family Limitation*.

In contrast to some feminists, Sanger demanded a more fundamental right for women: the freedom to control their own bodies. In 1920 she published *Woman and the New Race*, in which she asserted that the most far-reaching social development in modern times was "the revolt of woman against sex servitude" (p. 1). All the international programs, alliances, hegemonies, spheres of influence, even the League of Nations were to no avail, said Sanger, if women continued to produce explosive populations. These would convert men's pledges to scraps of paper.

To Sanger, men assumed and women accepted women's positions; even feminist demands for suffrage, legislative regulations of working hours, and equal property rights would not free women if they had no control over their own bodies. Although other feminists had made the claim prior to Sanger, few had emphasized it so eloquently and centrally. Woman, unconscious of her inferior status, was bound to her lot as a "brood animal for the masculine civilizations of the world" (p. 2). Tyranny, famine, plague, and poverty were founded on a "submissive maternity" that led to overpopulated nations too large for their boundaries and natural resources. In ignorant resignation, most women knew nothing about reproduction and the consequences of excessive childbirth; some revolted, using infanticide and abortion, but individuals could not create the fundamental revolution in which women were now engaged. The key to liberty, said Sanger, is to control whether, under what conditions, and when women will be mothers. Palliatives, "child-labor laws, prohibition, regulation of prostitution and agitation against war" (p. 6), are superficially useful, said Sanger, but do not touch the source, the cheapened value of life in overpopulation. Woman must know her reproductive nature and rid herself of ignorance of the extent and effect of her submission. To do this "means warfare in every phase of her life" (p. 7).

Women's goal was to remake the world, to create a new race. An "incubated" race brought quantity, not quality, but women's choice could lead to greater influence on fewer children. In an evolutionary argument for eugenics, Sanger claimed that full development of womanhood must precede motherhood. Liberation of the feminine spirit would enable women to enfold not merely their own children, but humanity's children. Unequivocally, Sanger stated, "An abused motherhood has brought forth a low order of humanity. . . . Fearless motherhood goes out in love and passion for justice to all mankind. It brings forth fruits after its own kind" (p. 234). The clarion call for women to control their own bodies is now fundamental to the current philosophy of feminism. The issues as posed by Sanger are still appropriate today: the unfinished task for women is to take charge of their biological "destiny." Sanger claimed: "The basic freedom of the world is woman's freedom. A free race cannot be born of slave mothers. A woman enchained cannot choose but give a measure of that bondage to her sons and daughters. No woman can call herself free until she can choose . . . whether she will or will not be a mother" (p. 94).

Sanger's theoretical base extended beyond socialism to a radical feminism that demanded full freedom, a mastery of sex through birth control, providing an autonomy that was the basis of a new morality, spiritual growth, and familial harmony without a sexuality based on fear and guilt. Ruffing-Rahal (1986) contrasts Sanger, who challenged the system, with Nightingale, who worked within the system. But, had Nightingale's book that included the *Cassandra* essay been published, it is questionable how much she would have been seen as working within Victorian social and religious norms. To Ruffing-Rahal, Sanger's life "demonstrates that nursing interventions concentrated at the level of individuals and personal systems are not enough. . . . We must venture beyond client advocacy and personal service into the realm of social and political change" (p. 249).

It is important to understand that, working as a nurse, Sanger could not realize her goals of emancipating women from society's reproductive expectations because of constraints on practice imposed by male medical and governmental authority. She realized she could not function effectively as an advocate for her patients under these restrictive conditions. Thus, Sanger was forced to go *outside* of her profession to fight for the rights of women and to effect change. Perhaps this is why her work is usually portrayed as unrelated to nursing, and why some in the profession are not aware that she was a nurse.

PROGRESSIVE REFORMER AND HUMANITARIAN: LILLIAN WALD

At the same time that Sanger called for women's biological freedom, Lillian Wald, an outstanding progressive nurse activist and a supporter of feminism, founded, with Mary Brewster, the Henry Street Settlement House in New York City, where she crusaded for improving the health of poor people from all ethnic and racial groups. Wald's activities provide a notable example of the essential relationship between humanitarian and feminist concerns. She involved herself in trade unions, established the Children's Bureau, and became a suffragist, though "not an aggressive one," according to Robert L. Duffus (1938), who restated the feminist position: "It did seem absurd that she (Wald) and 'Sister' Kelley and Jane Addams and a multitude of women who were carrying the world's burdens on their shoulders shouldn't be thought capable of casting a ballot wisely, while drunkards and gamblers, procurers and bums, the ignorant and debased of the male sex, were welcomed at the polls" (p. 113).

Wald devoted her life to the Henry Street Settlement; but she also gave much for the suffrage battle. She took a clear position on women and war: "Never before, during the time of any great conflict, have women been so organized or self-conscious as now" (p. 148). Speaking of women in 1915 during World War I, she exclaimed: "It is fitting that the world should ring with their outcry against this blasphemy upon all the things that they hold most sacred. . . . The voices of free women rise above the sounds of battle in behalf of those women and children abroad, for it is against women and children that war has ever been really waged" (p. 148). Wald recognized not only the inherent conflict suffered by nurses as healers caught up in wartime expectations, but also the devastating effects of violence on women and children.

As Duffus stated, Wald did not expect a political utopia as the result of women's suffrage. "Neither did she have that dread of a growing antagonism between the sexes. . . . The suffrage, for her, was a practical way of getting things done that needed to be done" (p. 171) and, although she was not "militant" for suffrage, she understood and had deep affection for many who were; for example, she knew and admired the radical feminist Pankursts in England. "She took endless delight and satisfaction in the enthusiasm which Lavinia Dock and Florence Kelley had for the cause, and the characteristic ways in which they showed it" (p. 172). Although Duffus takes great pains to prove that Wald was not a militant feminist, his perspective has been questioned by later scholars.

Teresa E. Christy's 1970 article on Lillian Wald presents a different view of this fascinating woman and nurse, recounting Wald's nursing experience and life in the Lower East Side of New York City. It is clear that Wald's daily life was a living example of the independent woman, who fought against the suffering of women and their children. Christy does not focus directly on Wald's feminism, and some writers have downplayed and excluded the feminism expressed by both Wald and Dock. Other views, however, are offered by Resnick in her 1973 dissertation on Wald and her years at Henry Street, by Doris Daniels in her fine 1976 dissertation, *Lillian D. Wald: The Progressive Woman and Feminism*, later published as *Always a Sister: The Feminism of Lillian D. Wald* (1989), and by Coss (1989). Daniels' work is more centered on gender issues, and she recognizes that Wald's world was essentially a woman's world.

Daniels (1976) claims that Wald's pragmatic nature did not permit her to take a doctrinaire stand or to develop a comprehensive and consistent philosophy extended to feminism; thus, her writings on women seem contradictory, being more overtly feminist in private letters to other women than in public speeches. Daniels also asserts that Wald changed her thinking over time: "Before suffrage, she emphasized woman's traditional relationship to the home. In the 1920's and 1930's, she stressed more the right of " 'each one to decide for himself or herself what he or she wants to make of life . . . [and] the professions, the vocations and avocations should be and ought to be the privilege of the individuals . . . irrespective of sex' " (p. 158). Daniels contends that Wald was not able to resolve the dichotomy of home and profession or occupation. It is also likely that the originator of an experimental "commune" for women knew what the public could accept. Wald asserted that the age-old desire to cherish and dignify life still sustained women, but that they had to expand their interests from home to community; to increase their social self-consciousness in the struggle for social and political freedom; to obtain the education needed to readapt their social interest to a changed environment.

According to Daniels, Wald, an optimistic, liberal reformer, believed that women's involvement in the public sector would enlarge, slowly but inevitably. Wald knew that she and others accepted by the public had established precedence and had a responsibility for removing barriers to employment. But she deplored the emphasis on appearance and the indignities endured by women who wanted government jobs. For example, she brought her power to bear on Chicago officials who required vaginal examinations for nurses employed by the health department. With humor, Wald told of shocking some inmates in a girls' reformatory who refused to accept women as police officers, claiming, instead, that a woman's place was in the home!

Wald welcomed the end of the " 'restricted, secluded, non earning woman . . . the clinging vine . . . who rejoiced in the place assigned to them' " (p. 160). She admitted that women differed in their devotion to home, but this was only a question of degree, since both men and women have an identical stake in life and sources of happiness and security. Still, Wald considered the care of home and protection of children the most important work that visiting nurses could help sustain. She fought for aid to dependent children of widows, and rejected the right of the New York City Board of Education to deny leaves of absence for pregnant women teachers.

Wald was not able to be too vocal, but favored instructing children in sex education and hygiene, particularly since her nurses could not avoid their patients' ignorance of contraceptive matters and the resulting problems this caused. Though unwilling to confront the medical "fraternity" on the issue of contraception, she was supportive of those physicians who were willing to investigate the practice of contraception. Wald watched Margaret Sanger's work closely and regretted that her individual inclinations to support Sanger must be subsumed in order to secure the resources necessary to sustain her nurses, many of whom were already criticized for their attitude on the issue. In 1921 Wald allowed her name to be used as a committee member to organize the first American Birth Control Conference. Still, she differentiated her endorsement of contraceptive information as a personal position only and assured a Catholic monsignor that her nurses were not giving contraceptive instructions nor encouraging abortions. In other correspondence, however, Wald implied that the nurses were involved in contraceptive actions to help women.

According to Daniels, Wald, in not questioning marriage and motherhood, was similar to most other feminists of the period who, themselves, had rejected marriage, even expressing hostility toward it. The enslavement of womanhood by the "master of the house" was even a more cruel trap for emancipated women. It is obvious that Wald could not publicly attack, but privately considered marriage and maternity as blocks to a public career. She said to Lavinia Dock: " 'I can't bear to think of your gallant spirits held down to household drudgery' " (p. 168). Certainly, Wald's feminist philosophy was coherent if it is traced in her actions, not simply her words, in the experiment with nurses to free women.

In 1993 Barbara A. Backer connected Wald's activism with caring, translating the latter into health and social policies and practices, the more impressive given the fact that women did not achieve voting rights until 1920. Born in changing times, Wald was a product of her time: the shift from rural to urban, the migration of nearly 30 million immigrants between 1820 to 1910, the struggle of African Americans to change from slaves to free people, the shift to industrialization and its product, wretched living and working conditions—all these were associated with extraordinary changes in women's lives, including a decline of fertility of White American women and their increasing entrance into higher education. Oddly, Backer makes no direct mention of the earlier women's movement beginning in the mid-19th century, which strongly influenced Wald and her generation.

Backer, however, is clearly aware that Wald's Henry Street Settlement provided women the opportunities to express leadership and power, opportunities not readily available for women at the time. Wald's leadership style was participatory, but her own authority and the nurses' needs for autonomy were both recognized. Backer accepts Daniels' emphasis on Wald's pragmatism rather than theory and her desire to dignify homes, mothers, children, and families, but in the real sense of the word—through health, housing, and protection. In addition, Backer shies away from Wald's private self, believing her personal feelings, relationships, and thoughts were not well known.

Backer's major interest is in Wald's capacity to establish caring, not simply curing, and she uses her success as a model for nurses today. How do nurses who value caring function in bureaucratic and technological systems that do not reward caring values, and how do they transform these values into activism to create a more humanistic system? Relying on Susan Reverby's work (1987a; 1987b), Backer also concludes that caring, traditionally associated with women's work, forced nurses to deal with gender and class in the broader society and into coalitions with other professional, occupational, and consumer groups to initiate change. Interestingly, however, Backer excludes mention of feminist groups, those who most strongly supported Wald and her family of women nurses in the early 1900s.

NETWORKS OF FEMALE LOVE AND SUPPORT: CRUCIAL TO WOMEN IN A HOSTILE WORLD

The female support networks of early political activists captured the interest of several women's studies scholars during the 1970s. Blanche Wiesen Cook (1977), for example, analyzes two nurses, Lillian Wald and Emma Goldman, and lawyer/journalist Crystal Eastman. While men's friendships have been historically glorified and acclaimed, the friendships of women, according to Vera Brittain (1947), have been unsung, mocked, belittled, and falsely interpreted. Cook deplores the traditional historian's emphasis on the great-men tradition, espousing instead the inseparable connection between personal choices and relationships and political, public efforts. In Cook's ten years of historical research on the earlier peace movement, she had focused on women's political contributions and not on their personal lives; for example, when she came upon a love letter by Lillian Wald, she would simply note "love letter" and move on. In her 1977 article, she corrects this approach to women's history, recognizing that "networks of love and support are crucial to . . . women [who] work in a hostile world" where they are not expected to prevail or even survive (p. 44).

Jane Addams and Lillian Wald, progressive reformers, founded the most famous of all settlement houses—Hull House and the Henry Street Settlement, respectively. Attorney Crystal Eastman, a generation younger, authored New York State's first workman's compensation law; founded with Alice Paul the Congressional Union for suffrage; helped found the Women's Peace Party, later named the Women's International League for Peace and Freedom; and was president of its New York branch. Emma Goldman, anarchist immigrant, visited the Henry Street Settlement in New York where she found, in her words, " 'women of ideals, capable of fine, generous deeds' " (p. 44), but who, she feared, would foster snobbery among the people whom the nurses were trying to help. Goldman and Eastman worked on behalf of birth control, legalization of prostitution, and free speech in wartime. Wald, Eastman, and Goldman all worked to avert war, but only Goldman was deported.

With very different political strategies and visions, all four women were centrally devoted to the full development of women based on absolute equality guaranteed by economic security. Their lifestyles were dramatically different, but only Goldman relied predominantly on men for emotional and political support; nevertheless she "'longed for a friend of my own sex, a kindred spirit with whom I could share the innermost thoughts and feelings I could not express to men . . . [but] there was no personal, intimate point of contact'" (p. 45). Eastman, surrounded by men committed to social change, also had a feminist support group composed of the "new women" of Greenwich Village, who considered men "splendid lovers and friends" but turned to women for more "egalitarian support" (p. 45). In contrast, Jane Addams and Lillian Wald were "involved almost exclusively with women who remained throughout their lives a nurturing source of love and support" (p. 45).

Cook laments the exclusion of women's private lives from historical inquiry, which, when connected to the bigotry of homophobia, has erased women's capacity to deal healthfully with a variety of role models and creative communities of women. Thus, many women were branded "lonely spinsters," and the papers and letters they wrote, revealing life-long love and companionship with other women, have been suppressed, excluded, or ignored. The forty-year relationship between Jane Addams and Mary Rozet Smith has been called by historians one of "spouse-surrogates." Addams, without a man, marriage, and children, was, according to one man, "'largely untouched by the passionate currents that swirled around her'" (p. 47). According to Cook, male historians have pictured Jane Addams as a conventional lady with pearls; thus, they could exclude her intense, romantic attachments to women, avoiding any suspicion of "perversion."

Of nursing leader Lillian Wald, historical facts show that she made no denial nor discouragement of female affection, but this is explained away by claims that she was too busy for social relations, or that the lesbianism inherent in the warmth and strength derived from other women is "irrelevant" (p. 47). But Cook states: "Not until our society fully accepts as moral and ordinary the wide range of personal choice will differences be 'essentially irrelevant'" (p. 47). Difference arouses fear and condemnation, causing serious methodological problems in writing about women who were forced to hide their sexuality to avoid both psychoanalytic "treatment" and criminal prosecution. The question of who is a lesbian is answered by Cook: "Women who love women, who choose women to nurture and support and to create a living environment in which to work creatively and independently, are lesbians" (p. 48). To define lesbianism by sexual behavior alone is ridiculous since it is only "one expression of a whole range of emotions and responses to each other that involves all the mysteries of our human nature" (p. 48).

If one must rely on physical evidence, Cook contends there *is* evidence of Wald's sexual intimacy with women in her two volumes of memoirs and over 150 boxes of correspondence. Wald and her long-term supporters at the Henry Street Settlement worked, lived, vacationed, and traveled together for over 50 years. Yet Cook admits that the specifics are missing in, for example, Lavinia Dock's 10-year hiatus in corresponding with Wald, and Dock's unexplained departure from the Settlement house in 1915. Cook wonders whether the Dock–Wald estrangement was caused by different political orientations of the two women. Dock joined the Advisory Council of the Congressional Union but informed Alice Paul that Wald could not ally herself with any one feminist group because she had friends in all of them. While Wald was negotiating on peace with President Wilson, militant suffragists were being arrested for their demonstrations. Dock was furious with criticisms (including those of Wald's) of feminist confrontational tactics as harmful to both the suffrage and peace movements. Still, Wald wrote of Dock, " 'Everyone admired her. . . . Reputed a man-hater, we knew her as a lover of mankind' " (p. 50).

Cook points to the irony of current attacks on homosexuals, particularly as teachers, claiming that Anita Bryant, then crusading (in 1977) against homosexuals as educators, would no doubt demand that our children be saved from such as Wald and Addams, both of whom helped establish the U.S. Children's Bureau, which set up programs for battered women and children, fought against child labor, and promoted humane child care (p. 48). What would Bryant and other homophobics say if they knew that Addams "slept in the same house, in the same room, in the same bed with Mary Rozet Smith for 40 years. . . . And when they travelled . . . even wired ahead to order a large double bed for their hotel room" (p. 48)?

Cook contends that the criminal stigma attached to homosexuals, en masse, is largely a product of this century. From 1740 to 1895 the *Index Catalogue of the Library of the Surgeon General's Office, U.S. Army,* contained only one article that dealt specifically with lesbians; but Nancy Sahli finds that between 1896 and 1916 there were over 90 books and 566 articles about women's so-called "perversions," "inversions," and "disorders"—emerging from pseudomedical "science" or more precisely psychoanalysis (p. 48).

According to Cook, woman-related women do not respond only sexually, but "feel attraction, yearning," and emotional and intellectual "excitement" with women, none of which has been successfully explained by any existing theories (p. 48). Lillian Wald, unlike Jane Addams, had several companions who were her friends for life; first, her nurses at the Settlement house; second, society women who attempted to influence and monopolize her; and third, affluent women, such as Alice Lewisohn and Rita Morgenthau, who, with Jacob Schiff, contributed much to the Henry Street Settlement. These women were also co-workers in the Women's Peace Party. Alice's sister, Irene Lewisohn, in one letter to Wald, expressed her love and gratitude for cherished memories: " 'A fireside romance and a moonlight night are among the treasures carefully guarded'" (p. 50). Wald's influence was profound. Morgenthau wrote that everything that stood for beauty had been inspired by Wald, for whom thankfulness could never be whispered. Wald's inspiration to others was, according to Dock, due to Wald's absolute belief in human nature and her ability to develop perceived strengths in people that had been dormant. Dock remembered being greatly impressed by Wald's "'inner vision'" (p. 50).

Society women, such as Mabel Hyde Kittredge and Helen Arthur, were encouraged to think politically by Wald, but social change was not their primary commitment. According to Cook, Kittredge's demands seemed on occasion to be outrageous, but Wald was smitten by her, relied on and deeply trusted her. Supporting Wald, who was grieving about a friend, Kittredge wrote:

> I seemed to hold you in my arms and whisper all this. . . . If you want me to stay all night tomorrow night just say so when you see me. . . . Please don't feel that I keep before me the signs of sorrow that you trusted me enough to let me see—of the things of Thursday evening that are consciously with me are first the fact that in a slight degree I can share with you the pain that you suffer. Then I can hear you say 'I love you'—and again and again I can see in your eyes the strength, and the power and the truth that I love—but the confidence in yourself not there. All this I have before me—never a thought of weakness because you dared to be human. Why dear I knew that you were human before Thursday night—I think though that our love never seemed quite so real a thing before then. Good night. (p. 51)

It is clear, according to Cook, that Wald's nursing and social commitments took priority over her personal relations, and even Kittredge realized that Wald really did not have much time for her. In 1906 Wald vacationed with another society woman, Helen Arthur, an attorney who understood the demands on Wald but still yearned to be with her: "I think so often of the hundreds who remember you with affection and of the tens who openly adore you and I appreciate a little what it all means and I'm grateful to think that your arms have been close around me and that you did once upon a time, kiss me goodnight and even good morning, and I am your lonesome little/Judge" (p. 53). Such letters, according to Cook, representing only a fragment of Wald's life, leave unanswered questions because intimate details cannot be known if they are "censored, withheld, or destroyed"; nevertheless, Cook concludes that the evidence is clear: "Wald lived in a homosocial world that was also erotic" (p. 53). Thus, it is unnecessary to provide evidence of a specific type of sexual contact. What is important to establish is the truth of the multiple variations in lifestyles and of role models actually available to women.

Cook contrasts Wald and Eastman with Goldman, whose devotion to the men in her life was discussed earlier. Goldman decried the brutally deforming institutions—the family, state, moral codes—which see " 'in every strong, beautiful uncompromising personality a deadly enemy' " (p. 54). Both Goldman and Eastman, though identified with men, refused to be trapped by conventional or legal arrangements such as traditional marriage. An advocate of "free love," Goldman had long-term, tender, and nurturing relations with the men she loved; they did not possess, control, or dominate her, but expected free giving from her because she loved as a free woman. But, says Cook, "The refusal of Eastman and Goldman to separate the personal from the political, their contempt for sham and hypocrisy, and their unfaltering openness about the most intimate subjects horrified their contemporaries" (p. 54). Ironically, Addams barred Eastman from an international women's meeting in the Hague in 1919 because of her radical socialism and advocacy of "free love." Dependent on the rich to help the poor, social-reform women had to make "political decisions which were not in harmony with their lives and which locked them into a conservative public position regarding such issues as sexuality" (p. 54).

Goldman temporarily received support from the two women editors of *The Little Review*, but she scorned American feminists as class-biased and of no interest except as amusing examples of feminine intellectual homosexuality. Ironically, she was also the only woman in America who, according to Cook, publicly defended homosexuality and decried the conviction of Oscar Wilde. When criticized by friends, she said, " 'I minded the censors of my own ranks as little as I did those in the enemy's camp' " (p. 56). Cook claims that Goldman's ambivalence toward lesbianism could be understood in her relation with Almeda Sperry, with whom she was probably involved, but about whom she does not speak; nevertheless, Cook concludes that Goldman felt the right of any woman to be a lesbian was absolute, but somehow this made her less than a full woman. Goldman wrote to her lover, Sasha Berkman, in 1925 that a woman needs a person who really cares, and that with age, " 'it is doubly tragic not to have anyone, to really be quite alone. . . . I am consumed by longing for love and affection for some human being of my own' " (p. 58). Goldman never found the one great friend "who could understand her empty places, and . . . never acknowledged the value of feminist alliances" (p. 59).

To Cook, these four women—Addams, Eastman, Goldman, and Wald—presented a "range of choices and affinities that were charged with courage, experiment, fulfillment, and intensity" (p. 60). Rather than assuming that women social reformers were asexual, self-denying, or puritanical, or that they were, without men, lonely, bitter, and without community, Cook finds that they were often supported by strong female networks and communities, with personal relations marked by passionate loyalty and love.

Daniels (1976), too, in her earlier research, found that although Wald had extensive ties with influential men, she could say of women that they were more than friends. Men were included, however, and Wald saw her "family" as more balanced, but as Daniel notes, the nurse-female influence was so extensive that Yssabella Waters asked permission to bring men to Christmas dinner, assuring Wald that they would leave shortly after, but explaining that it would be "'heathenish to shut them out in a night like this when they have no home to go to'" (p. 133).

Far from feeling like lonely spinsters, the women of Henry Street, freed from "divisive competition for men and the usual competition from men," considered themselves fortunate in their "camaraderie and commitment" to their social causes (p. 133). To one observer, Wald was seen as stateswoman, the "Great Mother" of a new order that would not function through the old, rigid, patriarchal system. Daniels catches the exhilarating sense of belonging, the sisterhood allowing self-realization and more power than is possible in "'more fixed and older institutions'" (p. 134). The women worked and played hard, writing skits for evening entertainment; in one of these, Wald was elected mayor of New York City and chose her "cabinet" from the nurses. This happy environment was achieved by talking "'suffrage loud and suffrage long, at every chance you get'" (p. 134).

Daniels claims that entrance into the "family" was based on common interests and goals, and the fact of womanhood rather than ideology and class. Not only nurses, but all "kindred spirits" were included, working class women and those from other nations. These women were activists, who acted and accomplished change for the improvement of life, feminists in a women's network that stretched across states; they mutually supported each other in a feeling of sisterhood. As family members, they ran errands, purchased gifts, helped blood relatives, accepted "souls" sent by friends, worried about health and medical problems, gloried in each other's achievements, particularly when "mere females" secured good positions. Wald exulted when Alice Hamilton was appointed to the Harvard Medical School, which could not avoid doing so since she was the foremost authority on industrial hygiene: "'I think she would disarm any anti-feminist'" (p. 136). This generosity was extended to the younger generation of women. For example, Wald recommended Grace Abbott to head the Children's Bureau, and later campaigned for her to be Secretary of Labor under Hoover, arguing that women had proved their "'ability and suitability . . . for high office without prejudice of sex'" (p. 137). Although unsuccessful in her efforts for Abbott, Wald and her friends did succeed in getting Frances Perkins appointed as Secretary of Labor under Franklin Roosevelt.

Lillian Wald and Jane Addams worked together on scores of projects over the years, even though they had difficulties at times in agreeing on tactics or goals. Attorney Florence Kelley, very different in personality and temperament, shared the same principles and worked well with Wald for many years. Kelley was not, in Wald's words, a "'gentle saint'" but an inspirational influence; intolerant of inaction, she was "'a terrifying opponent'"

(p. 140). Kelley married, had three children, divorced her husband, lived at Hull House in Chicago, and was excluded from socialist circles; but she was appointed the first female chief inspector of factories in Illinois, setting legislative standards against child labor and sweatshops. Daniels notes that the women at both Hull House and Henry Street became "surrogate mothers" for Kelley's children, and eventually, Kelley moved to New York and lived at Henry Street for 24 years. Daniels concludes: "The bonds of friendship and love that existed between Addams, Wald and Kelley are documented by their correspondence. The support they provided one another, even when they differed should never be underestimated. Wald was the politician, Kelley the passion and Addams the philosopher and symbol of the women of the Progressive period" (p. 142).

Daniels confirms the trust and respect that Wald and Goldman expressed to each other, although, as previously noted, Emma considered Wald's work only palliative, though sincere. Still, Goldman called on Wald for help; however, in one case, Wald refused to help Emma place ads in the nurses' *Journal* when she wanted to represent herself as a "Vienna Scalp and Face Specialist" (p. 144). Wald did contribute money to Goldman so she could write her autobiography, and Goldman welcomed Lavinia Dock as a fellow convict after Dock was jailed for her feminist activism.

In contrast to Cook, Daniels rejects the claims that the Settlement House women were, as James R. McGovern said, critical of men and lacked sexual contacts with them. Daniels acknowledges that there is evidence that the women's relations were not "genteel," a curiously Victorian expression, and that the evidence comes from "their sentimental and emotional personal letters" (p. 144). Daniels admits that the letters do imply intimacy, and superficially they might prove homosexuality not uncommon; however, she finds it inconceivable that Wald's flowery style in many letters to both women and men could all indicate intimacy. Furthermore, Daniels cannot believe that Wald would have allowed these letters to be used for her 1938 biography by R. L. Duffus if indeed they contained evidence of physical intimacy. In 1963 Alice Hamilton denied open lesbian activity occurred at Hull House, but agreed that there was unconscious, although unimportant, sexuality. However, it seems quite impossible that women at the level of intelligence of Wald and Addams could be totally unaware of their own sexual proclivities. Daniels argues that sublimation of sexual interests did not mean the end of romance or of significant personal relations. But, it is quite impossible to miss the fact of physical intimacy in the letters and lives of these women. Perhaps Wald believed her letters innocent in the true sense of the word: love for other women was seen as pure, decent, and even desirable. Certainly, being "genteel" was not high in Wald's priorities for social change.

Whatever the truth, it is clear that the Henry Street Settlement housed a close family of women. Wald favored women workers and Jacob Schiff, a primary benefactor, would not tolerate men in residence. Even Backer, who seems to believe that not much was known about Wald's personal life, agrees with Cook that the emotional ties with other women were important to Wald. Avowals of love in women's letters to Wald are mentioned by Backer, but the possibility of homoerotic relationships is excluded from her analysis. In fact, Backer makes a point of Wald's positive relations with men, her programs for boys and men, and her mentorship of both young men and women. Wald's decision not to marry was related to her dedication to her career. Certainly, other settlement women also chose not to marry or abandon their careers. Backer considers no other alternatives for the women's choices, such as simple preferences for the company of other women with or without sexual involvement. Nevertheless, Backer agrees with Poslusny (1989), discussed later, that the Settlement house served an important dual function for women: "It was a source of personal liberation and autonomy, and it provided a secure, supportive, environment consisting mainly of other women that allowed them to develop their abilities while still enjoying the close ties of feminine companionship they valued and had nurtured in their lives" (Backer, 1993, p. 127).

THE STRONGEST FEMINIST VOICE IN NURSING: LAVINIA LLOYD DOCK

Although Wald has been widely recognized for decades as the founder of public health nursing, Lavinia Lloyd Dock, the dedicated nurse feminist, began to receive the broader attention she deserves only with the recent reemergence of feminism. Several views of her can be seen in six articles, published over the past fifty years. In 1932 Dock presented her own self-portrait, responding to a request from the *American Journal of Nursing* (*AJN*); this was reprinted in *Nursing Outlook* in 1977. Dock delighted in recalling many of the activist happenings in her life, her close relationship with Lillian Wald, her spiritual feelings and outlook, her beliefs about legal and economic issues in relation to women, and her interest in national and international affairs in nursing. An article by Mary Roberts (1956) is a tribute to Lavinia Dock as she was nearing her 100th birthday. Noting Dock's incredibly modest assessment of her own achievements, Roberts chronicles the activities in which Dock engaged, the many publications she produced, and her remarkable influence on the development of the nursing profession. In analyzing Roberts' article, however, one notes that Dock's feminism is downplayed, or at best remains vague. Another portrait of Lavinia Dock is presented by Teresa E. Christy (1969), who remembers Dock for her outspoken stance on the taboo subject of venereal disease. True to her concern for women, Dock caused a ripple of notoriety because she insisted on discussing syphilis at an open meeting in London in 1910. Dock, the crusader, believed that nurses ought to be openly informed of this disease; otherwise their own health might be placed in jeopardy.

In a later 1971 article, "Equal Rights for Women," Christy corrects her earlier omission of Lavinia Dock's feminist accomplishments: "She became more and more disillusioned by the indifference of elected state legislators, and soon realized that a woman's occupation, such as nursing, could not exert influence nor expect support until women had bargaining power to wield. Lavinia Dock knew that this power was the ballot and concentrated her efforts to gain for women the right to vote" (p. 288).

This view of Lavinia Dock was reconsidered 14 years later by Peggy Chinn (1985), who uses Dock as a model for political activism in nursing. "Contrary to popular belief, political action in nursing is not a new or recent phenomenon. Nor have nurses been weak and ineffective in political action in the past" (p. 29). A sexist system, says Chinn, covers up the historical evidence: "Given that women are silenced or at best only valued to the extent that we serve men's interests, and that the values we espouse are given little if any priority in the public sphere, how are we to proceed in gaining a public voice and public influence?" (p. 31). In large part, Chinn is accurate in blaming the sexist system for veiling the significant contributions of early nursing activists. Nevertheless, why have nurses *themselves* not recognized their forebears' contributions? Their lack of knowledge or outright denial of their nursing pioneers is insufficient excuse. However, history informs and Chinn turns to the early politically strong allegiance between Dock and Wald, which produced a wide range of actions directed toward social reform but little agreement on political tactics. Deeply committed to social justice, Dock at times used confrontational tactics. A sharp and vocal literary voice, Dock chided Sir Edward Cook on his biography on Nightingale, considered in Chapter 1, for failing to recognize that she had wrested authority from men in the administration of hospital nursing. Concerned with international feminism, Dock attacked war's "colossal outrages on humanity." Clearly Chinn, in contrast to earlier writers, sees Dock, the strong activist, as the best model for current political action.

Writings on Dock have appeared in various biographical collections, such as *Notable American Women: The Modern Period* (1981), edited by Barbara Sicherman and Carol Hurd Green. Janet Wilson James' article from this collection is reprinted as a "Biographical Introduction" to a long overdue book, *A Lavinia Dock Reader* (1985), which brings together Dock's writings so that nurses can finally see an early model of a strong feminist woman. James credits Dock (1858–1956) as a leader in the organization of the nursing profession, a Settlement house worker, nursing historian, and suffragist. Dock described her parents as liberal, but asserted that her father had "'masculine prejudices'" although her mother was "'broad on all subjects and very tolerant and charitable toward persons'" (p. vii). In 1884 "Vinnie" attended Bellevue, the first American nursing school modeled on Nightingale's principles; she survived 12-hour work days, the "skimpy" evening instruction, and graduated in 1886. She then worked as a visiting nurse among the poor; ran a ward during the yellow fever epidemic in Jacksonville, Florida; worked with patients during the Johnstown, Pennsylvania flood where she met Clara Barton; and served as Bellevue night superintendent, compiling the first nurses' drug manual, *Materia Medica for Nurses* (p. viii).

Dock became assistant superintendent of nurses, under Isabel Hampton, at Johns Hopkins Hospital, Baltimore, where Adelaide Nutting was a student. All three women were to become preeminent leaders in nursing. At the 1893 Chicago international conference on hospitals, Dock spoke on the separation of medical and nursing spheres of authority, and Hampton organized the nurse administrators into the American Society of Superintendents of Training Schools (p. ix). Dock stayed in Chicago to become superintendent of the Illinois Training School, Cook County Hospital. Later, in 1896, she moved to New York City and joined the nurses at the Henry Street Settlement. The nurses were virtually independent practitioners in sick and preventive care, health, education, and school nursing.

James notes that Dock rejected Social Darwinism, focusing instead on theories of social evolution through mutual aid and cooperation, the latter now important to modern feminist theory. She acted on her theoretical understanding by organizing with Leonora O'Reilly the women's local of the United Garment Workers of America. According to James, Dock's experience "fortified the feminism Dock had absorbed by the time she was twelve from reading 'some of the earliest challenges thrown out by defiant women'" (p. xi). Again, she acted on her feminism, researching the structure of the American Medical Association and women's organizations to establish the framework for the Nurses Associated Alumnae (later the American Nurses Association [ANA]). As contributing editor to the *AJN*, Dock brought a socialist, feminist, and international perspective, the latter derived from her founding in 1899, with English nurse Ethel Gordon Fenwick, the International Council of Nurses, following the International Council of Women conference in London. Thus, it is clear that worldwide feminism at the turn of the century directly influenced the international connections of women in nursing. Dock urged her European sisters to challenge male medical authority and reported to American nurses, through her *AJN* "Foreign Department" column, the overseas progress of nursing, public health, and social legislation.

Together, Dock and Nutting created nursing history as an integral part of women's history in two volumes published in 1907. Dock actually wrote all but two chapters of *A History of Nursing*, a social history of the "usual and homely," and a feminist history that traced the care of the sick from primitive civilizations through the ages: "Women's autonomy, she found, had been lost when men took control of health care systems in the seventeenth century, bringing 'general contempt' to the nurse and 'misery' to the patient until Florence Nightingale came to the rescue" (p. xiii). In 1912 two more volumes were added, recording the experiences of Dock's own generation on four continents. The thoroughly documented books "conveyed the excitement of Dock's discoveries of women's past in libraries in France and Germany and the United States surgeon general's library in Washington" (p. xiii).

Though Dock stopped practicing nursing when she neared fifty, she helped Adah Thoms and other Black nurses organize a national association, and as a member of the New York Women's Trade Union League, she walked the picket lines in the shirtwaist strike of 1909. Dock increasingly saw nursing problems as "only a part of the larger question of women's economic, sexual, and political bondage" (p. xiii). She was nursing's primary crusader against venereal disease, joining physicians in bringing the subject to public attention, and was one of the few women members of the American Society of Sanitary and Moral Prophylaxis. Dock campaigned against " 'any treatment which would make it hygienically safe for men to continue a brutal misuse of women.' " In 1911 she published *Hygiene and Morality*, a manual for nurses and others in which she demanded the "abolition of the double standard of morality" (p. xiv).

James traces some high points in Dock's feminist career. She was arrested for attempting to vote in 1896, enlisted in the Equality League of Self-Supporting Women in 1907, and ran a suffrage newsstand in front of their office. Dock was assaulted by police as a pioneer poll watcher and was one of five women who, in 1912, made a thirteen-day suffrage hike from New York City to Albany. She sold suffrage papers in Picadilly while in London on International Council of Nurses business, organized the contingent carrying banners in ten different languages for the 1913 suffrage parade, and was interviewed in 1915 while campaigning in a Bowery flophouse. She was a militant campaigner with Alice Paul, leading, in 1917, the first group of suffrage pickets from the National Woman's Party headquarters to the White House, and she was jailed three times in that year for participation in militant demonstrations.

Suffrage was finally granted, but war, "the monster twin of poverty, spawned by men's greed and competitiveness" (p. xvi), moved Dock to refuse to mention it, except to condemn it, in her *AJN* columns. Quite accurately, she predicted mass slaughter and even germ warfare. She alienated some nursing leaders by her stand against war, her support for the Equal Rights Amendment, and her support in 1921 for Margaret Sanger for conserving life through birth control, " 'for teaching to poor working women what all well-to-do women may learn from reliable authority, if they wish it' " (p. xvi). By 1922 she had retired, and thus was lost the strongest feminist voice in nursing.

In 1991 Dock's connection to Teachers College, Columbia University, was briefly acknowledged by Sandra Lewenson, who notes that Dock was one of the early volunteer faculty members and who, in her active role in the American Society of Superintendents, had influenced the establishment of the first postgraduate course in nursing education at Columbia. Lewenson stresses

Dock's scholarship, noting that her first book, *Materia Medica for Nurses*, was purposely written to provide information to nurses about the medications physicians were prescribing. This was important because physicians in some hospitals even numbered medications, removing names, in order to limit nurses' information and knowledge. Thus, Dock's work served to empower nurses. Ironically, a publishing house refused to publish her work, and she paid for the publication herself. The book was a success, used by both nurses and medical students. With Adelaide Nutting, Dock's four volumes on the history of nursing, begun in 1907, was followed in 1910 by *Hygiene and Morality*, again a book to empower nurses; in 1920 she published *A Short History of Nursing* with Isabel Stewart, which, like her earlier work on nursing history, provided nurses with a sense of their own identity. Lewenson stresses Dock's concern with power through her founding of several national and international organizations; her championing of women's rights and suffrage; and her connection of the development of nursing to the women's movement. In 1956 this remarkable woman died, leaving an almost forgotten legacy of a feminist woman, independent practitioner, Black women's advocate, social reformer, and international peace advocate. Yet to Lewenson, "Dock's ideas, rhetoric, and words have never retired or died for her name continues to evoke the ideas of suffrage, nursing, and reform" (Lewenson, 1991, p. 11). We have yet to see her full reincarnation in any "modern" nurse.

BATTLING THE PATRIARCHY: ISABEL HAMPTON ROBB, LAVINIA LLOYD DOCK, AND M. ADELAIDE NUTTING

As part of a series of "portraits," Teresa Christy (1969) presents a picture of another nursing leader, Adelaide Nutting, a close friend of Lavinia Dock. It is Christy's opinion that Adelaide Nutting was second only to Florence Nightingale in overall contributions to nursing in general, and second to none in the annals of American nursing. Whether one agrees with Christy's assessment, Adelaide Nutting was the first nurse ever to be appointed to a professorship in a university. Appointed professor at Teacher's College, Columbia University, Nutting headed the Department of Nursing and Health, the first in the nation. An excellent administrator and farseeing educator, Nutting believed that economics was the root of the problem in nursing education and felt that only separately endowed schools could ever truly be independent and, therefore, broadly educational.

A strong advocate of research in nursing, Nutting had a great desire to see improved educational opportunities for women and for nurses, always seeking to attract more intelligent and able women into the profession. She served on the Committee for the Study of Nursing Education, which produced the famous Goldmark Report of 1923 that delineated the economic and educational problems facing a woman's profession. As Christy notes, it is not well known that Nutting labored valiantly for more than a decade to force the production of the Report. Though implied, Christy does not make clear Nutting's position on specific feminist issues.

More recently, Susan M. Poslusny (1989) published "Feminist Friendship: Isabel Hampton Robb, Lavinia Lloyd Dock and Mary Adelaide Nutting." To Poslusny, the women's relationship was "an important part of the context in which feminism, social reform and nursing came together at the turn of the century" (p. 64). As part of the current efforts to understand the social networks of women, Poslusny looks at the social context that structured the professional interests and personal relationships of Robb, Dock, and Nutting in an article quite different from Cook's.

Poslusny claims that "Women who entered nursing often saw it as a way of entering the battle against male-dominated social structures" (p. 64). In fact, nurses were the first women to organize into professional associations, to publish a professional journal, and to establish an international federation of health workers. Further, Poslusny asserts that Florence Nightingale and Clara Barton were social heroines, and Wald, Dock and Sanger were leaders in social reform, women's suffrage, and voluntary motherhood: "Yet nurses are rarely recognized as being feminists and leaders in the fight to obtain equal rights and position for women" (p. 64). To Poslusny, liberal feminists worked for parity in a man's world, but nurses strived simultaneously for separate recognition through a women's profession. Today, notes Poslusny, this historical legacy is apparent in the problem of finding a cause or issue that can unite women and nursing organizations and memberships.

To achieve unity and progress, interpersonal support among individual women is essential. Relying on feminist writer Lottie Pogrebin (1987), Poslusny defines such support as feminist friendship, which is the "dialectic between struggle and victory, between nurture and empowerment" (p. 64). Such friendship reflects women's efforts to achieve influence and recognition in the context of mutual support. Using this definition, Poslusny believes that it was feminist friendship that created the framework for unity and progress of nursing at the turn of the century. At Johns Hopkins, Robb as head superintendent, Dock as assistant superintendent, and Nutting as a newly entered student, formed a triad eventually responsible for the creation of new nursing organizations and educational preparation.

The post-Civil War context is characterized by Poslusny as one of increasing disparity between the social classes associated with social, economic, and political shifts that affected women more because of their traditional dependence on men. Victorian society emphasized gender segregation; exclusion of more advantaged women from public work; repression of sexual or even anatomical discussions of or expressions about the body; the cult of female invalidism; and female responsibility for the care of the sick. Repression and segregation produced a culturally distinct homosocial world of women, marked by elaborate rituals of passage and a subculture in which, Poslusny claims, "Unabashed expressions of love and endearments between women were a reflection of the Platonic ideal" (p. 65). Certainly, Cook (1977) would not agree with this assertion. To her, unidimensional analysis of women's love and friendship impoverishes multiple role models and limits historical understanding and accuracy.

Nonetheless, in tracing the effects of industrialization, urbanization, and immigration, which led to the public health movement, Poslusny recognizes that settlement houses provided "the first viable option for secular women to live communally for the purpose of mutual support and aid" (p. 65), serving to recreate the homosocial world of intimate support and affection to empower women. According to Poslusny, Dock, Nutting, and Robb "shared a sense of history, a common frustration with the exploitation of nurses, a mutual concern for the rights of women, a common goal of unity for the profession" (p. 65).

Isabel Robb was the visionary leader whose mind, Dock claimed, was truly original and creative, and whose ideas "'are now embodied in living groups . . . and in broad lines of organization'" (p. 66). After meeting Dock at Bellevue, Robb asked her to help establish the nursing school at Johns Hopkins. She later supported Nutting as her replacement as Superintendent and eventually became both an administrator and a faculty member at Columbia University. Dock and many others were dismayed with Robb's marriage because they knew, as societal norms demanded, that this would restrain her from working fully in the public world.

Lavinia Dock, the revolutionary spirit of the trio, saw nursing and women's issues as inseparable. While at Columbia, Isabel Stewart recalled Dock, not as "'tall and angular and intellectual looking . . . but this small, short sort of roly-poly little person with curly hair'" (p. 66). Dock, having been invited by Stewart to speak to her students, had just come from a suffrage meeting, with "Votes for Women" emblazoned across her chest and hat. "'Now what am I going to talk about?'" she asked. Stewart reminded her that she was to talk about nursing on the Continent. "'Oh,'" Dock said, "'very bad. It'll not be any better till they get the suffrage. I'll talk about suffrage'" (p. 66). Dock challenged the newly formed Society of Superintendents of Nursing to recognize their political power: "Yet this society, as one body, would often be astonished at the actual extent and weight of its influence if its whole latent and at present unsuspected power were actually to be systematically exerted in an intelligent and energetic manner" (p. 66).

Adelaide Nutting was the administrative leader, and so involved and dedicated to nursing education that she was unable to join her friends in the suffrage movement. One wonders if Nutting, as the youngest of the trio and newest to nursing, did not represent the emerging institutional nursing leader, concerned primarily with leadership *within* the profession rather than broader society.

Despite their differences, these three women maintained a close, interdependent, professional relationship of collaboration and support, promoting unity and esprit de corps in nursing. But the joy expressed by Wald and Dock in their Settlement house relations is not evident in Robb's rejection of "cliques": "Sentimental, intense personal friendships are a mistake, and are rarely productive of good. In some instances they must be regarded as forms of perverted affection; they are always unhealthy, since they make too great demands upon the emotions and nerve force, and are likely to assume undue proportions, so as to interfere with the proper discharge of one's duties" (p. 67). This institutionalization of female friendship and fear of female closeness—all in the name of duty—are far removed from the feminist delight in each other expressed by independent nurses in the Settlement house.

According to Poslusny, friendship for nurses had become a question of ethical behavior, located "somewhere between the Victorian tradition of romantic friendships and the Platonic ideal" (p. 67). To her, unity of the profession became the new purpose for women's friendship. Perhaps this is why the interpersonal relations among the three women, as presented by Poslusny, seem so stiff, devoid of the actual emotions of everyday reality. Poslusny does state that the personal needs of these women were as important as social context, political climate, or altruism. Indeed, it is personal needs that create these three, and in turn feminist friendship provides a political context for expressing social change. By restructuring nurses' friendships in feminist terms, Poslusny asserts that this can change the nursing tradition of service and dedication to morality and public welfare to one that involves politics and the dialectic of power relations.

Mentoring, collaborating, and networking, all apparent in the nursing literature, are indications of interpersonal support, but Poslusny asks nurses to learn from history that feminist friendships can help them establish a framework for unity and progress in the empowerment of women. We must add that central to politicized friendship is the sheer delight in the enjoyment of other women, the deep respect for their personal and political achievements, and the dedication to their welfare. These deeper aspects of feminism seem lacking in the relations described by Poslusny. It is as though she resurrects three women as sacred icons, but does not realize that Robb's injunction against emotional intimacy, for example, rules out the essence of the phenomenon. It is precisely the intensity of emotional commitment to other women that fortifies them in their struggle for equality. It is basically love itself, whether or not physically expressed, that empowers and is central to making personal and social change. This concept was understood by Nightingale, Barton, Wald, and Dock in different ways and at various levels of comprehension.

JEWISH WOMEN LEADERS AND NURSING

Love and respect between women from different religions and ethnic backgrounds emerged early in the development of national and international nursing. However, seldom has anyone specifically considered the relations with and contributions of Jewish women to nursing. Correcting this oversight, nurse administrators Evelyn R. Benson and Janice Selekman (1992) note that training schools in Jewish hospitals were founded in the late 19th century at the prodding of women's committees, and many Jewish women attended these institutions. Rose Frank, for example, was central to the nursing school established at the Jewish Hospital in Philadelphia in 1892; Maud Nathan, a progressive social reformer, influenced the founding of the school of nursing at Mount Sinai Hospital in New York.

Lillian Wald's family immigrated from Germany in the mid-19th century. Despite their disapproval Wald went to the New York Hospital School of Nursing, which had previously graduated few if any Jewish nurses. According to Benson and Selekman, Wald was a universalist, not a religious Jew, but maintained strong relations with the Jewish community from which she gained financial support from wealthy German-Jewish families in New York, most notably Jacob Schiff. Of the large numbers of Eastern European Jewish immigrants, the women were the most eager to become Americanized, experiencing a degree of freedom infrequent in the 3000-year-old Hebrew tradition of women staying home and caring for children. Despite prejudice against them as women and Jews, many entered the garment industry, becoming trade union activists; some were involved in the women's movement as well. In nursing, the interconnections between Jewish and non-Jewish women, for example, at the Henry Street Settlement, were laudatory, exhibiting not only respect but love.

Wald's contributions and her public health nursing model, say Benson and Selekman, inspired Henrietta Szold's plan to create health services in Palestine before the First World War. The founder of the Zionist organization Hadassah, Szold obtained financial support from Nathan Straus and his wife and recruited two Jewish nurses, Rose Kaplan and Rae Landy, who, in 1913, left their positions in New York and established a district health program in Jerusalem. This was interrupted by the war, but laid the ground work for current programs in Israel.

Josephine Goldmark, although not a nurse, was the author of the first major study of nursing in the United States. Published in 1923, the Goldmark Report strongly influenced nursing education. Of course, Emma Goldman, too, was a Jewish woman and a respected nurse and midwife. Benson and Selekman are to be credited with trying to fill a gap in nursing history by providing an initial overview of Jewish women leaders in nursing.

THE DOUBLE-EDGED PREJUDICE:
BLACK WOMEN LEADERS IN NURSING

How far love can be extended as a true measure of radicality is tested most severely in race relations. An important part of the history of nursing centers on the relationship between sexism and racism. The struggle of Black nurses to be equal to White nurses was presented in an early article by Adah Thoms in 1929 and more recently in 1976 by Joyce Ann Elmore. Both demonstrate the historical progress of African American women as nurses, their service to the profession, and the difficulties they have encountered. Lillian Wald wrote the supportive introduction to Thoms' book, which presents a history of the entrance of African American women into nursing and a summary of their progress in the profession. As with White nurses, famous Black women nurses have not usually been recognized as nurses, but as political activists. Few acknowledge or remember, for example, that the abolitionist and feminist, Harriet Tubman, was a Civil War nurse, known as "Aunt Harriet." Few know much about Mary Mahoney, the first professional Black nurse. Thoms does not connect the efforts of Black nurses to fight against both racism and sexism. Nor is there a good historical account that interconnects the work of women activists, such as Wald and Dock, in supporting the efforts of African American nurses.

Elmore's 1976 article, "Black Nurses: Their Service and Their Struggle," points out little known facts about feminists Harriet Tubman and Sojourner Truth, but fails to interconnect their fight against both racism and sexism. Elmore does, however, make it clear that these women, known for activities other than nursing, were indeed nurses during the Civil War. Sojourner Truth was well known as an abolitionist speaker, but her ringing feminist declarations have only recently been resurrected. Harriet Tubman was acclaimed for her dangerous work in the underground railroad for escaped slaves and her activities as a Union Army spy.

The activism of African American women nurses did not stop with these earlier feminists. There were Black nurses in the Spanish-American War; Adah Thoms worked to open army nursing to Black women; however, it was not until after World War II that Black nurses were finally accepted and integrated in all the military services. All women, Black or White, struggled to gain recognition for nursing, and in this way, improve their status as women; but Black nurses had a triple struggle: to improve their status as women; to fight discrimination because of their race; and to work to improve their place in the profession, while simultaneously increasing its status. Thus, the meaning of feminism to Black nurses has been significantly different from that of White nurses. The full ramifications of African American experience in nursing has yet to be clarified. Similarly, the experiences of women in nursing from other racial and ethnic groups are only beginning to be fully considered.

In 1908 Black women, aided by Dock and a few others, created the National Association of Coloured Graduate Nurses, which existed until 1951. Mabel K. Staupers, early Black nursing leader, influenced younger women, such as Mary Elizabeth Carnegie, to fight for full recognition and opportunity. Carnegie (1962), in "The Path We Tread," credits Staupers for bringing Carnegie and other African American student nurses "full face with the many obstacles that we could expect as Negro nurses—and yet, simultaneously, we were led to the realization that we were capable of meeting the challenge" (p. 25). In her 1936 speech to the Black student nurses, Staupers traced the struggles encountered to become members of the nursing profession, to be admitted to schools, hospitals, and public health agencies. As Carnegie recalled, Staupers received a "round of applause . . . such as we had never before given a guest lecturer" (p. 25).

Graduated from one of two all-Black nursing schools, Carnegie's class of 1937 could seek employment in only four of about 200 New York City hospitals, or in only two federal hospitals where nurses could be assigned in the entire nation. On a segregated train, Carnegie traveled to her first position at one of these, a Veterans Administration hospital in Tuskegee, Alabama, where the county health department employed one White and one Black nurse, each to care for patients of their own races. Eventually, after further education, Carnegie became a clinical instructor at St. Philip Hospital School of Nursing, Richmond, Virginia. Working in the Black school and hospital, Carnegie learned what it was like to be a "Negro" nurse in the South: White nurses were addressed as "Miss," Black nurses as "Nurse." Carnegie rejected this usage, urging her students to address each other as "Miss" and to use formal titles, not first names, with their Black patients. An unnamed White director of nursing had "the courage to insist on respecting the Negro nurses and patients" (p. 27), and thus, the system changed.

By 1941 the U.S. Army allowed Black nurses to serve in World War II, but only in segregated units and facilities. However, Carnegie could not be accepted at all in the Navy Nurse Corps, whose recruiting was done by the American Red Cross (ARC). It is strange that the organization founded by Clara Barton, who in the 19th century would give up her right to vote in preference to Black men, who, she said, had suffered deeper wrongs, could have told Carnegie in the 20th century that she could not join their ranks of navy nurses. In 1945 the navy finally accepted Black nurses; however, they could not share a room with a White nurse. In 1948 President Harry Truman issued the order for full integration of all armed forces.

Most schools for Black students were still administered by Whites, although Hampton Institute in Virginia established a collegiate nursing program in 1943 to prepare Black nursing leaders and Carnegie, acting as assistant director, established the program until a White director was hired. Carnegie next moved to Tallahassee, Florida, to start a collegiate nursing program at Florida Agricultural and Mechanical College, one of two Black schools in the state.

To obtain clinical experience for her students, Carnegie wrote to White directors of nursing at several hospitals. All replied cordially by mail, but on seeing Carnegie, who extended her hand in greeting, left the issue "dangling in every instance!" (p. 28). Finally, she found one White director who accepted her extended hand and supported her. Carnegie left, "feeling that here was hope, not only for the future of our school, but for the race of man" (p. 28), an affirmation she needed badly. Later, this same director, at Carnegie's request, changed the system of addressing the Black students as "Nurse" to "Miss." A threatened strike by White nurses was averted, and eventually all services in the hospital were opened to Carnegie's students.

By 1946 Carnegie and others were fighting for full-fledged membership in the Florida State Nurses Association (FSNA), the only avenue to the American Nurses Association. The Black nurses' association, which White nurses had helped form, led the effort to join the FSNA, but at a convention in 1946, the two races met separately. Carnegie notes that the Florida branch of the National League for Nursing had already accepted Black nurses on an equal basis. In 1948 Carnegie spoke to an open session of the FSNA and the "ovation was overwhelming" (p. 31); she was subsequently elected to the FSNA board of directors. Shortly thereafter, the separate Black nurses' association was dissolved and Black nurses were integrated with the White nurses, eventually attending all meetings. Still, the game of "musical chairs" had to be dealt with. At meetings the White nurses would wait until the Black nurses were seated, then sit opposite to them. Finally, the Black nurses waited for the White nurses to be seated and scattered themselves throughout the meeting hall; before long, "no one paid any attention to who sat where" (p. 32). Unfortunately, a plan to integrate an extension program for nurses had to be shelved when the White state attorney general ruled against educational integration. Still, Carnegie concluded that "Negro nurses, with the co-operation and support of democratic white nurses, have scaled innumerable hurdles, and there are many more to be crossed" (p. 33).

From Carnegie's account in the 1960s, there is little evidence of overt consciousness of the relation between racism and sexism, but in 1988, Darlene Clark Hine interconnected both. In her consideration of Black nurses from 1890 to 1950, Hine states that there have been two images of the professional African American nurse: first, one of an essential and competent provider of health care in Black communities, with "an uncompromising voice speaking out for the best interests of blacks"; second, as an "inferior member of the nursing profession when compared to her white counterparts" (p. 177). Hine accuses the ARC of discriminatory treatment, beginning with Frances Elliott Davis, the first Black nurse in the ARC, who, at the end of World War I in 1918, received a pin marked "1A," denoting her as the first ARC Black nurse. This practice continued until 1949: all Black nurses received pins with "A" inscribed on them. In Tennessee, Davis objected to the designation of her by her first name and refused to enter the hospital through the back door. But it was Mabel Staupers who orchestrated the pressures and protests about discrimination during the Second World War that led to integration; she met with White nursing groups, top military officials, Black civil rights leaders, newspaper editors, women's clubs, and philanthropists. Because of the personal appeals by Eleanor Roosevelt, the protests of the National Nursing Council for War Service, and the critical nursing shortage, Black nurses eventually won inclusion and integration.

Hine contrasts this fight for status in the White world with the high esteem Black nurses enjoyed in their own communities where their importance was emphasized by the unavailability of health care to large portions of the population, particularly in rural areas. Black nurses have acted as mediators between racial groups, but because of sexist subordination, have not, as facilitators, always improved the health of African Americans. For example, in the highly questionable Tuskegee syphilis experiment (1932–1972), in which some of the men unknowingly received *no* treatment, Black nurse Eunice Rivers was the facilitator, bridging the educational and cultural gaps between physicians and patient-subjects. Rivers states: "It was up to you to help that patient carry out [the doctor's] orders. . . . The doctor said you do so and so. . . . Patients . . . get to the point where if they're not sure, they're going to ask you. They get you in the middle" (p. 181). Without Rivers, says Hine, the White doctors would not have been so successful in "engaging so many black males in such a detrimental and ethically bankrupt experiment" (p. 189). Their faith in the Black nurse made them believe the experiment was legitimate. Certainly, as a "female in a male-dominated world, deference to male authority figures reinforced her ethical passivity" (p. 190). This was further reinforced by southern racism in which Blacks, and certainly not Black women, could not question White authority.

Hine asserts that traditional nursing histories pay little attention to African American nurses, yet their struggle in many instances mirrors the efforts of all nurses. However, sexist images of a Black woman as a "defeminized beast of burden, a sexually promiscuous wanton, or a domineering mammy" (p. 182) created special problems, which, according to Hine, were exaggerated in nursing by the desire to distance it from the image of the domestic or servant. This coincided with hardening of the color line: "As segregation pervaded the country, all southern and most northern nursing schools barred black women" (p. 183). Even liberal northern schools set quotas: "The charter for the New England Hospital for Women and Children . . . stipulated that only *one* Negro and *one* Jewish student each year would be accepted" (p. 183). One could argue that these two were two more than the men allowed in their institutions, which was usually none; however, this hardly exonerates the practice of racial exclusion.

According to Hine, African American men, such as Booker T. Washington, spearheaded the education of Black nurses. Unfortunately, they merged the sentimental Nightingale icon with their own views on the "proper" woman—a woman responsible for proving the humanity of Black people by showing herself as a "self-sacrificing, warm, and devoted mother figure," downplaying the "efficient, autonomous, and assertive professional" (p. 184). Daniel Hale Williams, founder of two Black nursing schools, extolled the nurse as having fidelity, tenderness, and sympathy; women were nurturing and noble, expected to be object lessons for the community. Booker T. Washington thought nursing a valuable career before marriage, which in emergencies after marriage could provide additional money. As Hine notes, Washington "wedded nursing training firmly to vocational work" (p. 185) and to stereotyped notions of what a female is. Black men, as administrators and physicians, shared these sentiments and lauded the womanly virtues of "'devotion, endurance, sympathy, tactile delicacy, unselfishness, tact, resourcefulness, and willingness to undergo hardships'" in order to persuade more Black women "to enter into the backbreaking, endless toil euphemistically referred to as nursing training" (p. 185).

According to Hine, the African American nurse was caught in the sexist and racist currents that prevailed in the thinking of both Blacks and Whites. She admits that White women were also caught in the ideology of gender segregation; but even women's jobs, when hooked to formal training, were beyond the Black woman's reach. Though educated in African American institutions, Black nurses shared the White women's search for professional acceptance and recognition, but also bore the burden of lifting up their entire race. In actuality, the excessive production of nurses in the 1920s by hospital schools controlled by male administrators, and the use of unpaid students in hospitals rather than graduate nurses, forced Black nurses to work longer hours for lower wages, and to perform more household and childcare chores as private-duty nurses. This in turn led White nurses, in at least one survey, to see Black women as less committed to professional advancement and lacking leadership potential, particularly when Black institutions were viewed as substandard. Obviously, both Black and White women were being manipulated by the men in power. In public health, Black nurses were allowed to work only with Black patients, while White nurses could work with both. In contrast to the usual derogatory assumptions made by agencies about Black nurses, nurses such as Lillian Wald employed Black nurses, paid them equally, and gave them the identical professional courtesies and recognition expected for White nurses; yet, as Hine notes, Black nurses were not sent to White families or placed in supervisory positions. Nevertheless, Hine lauds women such as Wald as being staunch friends of Black nurses.

Hine concludes that the image of the Black nurse was formed by the twin realities of racism and sexism. One can question whether the majority of Black nurses in the 1950s were any better able than White nurses to recognize gender-stratification systems, given the collapse of militant feminism by the early postwar period. However, by the 1970s, Black women clearly understood the "double-edged prejudice" and once again formed a National Black Nurses Association to fight injustices of all kinds.

INTERNAL INFLUENCE, EXTERNAL ANONYMITY?

This action by African American nurses was necessary, despite the fact that nursing was not only the first to organize a professional association for women, but the first major professional group to integrate Black members. According to Bonnie and Vern Bullough (1984), nursing is still the best integrated at every level of any professional national association. However, despite the "long list of successful battles that nurses have fought and won for women . . . most of the bibliographies dealing with women's history ignore nurses" (p. 42). This ignorance of both Black and White nurses, the Bulloughs claim, is not just a feminist put-down; women, who were denied power in the male world, coped by making their own place in a "ghettoized" female world and were shunted aside by women focused on male power domains. To the Bulloughs, "the traditional heroines of organized nursing have not been Sanger, Wald, or Goldman who fought for and gained power in the world at large, but the women who did their fighting within nursing to help it advance: Adelaide Nutting, Lavinia Dock, Isabel Hampton Robb, Annie Goodrich, and others" (p. 42). Though Dock's feminist concerns and activities went far beyond nursing issues, it is true that these women and Thoms, Staupers, and Carnegie, are relatively unknown to the non-nursing world and have largely been ignored by feminist historians.

The Bulloughs refer to sociological theorist Robert Merton, who distinguishes between professional power in local or parochial, and national or cosmopolitan settings as a useful dichotomy for analyzing male professions; however, the Bulloughs assert that this dichotomy is relatively useless for nursing or other women's groups, because women have been denied the cosmopolitan level of power to influence the larger world. To offset this, female nurses concentrated on nursing in an "attempt to gain internal influence in areas where external influence was difficult, if not impossible, to achieve" (p. 43). Thus, nursing leaders are known to nurses, but generally not to those external to nursing. The Bulloughs claim that "Wald, Sanger, Goldman, Kenny, et al., were externally-oriented nurses who chose to work in the world at large, while those recognized as leaders of the profession were those who worked from within" (p. 43). The internalist strategy is difficult for feminists to accept, because "success in the internal world of women might well demand different qualities than in the external world so controlled by men in the past" (p. 43). For nurses, communication about their concerns is difficult, not only because of male unwillingness to deal with predominantly female groups, but also because professional nursing associations, according to the Bulloughs, have not yet come to terms with the non-nursing world.

Organizational problems in a women's profession are apparent because only a few nurses have taken leadership roles in developing the profession. Historically, most nurses were young and unmarried and most nursing leaders were older and unmarried. Because of gender stereotypes, married women were not allowed or expected to work; they were even legally constrained from doing so. But single women were stigmatized, preventing them from attaining power in the external cosmopolitan world. The Bulloughs note that even if legal and social strictures were relaxed, the 12-hour working day, common until the Second World War, excluded most married women from working; thus, male control of hospitals and agencies forced the disparity between most nurses and their leaders. The role of public health or school nurse was often legally restricted to the unmarried woman. Even private-duty nurses, who could not take a case immediately, went to the bottom of the list and had to wait for a case to come up again. Since men in hospitals often indirectly controlled nurses' registries and cases were controlled by male physicians' referrals, both single and married women were subject to control beyond their own profession.

The Bulloughs claim that the career-oriented woman was often perceived as a lesbian or a "dedicated spinster," clearly distinguished from the woman who, as wife and mother, had shorter-term commitments, usually because of sexist constraints. Reviewing biographies of dominant nursing leaders, the Bulloughs could find, until after World War II, "almost no married women influential in the internal affairs of nursing" (p. 44), although there were some widows and divorcées. Most early leaders came late to nursing, often as a means of gaining independence and to work for the advancement of women. In seeming contradiction to this assertion, the Bulloughs claim that this small group of dedicated professionals made decisions often concerned with their own interests. It is equally likely that the leaders were more advanced in their understanding of sexism and, sometimes, racism, and that their decisions and actions were based on a much more liberal view of women's roles than the rank and file.

Over time, the original feminist goals became diluted and the professionalization of nurses was concentrated primarily in Eastern urban centers, beginning with Teachers College, Columbia University, in New York City. Here, the leaders created not only general internal agreement on goals, as the Bulloughs note, but also an increasing distance from activism in social, and more particularly, feminist issues. It is difficult to prove simultaneously that nursing is an objective, scientific profession, suitable in institutions of higher education and, at the same time, expose the sexist nature of the institutions, hospitals, and universities, which the nurses needed for the legitimization and accreditation of nursing.

As a result of the need for men in wartime, the composition of nursing changed to include more married women, who were not ostracized because of sexist restrictions. The Bulloughs believe that women nurses coming of age after World War II are more externalist. One can argue the reverse: these women entered nursing in a most conservative period, when women were expected to leave their wartime jobs, return home, and have four or even more children. Thus, as far as feminism is concerned, many of these nurses may be less externalist, far less so than their grandmothers, who grew up, lived, and worked during the earlier phase of feminism. The distinction between internalist and externalist is an interesting one, but requires far more complex analysis to achieve a clarity that would accommodate women's and feminist history in relation to nursing in the context of patriarchal society.

LEAVING VISIONS THAT TRANSCEND WHAT IS: CONTEMPORARY ACTIVISTS AND LEADERS

Whether their spheres of action and influence have been internal or external to the profession, there is little doubt that many contemporary American leaders in nursing have struggled to overcome societal constraints, discrimination, and stereotypes in their search for professional identity. Gwendolyn Safier (1977) conducted oral histories of 17 nurse leaders in 1976. Of these women, 14 were retired and 3 were close to retirement; 15 of the women had fathers who had not completed college and were not in a profession. Their mothers had followed traditional expectations, working outside the home only if they were widowed, making work an economic necessity. Only one Black woman was included, reflecting a disproportionately low number in ratio to the population of Black nurses. The leaders entered nursing because of altruistic-humanistic reasons, common to female expectations; or to get an education, usually a poor woman's route, particularly given gender-segregated and inadequately funded opportunities for female students; or because of "rerouting," they were actively discouraged from medicine or science, so they entered a socially acceptable occupation for women.

In contrast to previous periods, 9 of the 17 were married, most of them very happily; 5 of them married after 30 years of age. Whether married early or later, only two had children. Eight never married and did not regret their decision, having rich and satisfying lives. More highly educated women are less likely to marry or to have children; although the majority of women marry, the rates vary among different professional groups. Safier gives no information about the leaders' lifestyles and networks of support and concludes that these women were forced to choose between marriage and leadership. It is highly likely, however, that a portion of these and other leaders have chosen both careers and nontraditional lifestyles.

Interestingly, the leaders were thrust into deanships and directorships because of the demands of World War II and advances in science and technology. From her research, Safier concludes: "These women were pioneers. They had a difficult time in getting their ideas accepted. Their work was not easy in that at times it provoked much controversy, and it took considerable courage and determination on their part to forge ahead. They worked tremendously hard, at times at very low salaries, and faced much resistance and many obstacles along the way; but they had strong convictions for which they fought" (p. 387). Described best by the words "courage, vision, humility," their main issues were education and expanded roles for nurses.

Safier admits that she did not originally intend to make an "explicit contribution" to feminist scholarship; nevertheless, she found that the leaders' experiences shed light on the status of women in American society. The obstacles confronted and strategies used to cope with overt and covert discrimination "parallel those of women in other professions . . . a suggestive model for oral history forays into feminist studies" (p. 388). Safier notes that the sexist pattern is obvious in the active discouragement of these women from traditionally male professions, such as medicine and the biological sciences. One White leader, after completing her BA and MS degrees in the biological sciences, talked to a bacteriology professor who informed her that women have a hard time in science and, though she had the ability, she would have to be much better than the men with whom she would have to struggle in the department. One Black leader, whose brother was a dentist, decided that she, too, wanted to be a dentist; however, her brother told her very emphatically that dentistry was *not* a profession for women. After entering nursing, she fought overt racial discrimination, but refused to back off. Estelle Massey Osborne said:

> See, it's one thing to say, "Yes, you can come. You can join." But when you get there, nobody sits beside you, nobody says hello. I've been in meetings where, when I have spoken, they would look at me with the amazement that you would get if you bought a dog and he suddenly spoke. They would look at you with such an amazement, and no follow-up on what you said; just let it hang. So the freeze-out is a very difficult thing to take. (pp. 389–390)

Ironically, research on female-male interaction in groups shows similarities to those processes described by Osborne.

Safier also points to sexist behaviors and inequitable salaries experienced by these women. Ruth Freeman, for example, refused to be victimized and turned down an offer to develop nursing at Johns Hopkins University because the men would not give her a salary equal to comparably educated physicians. Other leaders struggled against discrimination in educational opportunity. Mary Kelly Mullane, on the faculty of a midwestern university, decided to obtain her doctorate. In 1949, when she approached the president, he told her it was nonsense, but if she could bring the names of a half-dozen women in her profession who thought the way she did, she could do it. Mullane said she really had to dig to get the names, but found six nurses with earned doctorates. She gave this list to the president, who admitted he was wrong. There actually were women nurses who had doctoral degrees!

Safier notes still other barriers, particularly attitudes of male colleagues, some of whom were "people-minded" (you are a person first and a woman second), and some who were "stereotype-minded" (you are a woman first and a person second). Safier concludes: "More often than not they found themselves confronting the latter" (p. 391). Mullane, on being told she looked like a woman but thought like a man, did not argue, but to Safier she said, " 'I don't think that I think like a man at all. I think that I think like an intelligent human being. I think like a scholar, that's what I think like' " (p. 391). A by-product of the male-dominated milieu was that "it transformed female members into staunch upholders of sexism" (p. 391). Instead of solidarity, the women "met with vicious competition from female colleagues" (p. 391). The nature of female behavior, as constructed in the context of oppression, is now just beginning to be explored by nurses.

As in the past, some contemporary nurses have taken the externalist route. The early legacy of social activism and feminism, exemplified by Dock, was revitalized by Wilma Scott Heide, who represents, as Joan I. Roberts states (1994), the most recent nurse to provide national leadership in combating racism and sexism. Heide received her license as a registered nurse in 1945 and served as a supervisor, faculty member, and administrator in nursing education and public health in three states. Her early work in nursing led her to combat the low salaries and excessive hours worked by women nurses. She organized them and other health-care workers around issues such as an economic security program, which would reduce the 12-hour days and 72-hour work weeks of nurses and attendants in Pennsylvania State Hospitals for the mentally ill.

After receiving a Master's degree in sociology, Heide moved south in 1953 and directed a school of nursing in Orangeburg, South Carolina. She served as a night supervisor at a hospital, conducted sociological research, and engaged in community civil rights work, including a drive for voter registration of *all* citizens. Of this work, Wilma said, "An attempt at assassination was made on my life, but the assassin missed me and killed a black man who was with me. This happened in 1954" (Roberts, 1994, p. 17). Heide understood the need to integrate racial and feminist issues. After working in antipoverty programs and then combining her work against racism with feminism, she eventually became president of the National Organization for Women in the early 1970s. She later obtained a doctorate, moved toward women studies, and worked for international feminism, playing major roles in multiple national and international conventions, forums, and commissions. Before her death in 1985, she wrote: "Among my most important contributions are . . . leaving visions that transcend what is" (p. 1). Heide, like the women before her, saw beyond her times to a future free of prejudice and discrimination. However, like Sanger, she had to leave nursing in order to achieve her goals and, in her own words, "to retain my sanity."

The visions that most contemporary nursing leaders are leaving behind them are primarily characterized by attention to intraprofessional issues —increasing the sophistication of nursing education and research efforts, legislation on entry into practice and third-party reimbursement, the continuing struggle for autonomy in practice, and the like. Although nursing's professional organizations have developed and proposed a National Health Insurance model for the United States, other social and environmental issues critical to the health and survival of our society receive relatively minor attention from nursing as a whole. The outspoken activist and feminist postures of nursing's early leaders—Barton, Sanger, Dock, and Wald—have still to be fully replicated by today's nurses. Dock's commitment to "urgent social claims" must be resurrected if nursing is to meaningfully contribute to the survival of humankind.

Chapter 3

The Paradox: Nurses as Healers in "Men's Horrible Wars"

Nurses, along with other women, have had to deal continually with their exclusion from medical, political, economic, and social power structures. Even more than other women, nurses have also had to cope with the military structure, the most male-dominated societal institution, and this has had an important impact on the profession. This chapter considers nurses' historical involvement with the military, a structure whose ultimate purpose is organized killing, and the effects of war on female healers whose nurturing values, traditionally connected to the women's world, contrast most sharply with the values of warriors. While the strength of women's nurturing and healing values has been apparent in nurses' involvement during wartime, other values such as nonviolence have led many women, nurses among them, to actively protest war and its atrocities. Several of the nurse activists discussed in Chapter 2 were involved in wartime activities, while others called for noninvolvement. In this chapter, the thoughts and actions of these women during war are considered, as well as those of nurses who participated in later wars in the 20th century. How did these women become involved in men's war activities? What were their major roles? How did nurses' values of healing and preserving life mesh with men's wartime values of killing and aggression? Why were some nurses antiwar activists and pacifists? How were nurses' wartime activities perceived by the public, the military itself, the soldiers who were nurtured? Were nurses recognized for their work in wartime or have they been ignored, their contributions devalued and trivialized?

There is a long and complex history of women in relation to war that has never been fully examined. Often, more is known about early male nurses, particularly those in religious orders attached to military units. To make the issue even more complex, cross-cultural variations in women's roles in battle and wartime make it difficult to derive generalizations from primarily Western cultural and historical data. Even in Western cultures, the small numbers of fully educated and scientifically prepared physicians before the late 19th century further complicates the issue of what nurses actually did in wartime. This is particularly problematic since gender-typed descriptions of women's war-related groups may have little to do with their real functions and activities. One thing is certain: the exclusion and extreme subordination of women as nurses did not bode well for the welfare of men as warriors. Certainly, the wars dating from the mid-19th century on provide more than sufficient information to prove the inadequacy, for example, of both British and American medical and hospital systems. We know this because of the women who reported the facts and forced reform of these systems.

NURSES OR CAMP FOLLOWERS? SOME WOMEN HEALERS OF THE AMERICAN REVOLUTION

Little is known about women nurses and healers who were involved in armed conflicts prior to the mid-19th century. What is written is generally from a male and often a medical perspective that provides a view of women as nothing more than camp followers, washerwomen, cooks, or prostitutes. A less biased account, however, is given by Ida Cohen Selavan (1975), who notes that women in the American Revolution, such as Mary Ludwig Hays McCauley (or McKelly), under her more widely known name, Molly Pitcher, rendered valuable service as army nurses. Pitcher may have become a legend, but her actual nursing care remains unclear. Though Selavan seems to accept that medical and nursing functions in the 18th century were clearly separate, this sharp demarcation is unlikely, given women's involvement in *both* domestic nursing and medicine. Surgical procedures, however, such as amputations, were more likely medicine's function. Selavan describes the confusion over women's roles as nurses, housekeepers, and nutritionists. According to one surgeon, women dressed meats, prepared drinks, and washed patients. Whether these women were "camp followers" is unclear; the term itself requires feminist clarification. Now a degraded expression, it is not an unusual linguistic phenomenon for words describing or denoting women to experience "downward" drift in meaning. For example, "madam," a term of respect, becomes degraded to a "keeper of a brothel." Thus, it is unclear whether a "camp follower," who laundered, emptied slop pails, scrubbed floors, provided cooked meals, and washed dishes, would qualify as a housekeeper or a nurse or both. Furthermore, it is also questionable whether physicians' reports would admit to women doing more than bathing or feeding patients.

Selavan does not know the extent to which these women actually administered herbs as medicines, made poultices, or provided dressings, but she notes that keeping the sick clean, well-fed, or comfortable should not be undervalued. In the Revolutionary period, physicians were unlicensed and poorly or haphazardly educated; medical schools, libraries, journals, or societies and hospitals were practically nonexistent. Indeed, since physicians often engaged in purging, bleeding, and blistering, it is unclear the extent to which they actually contributed to the 20% death rate suffered during the Revolutionary War. Medical reports claim that malnutrition, lack of medicines and supplies, and hospital conditions were related to disease and caused 90% of the deaths. Actually, only one of every ten of those who died succumbed from battle wounds. Obviously, nursing care would be critical to survival since smallpox, typhoid, typhus, and dysentery could wipe out entire units. How these diseases affected the nurses themselves was not noted.

Selavan claims that Martha Washington and other wives were "camp followers" who mended uniforms, knitted socks, and dispensed foods and home remedies, presumably medicines, to the soldiers. George Washington, wanting to systematize health care, worked to pass legislation establishing a hospital for 20,000 soldiers, providing a nurse for every 10 sick men, at a salary of $2.00 a month. But poverty, inexperience, and lack of female military status made the scheme unsuccessful. It is equally probable, as physician William Shippen said, that no woman could be found to work for $.50 per week. Later, Washington recommended that nurses receive the same pay as the soldiers, reasoning that better pay would attract more women to care for the soldiers, and he could "'no longer bear having an army on paper and not have them in the field'" (p. 594). Despite inadequate or no reimbursement, many women nurses served during the Revolutionary War, but only a few appear on payrolls or pension lists. Sometimes, notes Selavan, whole communities tended the sick and wounded soldiers.

After the Revolutionary War was over, physician Benjamin Rush wrote of nurse Mary Waters that she was a skillful nurse, but disliked lying-in women; she was "'minutely acquainted with the characters, manners, habits . . . of all the physicians in town and always showed a disposition to support their influence in medicine'" (p. 594). Given Rush's erroneous theory of disease, one can question whether this recommendation of Waters helped the physician more than the patient.

EXCLUDED, SENTIMENTALIZED, AND TRIVIALIZED

During war, women have simply taken on public roles or forced physicians to accept nurses' services. If unpaid and unorganized, their services have sometimes been accepted, particularly in doing the drudge work. Only gradually have organized female nurses been accepted to care for sick and wounded men. The paradox of women as wartime nurses, healers who sustain life, and military men, warriors who kill as they go about the usual business of war, is obvious. Nevertheless, some women have forced the military to use their services as nurses to relieve the suffering of the wounded and dying;

others have refused involvement and actively rejected war as anathema to women's own values.

Nevertheless, in wartime, all women have been expected to take on all family obligations and to sustain agricultural and industrial production while men are away fighting. During wars, traditional gender expectations may even be temporarily transformed or reversed. Often, women's work in wartime is rewarded by later historical omission of their services and accomplishments. More particularly, nurses' contributions have often been totally excluded or, if acknowledged, sentimentalized, or worse, trivialized. For example, in the recently televised, highly acclaimed 1990 Ken Burns' production of *The Civil War*, a total of only *13 minutes* out of the entire several hours, 9-part production focused on nurses and their activities during the Civil War years.

Women as nurses have seen the worst of war as they cared for the results of it: the maimed, suffering, and dying. Nevertheless, "modern" nursing originated in war—in Clara Barton's work during the Civil War and Nightingale's during the Crimean War. Monica E. Baly (1973) says Nightingale's achievements would "shine like a beacon," but emphasizes that Nightingale's reforms were not limited to nursing the sick and dying; rather they extended to investigating and improving "the hygiene of barracks, the diet of the Army, recreational facilities for soldiers, military clothing, all came under her scrutiny and were the subject of her pungent reports" (p. 64). Thus, a complex interaction of women, war, social reform, and nursing emerges with the beginning of "modern" nursing. Baly redraws the mythic imagery to extend the boundaries of nursing to include a wide spectrum of activities in which power to solve social problems is central.

This focus on power is evident in Irene Sabelberg Palmer's (1976) emphasis on Nightingale's leadership: "[Her] astute handling of mismanagement in Free Gifts Stores during the Crimean War underscored her administrative ability. Miss Nightingale went to Scutari ostensibly to nurse the British soldiers, and while there encountered innumerable instances of administrative and managerial ineffectiveness and difficulties" (p. 370). The organizational mismanagement women uncovered in the Crimea led to major reforms by Nightingale, which stand, says Palmer, as examples for future medical and nursing organizations in military and wartime situations.

But what of the women on the other side of the battle, the Russian nurses in the Crimean War? Although J. S. Curtiss had already published on the Russian nurses in 1966 and 1968, Evelyn R. Benson (1992) has provided further important translated materials that elaborate on the earlier accounts, describing the organization of Russia's volunteer nurses in the tragic Crimean episode with its enormous cost in lives and human misery. Nightingale herself "mentioned the Russian nurses in her Subsidiary Notes as to the Introduction of Female Nursing into Military Hospitals in Peace and War (Nightingale, 1858): and one of the Russian nurses paid tribute to Florence Nightingale and to her team in her own memoirs (Bakunina, 1898)" (p. 65).

According to Benson, the Russians were not prepared to deal with huge battle casualties and the starvation, epidemics, and illness of both civilian and military groups. These facts, in the absence of a free press, remained unknown in Russia, except through the efforts of Dr. Nicholas Pirogov, who was appalled by the disorder in military hospitals and proposed a plan to recruit trained volunteer female nurses. As with the British top medical leaders, so did the Russian men resist, saying the women's presence "would lead to mass rape and to an increase in syphilis" (p. 66). To Pirogov, the real reason was that the competent nurses would expose the military-medical inadequacy and insufficiency. Despite opposition, Pirogov sought the help of a woman, the Grand Duchess Elena Pavlovna, the widowed sister-in-law of the czar.

Pavlovna was a woman with a keen intellect, who had a superb education and who dedicated her life to liberal causes, including the emancipation of the serfs. In 1854, believing her actions would create an opportunity for women to prove they could work close to the front lines and contribute to their country, the duchess established the Order of the Exaltation of the Cross, a semireligious group of volunteer nurses. She called on all Russian women to serve for a year as military hospital nurses; they were to wear a brown habit and work without pay, reaping their rewards from self-sacrifice and spiritual devotion. Using her private funds, Pavlovna sent several groups of volunteer nurses to work, not under a woman like Nightingale, but under Pirogov; however, Aleksandra Petrovna Stakhovich served as the first director of the order.

Women from all social classes responded to the call. In 1898 Ekaterina M. Bakunina, the daughter of a former governor of St. Petersburg, published her memoirs in the journal, *Vestnik Evropy*. Most of the women had no hospital experience or training. Traveling to the Crimea under the most primitive conditions, they arrived exhausted and weakened; some became ill and died. Under Bakunina's leadership, part of the first unit was sent to Sevastopol, which was under siege from several heavy battles that produced horrendous casualties, many of these left unattended on the field. Working around the clock, the nurses brought order out of chaos, despite being exposed to extreme danger in first-aid stations that were under fire.

Before the war was over, 120 women from the order served in the Crimea, plus others from the organization of Compassionate Widows. Bakunina noted that some nurses quarreled among themselves, spreading malicious gossip that required the intervention of the grand duchess. Despite military leaders' opposition, the volunteer nurses, on the whole, were serious and dedicated; withstanding the rigors of battle and acting heroically, they were admired by the soldiers and cared for both their own and the British wounded. Unlike the British nurses, the Russian women served under fire in the thick of battle.

When Sevastopol fell in 1855, Bakunina stayed until the wounded were evacuated. She was the last to leave. After the war, the order ran a hospital, clinic, and girls' school, all managed by a committee composed of the nursing director, the sister tutor, and two members of the city council. In 1894 the order was absorbed by the Red Cross.

"SOLDIERS! I HAVE WORKED FOR YOU":
NURSES IN THE CIVIL WAR

In the United States, the Civil War was also the scene of women's involvement and reform. As noted in Chapter 2, Clara Barton, credited with initiating military nursing with the support of women's groups, organized and developed the American Red Cross, struggling throughout her life to achieve social change. Marshall W. Fishwick (1966) noted that Barton was known for bringing nurses into the American Red Cross, but fewer people realize her strong support of women's rights: "I believe I must have been born believing in the full right of women to all privileges and positions which nature and justice accord her common with other human beings. Perfectly equal rights—human rights. There was never any question in my mind in regard to this" (National Park Service, 1987).

Clara Barton and Florence Nightingale were contemporaries, and each was important both nationally and internationally. Nightingale was born in 1820 and died in 1910; Barton was born in 1821 and died in 1912. Neither married. The reputations of both were born with nursing and war. Yet of war, Barton said: "Men have worshiped war til it has cost a million times more than the whole earth is worth. . . . Deck it as you will, war is Hell. . . . Only the desire to soften some of its hardships and allay some of its miseries ever induced me . . . to face its pestilent and unholy breath" (National Park Service, 1987). Both Barton and Nightingale broke gender stereotypes by entering into wartime nursing. Barton said: "I struggled long and hard with my sense of propriety—with the appalling fact that I was only a woman whispering in one ear, and thundering in the other, the groans of suffering men dying like dogs, unfed and unsheltered. . . . I said that I struggled with my sense of propriety and I say it with humiliation and shame. . . . When our armies fought on Cedar Mountain, I broke the shackles and went to the field" (Fishwick, 1966, p. 153). Barton was in constant danger, a shell once taking off part of her skirt while she tended a wounded man. Her courage was not, however, limited to the men's battlefield, but extended to the feminist fight as well.

In a more recent reworking of imagery, Ellen Langenheim Henle (1978) questions whether Barton was soldier or pacifist. Henle notes that now that women are admitted to West Point, Annapolis, and the Air Force Academy, they are being trained for combat despite legal prohibitions. Their antecedents are women in nursing service and the Red Cross, munitions industries, and female military groups, where some in the air force even piloted transport planes. To Henle, "Historians have done little to shed light on women's roles in war . . . partly because women's history was considered unimportant"

(p. 153). Those writing on women have had a pacifist bias, being concerned about the increasing role of women in the military, particularly their demands for combat training and assignments. The clash between women's and men's traditional values are inherent in this unease. According to Henle, Clara Barton, who was actively involved in three major wars, provides perspective on women's future roles in the military. As noted in Chapter 2, Barton, Civil War heroine, founder of the American Red Cross in 1881, and its first president for over 20 years, was a battlefield nurse, bringing medical supplies and food to the front lines. In the Franco-Prussian War, she organized a relief program for poor women after a month-long siege of Strasbourg by German troops. In 1898, at 76 years of age, Barton went to Cuba to direct Red Cross field relief during the Spanish-American War.

Henle claims that Barton saw war as a fact of life and was skeptical that the women's peace movement, organized by Julia Ward Howe at the outbreak of the Franco-Prussian War in 1870, would succeed. Barton agreed that "'Women should certainly have *some* voice in the matter of war'" (p. 154) and wrote to a relative: "'I can never see a poor mutilated wreck, blown to pieces with powder and lead, without wondering if visions of such an end ever flitted before his mother's mind when she washed and dressed her fair-skinned baby'" (pp. 153–154). To Barton, women's subordinated status was sustained because of their exclusion from war. Men's circular reasoning started with the premise that since women did not vote, they could assume no functions in war; this, in turn, justified men's denial of enfranchisement because women had no military responsibility. Thus, noted a frustrated Barton, women could not say there will be no war; they could not take part in it when it happened; because they did not take part, they could not vote; because they could not vote, they had no voice in the government, which could then initiate wars only by agreement among men. Henle claims that Barton's position on the vote and war was more radical than that of other feminists, such as Elizabeth Cady Stanton. When asked by Horace Greeley what women who voted would do in time of war, Stanton pointedly replied, "'Stay at home as you did and urge others to go to the front'" (p. 154).

Barton was proud of the women who went to the battlefield because they advanced the cause of women's emancipation. Henle states that Barton's pride was based in part on her confidence that women under fire could be as brave as men: "She herself was fearless . . . had little fear of death . . . relished facing and overcoming dangerous situations" (p. 154). While most women served in hospitals, Barton once held on the battlefield a wounded man who was actually shot and killed while in her arms. On lecture tours, people were impressed with her steady gaze that conveyed the "'magnetic power that always accompanies true courage'" (p. 155).

That women were not protected in war was brought home to Barton when she discovered that more than half of those wounded in the siege of Strasbourg were women. To this she said: "I see no reason why women have not the same privilege to be shot that they have to be protected, the same right to danger that they have to safety, and this is at least a practical demonstration that they have the same *liability*" (p. 155). According to Henle, Barton felt that war could be exciting and knew the letdown after returning to civilian life, later rushing to the scene of natural disasters. Henle contends that Barton identified with her father, a noncommissioned officer in the Northwest Territories, who coached her in military lore, taught her to work out winning strategies using red and white Indian corn for soldiers, related tales of his experiences, and encouraged her to revere military heroes, such as Andrew Jackson and Napoleon.

Barton loved athletics and physical exercise, activities in which "ladies" did not participate. She rode the wildest colts, used a hammer, and threw balls as straight as her brothers. "In her fifties, she (Barton) took up rowing and challenged a much younger woman to a foot race in a public park. In her seventies she went camping in Yellowstone with her relatives" (p. 156). In her final years, she still mended broken boards in the sidewalk outside her home. War allowed Barton an outlet for her love of physical activity. Henle believes that Barton's "view of herself as a soldier was central to her personality" (p. 156). At the age of ninety, she dreamed she was back in battle and, comparing her own pain to a soldier's, said, "'I am ashamed that I murmur!'" (p. 157).

Barton worked hard to involve women in the military, supporting moves to create a woman's auxiliary. Thus, the Women's Relief Corps of the veterans' group, the Grand Army of the Republic, was formed. This, along with the American Red Cross, were vehicles for women's involvement in civic, charitable, and military affairs. As Henle points out, Barton really wanted women to be more than members of auxiliaries, to be able to obtain a military education in academies for women so they could be active, brave, strong, fearless, and able to understand campaign plans. A soldier reared by such a woman would be worth "'one thousand drilled doughheads who had merely, without foundation, been run through West Point'" (p. 158). A radical recommendation! Still, it relied on motherhood to justify it.

As with Nightingale, the popular image of Barton is as a nurse, the nurturant, gentle, humanitarian female; but, states Henle, Barton actually fashioned an alternative to a military career, overcoming prejudice against women at the front, who, she hoped, would not be hindered, belittled, turned back, or thwarted. This aspect of her philosophy she kept more private, publicly stating her hatred of war. She genuinely believed she worked for peace, viewing the Red Cross as the most potent force against war, which to her was simply agony. According to Henle, Barton did not see the ways in which the Red Cross could indirectly contribute to war, merely "patching up" the wounded. A complex person, Barton was both attracted and repelled by war; she found it a challenge, but simultaneously "genuinely longed for peace" (p. 160), seeing the Red Cross as a practical way to deal with the inhumanity of war. Her reputation as a humanitarian is well deserved, but she wanted women and men to be equal in all things, including war.

It is fascinating to see how non-nurses downplay actual nursing, while nurse authors center their analysis on it. Mary Madeline Rogge (1987) focuses on nursing and politics, a forgotten legacy. She, too, resurrects Barton and the Civil War nurses, but for the purpose of reclaiming the lost tradition of power and politics in nursing. To Rogge, many nurses today see political power as a recent development: nebulous policies on patient care and working conditions are expressed by a few, while the majority still resist political activities. But to Rogge, nurses' political power is not a new phenomenon. To her, the Civil War revolutionized nursing care, allowing women to care for those other than family and friends, creating a demand for education and breaching the barriers to practice in hospitals. Despite only grudging respect from physicians, some nurses became regional and even national heroines. These women, who were considered intellectually "incapable" of political intricacies, challenged military medical authorities by achieving public support. In the carnage of the Civil War, "more than 600,000 men died, two-thirds of them from disease rather than from wounds sustained in combat . . . the troops experienced more than ten million episodes of illness, wounds, and injury" (p. 26). Attempts to alleviate the appalling conditions, in the absence of experienced nursing, failed: using cooks, bandsmen, convalescents, and civilian males did not alter the shocking conditions. In 1861 the government authorized employment of women nurses in the North, appointing Dorothea Dix as superintendent of nurses; the Confederacy legislated nursing care for its hospitals in 1862. Rogge credits Georgeanna Woolsey with noting that once the government had decided that women were to be employed, the army surgeons were "'unable . . . to close the hospitals against them'" (p. 26).

As Rogge states, the women, lacking strength in numbers and rank, individually undertook reform and lobbied powerful men to challenge the military medical bureaucracy. Clara Barton arrived in Fredericksburg, Virginia, and found deplorable conditions following a battle in which 21,700 soldiers on both sides were killed and wounded. Patients were not sheltered because people did not want to open their homes to the "'dirty, lousy, common soldiers'" (p. 27). Barton found 500 men in one old sunken hotel lying on bare, wet, bloody floors, begging her for a cracker or a cup to get water. She had no crackers or cups for them, nor for the men crowded into 200 army wagons, reaching so far down the road that she never found the end of it. Outraged, Barton went to Henry Wilson, chairman of the Senate's Military Committee in Washington; she described what she had seen, but the War Department doubted the reliability of Barton's or Wilson's reports. Threatened by Wilson, however, the quartermaster general and staff rode to Fredericksburg that night, and Barton noted with satisfaction that by noon of the next day the soldiers were fed and housed. This quick action occurred because of the trust and good working relations Barton had previously established with Wilson.

Rogge details Barton's continual use of political power "to accomplish what she alone lacked the authority to enforce" (p. 27). To take nursing care to the front in order to avoid men languishing up to five days without help, Barton relied on Massachusetts Governor John A. Andrew, who owed her a favor. Even then, the local physicians denied Barton entry to the battlefield, but she went over their heads and arrived at the Battle of Antietam, the bloodiest single day of the Civil War, where the nursing care she provided laid the foundation of her life's work.

Barton was certainly not the only women to engage in wartime politics. Rogge also recognizes Hannah Ropes, a nurse and abolitionist who used political pressure "to rectify flagrant abuses of the patients at her hospital" (p. 28). On learning from her patients that the hospital steward was stealing patients' clothing and hospital laundry soap, Ropes complained to the head surgeon, who virtually ignored her. She then wrote to the U.S. Surgeon General, but he returned the letter to the surgeon in charge who informed her that she, not he, had to prove the charges against the steward. To Ropes, these charges were obvious, "'plain in the kitchen, the larder, and every pinched face one meets on the stairs or in the wards'" (p. 28). No action was taken, but shortly thereafter, the steward assaulted a patient and Ropes telegraphed his father, who arrived the next day, followed by a general. Again, no action was taken. The following week, the steward put a patient in a cellar prison. Finally, Ropes and another nurse went to see a high-ranking friend, General Nathaniel Banks. He was out of town so the two women continued on to the surgeon general's office. Here, they were informed that the surgeon general was out, but at that moment he walked by without looking, nodding, or even raising his hat, and then vanished into his office where he refused to see them, referring them to the assistant surgeon general, who was also "engaged." Ropes declared, "'Two rebuffs seemed about enough for a woman of half century to accept'" (p. 28).

The two women then went to the U.S. Secretary of War, who heard their complaint, ordered the soldier out of the cellar hole, arrested the steward, and had him imprisoned. Rogge emphasizes that Ropes tried to follow the chain of command, but was treated with contempt by the medical men, who refused to protect patients. Astutely, she went to a man who was at odds with the surgeon general. The surgeon in charge was also jailed for a week and then replaced. He subsequently became a leading New York neurologist. Ropes contracted typhoid fever while engaged in her nursing duties and died three months after her meeting with the secretary of war.

Another Civil War nurse, Cordelia Harvey, petitioned President Lincoln directly to establish a facility in a distant northern state to enable soldiers to recover from malaria and other fevers contracted in the steamy environments and swamplands of the South. Previously, Lincoln and his medical authorities had rejected such a proposal, fearing desertions by the soldiers. Harvey argued that Lincoln would lose more soldiers to illness and death, and that citizens could not understand why " 'their friends are left to die when with proper care they might live to do good service for their country' " (p. 29). She refuted the evaluations of hospitals made by medical inspectors, who reported whatever pleased the president. The physicians, she contended, passed rapidly through the hospitals with cigar in mouth and rattan cane in hand, emerging as though from suffocation, reporting that everything was fine. In contrast, Ropes said: "I have visited the hospitals, but from morning until late at night. . . . I come to you from the cots of men who have died, who might have lived had you permitted. This is hard to say, but it is none the less true" (p. 29). Harvey's perseverance and plain talk were rewarded when Lincoln ordered the establishment of a military hospital in Wisconsin.

Although written evidence is more fragmentary for Southern women, Rogge claims that they, too, used their political connections to achieve better care for the Confederate soldiers. Juliet Hopkins, named superintendent of all hospitals established in Virginia for Alabama soldiers, remained in constant contact with the Alabama governor. Sally Tompkins was "one of countless civilians who opened private hospitals. . . . Operating [them] at her own expense, she established such a high standard of nursing care that the death rate . . . was less than 6 percent of admissions, the lowest of any Richmond hospital" (p. 29). This rate was achieved despite the transfer of some of the worst cases to her hospital. Blocking women from control, Confederate President Davis later ordered these hospitals to be run by commissioned officers with a rank no lower than captain. Upon a request from Tompkins, however, Davis gave her a commission as captain of cavalry so that she could continue to administer her hospital and provide nursing care to the soldiers.

Rogge argues forcefully for this heritage of nurses who used political processes to improve care and practice: "They commanded the attention, respect, and cooperation of governors, congressmen, cabinet members, and presidents" (p. 30). To Rogge, political power is not only a legitimate option but an essential strategy for today's nurses who must, both as individuals and in coalitions, influence governmental policies. She does not, however, suggest that nurses cultivate political relations with leaders in the women's movement. Yet it is the broader societal attitude toward women that affects their success or failure in political actions.

In 1962 Sister Henrietta Guyot analyzed the nurse in Civil War literature, capturing the sense of women who, like Louisa May Alcott, writing in 1862, realized that she " 'must let out my pent-up energy in some new way' " (p. 311). Alcott's *Hospital Sketches* in 1863 opened with the cry, " 'I want something to do' " (p. 311). She voiced a sentiment common to many women when she pleaded for an opportunity to engage in worthwhile work. She joined 3,000 or more women who left home to care for soldiers during the Civil War and about whom there is a wide array of information. Agatha

Young's (1959) *The Women and the Crisis*, portrays women as " 'restive, resentful of men, aware of their own vitality and dissatisfied by the limitations which their way of life put on their powers' " (p. 311). With the advent of the Civil War, these women lost little time in moving into the new and larger world. With men away at war, women could work outside the home for a cause, no longer restricted to teaching, dressmaking, millinery, and writing. Mary Louise Marshall (1957) noted that Southern women responded with similar alacrity. Indeed, these women faced even greater difficulties entering public service, and their success in overcoming prejudice and the hardships of war service " 'may well be considered the turning point in the status of Southern women. . . . They marked the path to a new way of life for the women of the South' " (p. 311).

For the women who remained at home, the relief societies allowed a public outlet for female energies. In forming the Women's Central Association for Relief, 3,000 to 4,000 women attended a meeting at which they began the organization that later evolved into the American Sanitary Commission, similar to its British counterpart, so effective in the Crimean War. George W. Adams, in his 1952 medical history of the Union Army, *Doctors in Blue*, said the women proposed investigating the organization and methods of recruiting forces by each state, inquiring into diet, cooks, clothing, tents, campgrounds, transports, camp police, and sanitary and hygienic matters. In addition, the women proposed a study of military hospitals, the possibilities of using women as nurses, the inspection of the quality and procurement methods of hospital supplies, and a consideration of ambulance and relief services.

A product of women's organizations, "The Sanitary Commission . . . successfully formed several thousand ladies' aid societies in the North and thereby united many women in a common front" (p. 312), an arena where women could work as equals with men. A British writer claimed the Sanitary Commission " 'created a union of women, who molded and directed the "wills of the strongest" ' " (p. 312). For example, with this backing, and her entire soul in the effort, Dorothea Dix installed several hundred nurses, rented large houses as depots for supplies sent to her, and provided houses of rest and refreshment for nurses and convalescent soldiers. Guyot cites Mary Livermore as saying that Dix employed two secretaries, owned ambulances, printed and distributed circulars, visited widely dispersed hospitals, adjucated disputes, settled problems of her nurses, took long journeys, and paid her expenses from her own purse: " 'Her fortune, time, and strength were laid on the altar of her country in its hour of trial' " (p. 313).

Dix's requirements and qualifications in her selection of nurses were rigidly regulated to avoid any hint of scandal; however, she was never able to bring all the nurses directly under her authority. In fact, as Guyot notes, some feminists such as Clara Barton and Mother Bickerdyke were independent of Dix's authority. Working for no pay or only 40 cents a day, the required recommendations of "good character" may have ruled out the most rebellious women. As one of Dix's nurses, Louisa May Alcott's recommendation said that she offered "'no difficulties of . . . romantic involvement . . . or militant jargon about rights'" (p. 313). In contrast to other nurses, Alcott was treated with courtesy and kindness, even though she expected humiliation, to be treated as a doormat, "'nurses being considered as mere servants, receiving the lowest pay, and, it's my private opinion, doing the hardest work of any part of the army, except the mules'" (p. 314). About one-third of the nurses were from roughly fourteen religious sisterhoods, and, as Ellen Ryan Jolly (1927) said, these women were often greeted with joy by the officers. The influence of these women pioneers eventually resulted in a nursing bureau in Washington, demands for improvements in hospitals, and insistence on schools of nursing. By breaking down severe prejudices, states Guyot, these women opened doors to worthwhile work to other women and began a series of events that led to a new profession for women.

This is apparent in Anne L. Austin's (1975) article on wartime nurse volunteers from 1861 to 1865 in which she further documents the efforts of Northern women to organize relief societies to provide material needs and nurses for the wounded soldiers. The first of these, the Women's Central Association of Relief of New York, was initiated by Dr. Elizabeth Blackwell and women managers of the New York Infirmary for Women and Children. At first rejected, their plan was later used to create President Lincoln's order for the United States Sanitary Commission, branches of which were established in several states. As noted by Guyot, Dorothea Dix led the nurses, called for women between the ages of 30 and 50, being of good health, endurance, matronly demeanor, good character, experience, and plainly dressed with no ornaments or hoops.

The New York women selected 100 women to be trained by staff physicians at Bellevue and New York Hospitals. Some physicians believed the ladies were too proper and delicate; others that nurses were too demanding. The physicians preferred religious sisters, who took orders unquestioningly and did not use political connections to change things. It was customary for "visitors" to bring delicacies, clothing, books, and newspapers to the soldiers; they wrote letters, talked of home and family, and sat with dying soldiers.

Nurses were assisted by the enlisted men in giving medications and care, and the men often resented these assignments. Religious orders such as the Sisters of Charity, Sisters of the Holy Cross, Sisters of Mercy, and the Lutheran Sisters were also involved. Women of widely differing backgrounds—reformers, newspaper publishers, wives of clergymen, daughters of senators—without being "avowed" feminists, expected and received some recognition. Some of them became founders of the new nursing schools. In the South, by comparison, a Women's Relief Society was organized by Felicia Grundy Porter and other women volunteers, but no official organizations ever developed from them.

THE WAR WITHIN THE WAR

It is illuminating to compare nurse and non-nurse perceptions of women in war. Nurses have long complained that others do not understand their work, which involves the most difficult and demanding issues of life and death—both exaggerated during war. Ann Douglas Wood (1972), an English professor writing on American culture during the 19th century, focuses on "The War Within a War," in which the struggle between women and men is described as a rhetoric of mothering, used to justify women's involvement in healing. It is necessary to place this analysis in the context of the horrors of war. Unlike Irene Palmer, who speculates on the effects on Nightingale of dealing with 2,000 deaths during the Crimean War (see Chapter 1), Wood does not deal with the overwhelming impact on women of human destruction, mutilation, and death during the Civil War, at that time the most mechanized chaos to be created by men. Yet Wood's perspective that a gender war was enacted within the context of men's battles is useful, even if it remains unclear that, as Lillian Wald said, war itself is waged continually on women and children. The extent to which the warrior mentality, as the major distinction between men and women, perpetuates war is inherent in Wald's thought, and, when combined with Wood's, leads to a two-tiered understanding of women in wartime.

Wood, first, lays out the historical conditions for women that preceded the Civil War. She claims that women were increasingly excluded from public life from the 18th to 19th centuries. Women as healers were also purposely excluded by medical men, but female nurses reemerged during the Civil War. Dr. A. Curtis (1836) damned the passing of women midwives because the emergence of male midwives was not a change for the better, resulting in the "'destruction of scores of modern women and infants, and the miserable condition of multitudes that escape immediate death'" (p. 197). From the 17th century, when males could be prosecuted for practicing midwifery, to the mid-19th century, the professionalization of medicine by men forcibly and purposely expelled women from public practice to the home, where their "silent, long-suffering ministry" was restricted to the house; even here they were "never in any circumstance to come into competition with the professional doctor's role" (p. 198).

Wood notes that a Boston physician, William A. Alcott, supported women being trained for the care of the sick at home. This would give the women tasks that would "save them from 'ennui,' 'disgust,' and even 'suicide'" (p. 198). According to Alcott, women were "formed" by days, nights, months, and years of watchfulness; thus, they were presumably capable of marathons of selflessness, particularly since they could anticipate men's needs and give cheaper care. Wood concludes that women exchanged "professional expertise and official recognition for a domesticated version . . . sapped by its distance from technological, scientific advance" (p. 198). Wood further asserts that inadequately educated physicians told the ladies that they had been third-rate professional doctors, but now were promised they could be first-rate amateur nurses. Thus, if they could not be midwives, they could be "madonnas." This mystique, according to Wood, was later inverted and used by the women themselves to attack their exclusion from professional activities.

During the Revolutionary War, the professional control of medicine by men was strengthened because of increased demands for men who could practice their skills on the battlefield. This was the death-knell of the woman physician, says Wood, who contends that the Civil War also increased male power, through discoveries made from the study of gun-shot wounds, the development of anesthetics, and basic principles of sanitation. Though ejected from "official" medicine during the Revolutionary War, the women in the Civil War, basing their efforts on Nightingale's work in the Crimea, used the myth of the bedside madonna's healing power and pitted it against male authority.

The majority of women stayed home during the Civil War. Wood notes that Elizabeth Stuart Phelps (1897) claimed that many of these women "seemed to see the war as an act of hostility committed by men against the all-too-delicate sensibilities of their women-folk . . . 'the helpless, outnumbering, unconsulted women . . . whom war trampled down, without a choice at protest'" (p. 199). The women actually *were* excluded politically and legally from decision making. In this sense, war *was* imposed on them, so it is hardly appropriate to view them as passively taking on the men's suffering. Indeed, Wood notes that some ten thousand Soldier's Aid Societies were formed by the women, and huge "Sanitary Fairs" netted $3 million, a very significant sum for that period. Furthermore, the women refused to allow the government to take the men from home and organize them in the army. Instead, the women waged their "own war on military professionalism and on the masculine establishment that tried to exclude them . . . they simply refused to let this be the old kind of war, fought by men, with the wounded tended by men" (p. 200). Thousands entered the war as volunteer nurses.

Wood claims the women were all without formal training. Since some had been trained in alternative schools, others had on-the-job experience, and most had provided home nursing and medical treatment, it is questionable whether this assertion can be so confidently expressed. However, it is true that most had to rely on experience at home, since there were few nursing schools and no women were allowed into the "regular" medical schools; thus, their ideal was the home, not the hospital or barracks. Although Wood sees the battle as one over professionalization, it is quite clear that the vast majority of physicians also had very little formal training. In fact, the women's actual healing experiences, in some cases, may have been more extensive. Though men *presumed* to be professionals, only a few were actually educated in European or American medical schools and those formally trained were still a minority compared to those who had on-the-job training.

Wood claims that a maternal code was used by women to fight the masculine military code; the women tried to extend the definition of home to the larger world, and in this process, progressed from female self-abnegation to competitive involvement. Wood stresses that motherhood and hearth were used as the bases for the emergence of organized nursing. However, it is clear that women such as Clara Barton had far more complex motivations than these. Nurses presumably were also guardians of morality; even Dorothea Dix was called a vigilance committee in herself, attempting to clean up the army as she had the jails and asylums. Non-nursing authors, too, often overlook the real horrors of these institutions that women such as Dix actually confronted. To refer to nurses as having "maternal lust" is hardly useful and quite condescending in tone and terms.

During the Civil War, some 400 women passed as men. These "actual Amazons" were few, but some of the "volunteer nurses showed sparks of the same martial fire" (p. 202). Indeed, more than a few expressed horror with war, but also excitement on passing the confines of hearth, home, and maternity to become participants in American history. Wood claims that many of the women leaders were fighters from birth, noting that Barton, on hearing of the beginning of the war, took a rifle and put nine balls in a target "within the space of six inches at a distance of fifty feet" (p. 203). Instead of seeing this action as simply an expression of assertive skill, Wood claims these "strongly aggressive, not to say belligerent gestures, [were] conspicuous in the careers of not a few of the most famous nurses" (p. 203). Such actions, says Wood, unmasked the women's competitiveness with men, whom they not only wanted to care for but to "take over" as well.

Given the horrible messes the women found both in the Crimean and Civil Wars, it is obvious that *someone* had to do something. One must question who was taking over from whom. Given Wood's earlier assertion that men had taken away healing, even midwifery, from women, and given the historical exclusion of women from formal education and the active opposition of undereducated physicians toward early and later nurses, it is peculiar to assert that the men's hostility was caused by the nurses' competitiveness. Indeed, medical hostility preceded rather than followed the nurses' actions in the Civil War.

Wood notes that various male officials continuously attempted to drive the women out of the army; even Barton was rudely ousted from her post at one point, and Dix's authority was permanently subordinated to the surgeon general's. Since the resistance to women nurses did not come from the ranks of the ordinary soldiers, Wood believes that lack of professional status was the issue. Again, it must be emphasized that most physicians were poorly educated at this time, that strong professional associations were yet to emerge, and that "heroic" practices of purging and bleeding were hardly indicators of a unified, educated, and professional body of men. Thus, simple professionalism could not be a sufficient cause for the hostility of physicians, who, according to one nurse, were " 'determined by a systematic course of ill-treatment . . . to drive women from the service' " (p. 205).

Admitting that some women were incompetent, but not stating the same of some of the physicians, Wood claims that even the skilled women aroused hostility because they were challenging male authority and comparing their work to the men's: "Naturally the military officials were antagonized and threatened by this challenge" (p. 205). Was this so natural? With inadequate help, equipment, supplies, and transportation for thousands of wounded and dying men, one would suppose the natural reaction should have been gratitude for the women's help. Furthermore, if women had not been excluded from public life by men, their presence would have been unremarkable. Again, it is important that non-nursing researchers grasp the actual work of women nurses. It takes astonishing courage to face hundreds of bloodied, mutilated, and dying men without the support of physicians, who, according to Wood, were especially antagonistic and "took an attitude of no-holds-barred in their resistance" (p. 205).

One nurse, Mary Phinney von Olnhausen, associated with Dix, stated flatly that surgeons were "'the most brutal men I ever saw'" (p. 205). Georgeanna Woolsey stated the surgeons were determined to make the nurses' lives "'so unbearable that they should be forced in self-defense to leave . . . how much ill-will, how much unfeeling want of thought these women nurses endured'" (p. 205). Woolsey asserted that hardly a surgeon treated the nurses with even common courtesy; the women were "'half fed in hospitals, hard worked day and night, and given, when sleep must be had, a . . . closet, just large enough for a camp bed to stand in'" (p. 205). To her, only the knowledge that they were pioneers sustained them. The war against sexism was, indeed, the war within the war.

Finally, Wood admits that many of the "contract" physicians were men who had failed in their home practices, "'to whose care we would not be willing to intrust a sick or disabled horse'" (p. 206). As Wood states, *medical*—not war—casualties were severe. Soldiers' lives were more imperiled, according to historical sources, by hospital medical treatment than by fighting the entire battle at Gettysburg. Despite this, or perhaps because of this, one observer claimed that the best physicians were almost like mothers, assuming not just technical skills but the identity of women themselves.

The women's motivation, according to Wood, was to overcome "being kept out, of medicine, of war, of *life itself*, by a complicated professional code that simply boiled down to men's unwillingness to let anyone—including themselves—know what a mess they had made" (p. 207). The women revealed the mess: Eliza Howland wrote that her hospital was a stable, covered with dust, nails, and shavings that the nurses shoveled into barrels. She wrote of crowded patients, soaked with malignant malarial fever, exposed every night to drenching rains. She damned the "'murderous, blundering want of precision and provision'" (p. 207) that caused these horrors.

IT'S TIME TO OBEY THE WOMEN!

With tremendous courage, the women marshaled their forces against the men in command. In one case, nurse Annie Wittenmeyer was shocked to find a military hospital director "reeling drunk" on the job. He ordered her off the premises, insisting he was boss. Wittenmeyer grimly decided that one of them would indeed go; eventually the surgeon left.

Wood claims that the nurses had previously failed to understand that the men were "incompetent despite the reassuring tokens of self-confidence, responsibility, training, in sum, of masculinity, which she and all her world were accustomed to accept as some kind of seal of approval" (p. 207). After seeing the neglect and maltreatment in the jails and asylums, Dorothea Dix *"doubted"* the men's competence. Whether Wood is correct in saying that Dix enjoyed her doubts, it is obvious that her lack of qualifications became her asset, leading her to feel that she was the "only wakeful passenger on a ship headed for certain wreck" (p. 208). To Wood, thousands of women in the Civil War saw and doubted and acted. Whether they felt "hysterical fear" or "righteous elation," as Wood claims, is questionable. More likely, they experienced grim determination and satisfaction when they succeeded in changing the horrors of the men's world.

Nurses led the opposition for change, insisting on their own authority over each other, cutting through the "red tape" to destroy the bureaucracy that kept them out and the wounded uncared for, the " 'Professional Etiquette . . . which kept shirts from ragged men, and broth from hungry ones' " (p. 208). According to Wood, Mary Ann (Mother) Bickerdyke exemplified the maverick; once a botanic doctor, she then practiced nursing on a large scale. She and many other women joined the war effort not to satisfy their maternal urges, but to use their maternal status to establish a professional legitimacy, an efficiency with a heart the men obviously lacked. To one irate physician, Bickerdyke said there was no use in his stopping her with his red tape (medical protocol) because " 'There's too much to be done down here to stop for that' " (pp. 209–210). Of her and other nurses, Wood states: "The underlying reproach to the dangerously silly men in command around her, unwilling to stop playing the games they have been trained to play even when life and death are at stake, is clear. Men can be allowed to play at authority in peacetime, she implies, but when a war comes, it's time to obey the women" (p. 210). Bickerdyke's natural leadership included simple justice and ready kindness, but when she found an officer stealing clothes from sick soldiers, she "stripped him publicly, 'leaving him nude save his pantaloons' " (p. 210).

In contrast, Clara Barton anticipated and forestalled needs, appearing at moments of crisis "when officialdom is always irrelevant" (p. 210). Barton obeyed physicians when appropriate, but greatly distrusted medicine and men's institutions. The Red Cross, as Barton developed it, was an anti-institution that could take instantaneous action, offsetting men's red tape in order to relieve suffering humanity. Interestingly, women leaders such as Barton and Dix believed they had the healing power that men had lost. These women, concludes Wood, did not make the world a home, but made themselves at home in the world. This is the legacy nurses give to other women: "The wartime nurses, it seems, had joined a bigger army than they knew" (p. 212).

With terrible irony, the work of the feminists during war legitimized, as Clara Barton claimed, new roles for both Northern and Southern women. Margaret E. Parsons (1983) rediscovers and illuminates the activities of several Confederate nurses, such as Kate Cumming, a Southern 26-year-old, who, referring to Nightingale, maintained that "'what one woman had done another could'" (p. 276). Cumming relocated with her hospital from Tennessee to Alabama and then to Georgia. In contrast, Phoebe Pember remained in Virginia as hospital matron.

These women, like their Northern counterparts, endured the worst of war, the wounded, the dying and dead. Cumming survived two hospital fires, frozen water in pitchers and buckets, and periods of sickness. Pember had one day free to herself in three years, and contended with rats, even using fishhooks to catch them. Both women dealt with intoxicated surgeons; Pember finally had to guard the whiskey barrel with a loaded gun. Like the Northern women, they faced the usual hostility, disrespect, and derision from those who expected women to remain in traditional roles. Black women, who cooked, laundered, and supported hospitals, were even less likely to receive any approbation. The "romance" of the Civil War nurse was not the reality during or after the war for most women. Thus, we see an interesting paradox emerge: the reluctance of men to include women in their military activities, the romanticization of women in war when they were included, and the eventual exclusion or trivialization of them in many subsequent military and medical histories.

The services of both Northern and Southern and White and Black women ended with the close of war. In 1887 Congress authorized the enlistment of men in a hospital corps to supply nurses and attendants in army hospitals, in camps, and on the battlefield. This medical or hospital corps was supposed to be equivalent to student nurses in civilian hospitals. At the outbreak of the Spanish-American War in 1898, the hospital corps consisted of only 723 enlisted men, an insufficient number to take care of health services during wartime. The Daughters of the American Revolution, through physician Anita McGee, established the groundwork for a female army nurse corp in 1898; thus, American nurses became involved in yet another war. Historian Phillip A. Kalisch (1975) analyzes the experiences of the female army nurses during the Spanish-American War, noting that the question of appropriate military rank for these nursing heroines arose as early as 1899, but the issue was not successfully resolved until many decades later. In refusing to grant rank to the nurses, men, in effect, were denying women power and sustaining their subordination.

A SPLENDIDLY COOPERATIVE SPIRIT:
AFRICAN AMERICAN NURSES IN WARTIME

The issue of utilizing African American women in nursing activities during times of war and catastrophes had been debated for many years. Adah Thoms (1929) provided an early in-depth look at the questions raised. Assigning Black nurses to a military hospital was carried out experimentally at Camp Sherman, Ohio, during the 1918 influenza epidemic: "The question of utilization of colored nurses had been the cause of prolonged discussion between the Surgeon General's office and the American Red Cross" (p. 155). At a 1911 meeting of the National Committee on Red Cross Nursing Service held in the Continental Memorial Hall of the Daughters of the American Revolution, it was decided that " 'Owing to the impossibility of securing proper quarters for them, it has never been the policy of the Surgeon General's office to consider the appointment of colored nurses' " (p. 155).

For the present, the motion that Black nurses could not be enrolled for service under the Red Cross was carried. By 1917, however, with involvement in still another war, this same group approved a plan for Black nurses to be organized for Black troops only. At their June meeting, it was decided that open enrollment for Black nurses was not possible unless the surgeon general found a way to use them. They would then be enrolled for that special service, " 'to go out in the uniform of the Red Cross nurse and to be given the Red Cross badge . . . when enrolled they would be on the same footing upon assignment to duty as were other nurses' " (p. 156). By September Thoms received a letter from Jane A. Delano, chairperson of the committee, who reported that she had met with a Dr. Squires and " 'assured him of our entire willingness to enroll colored nurses for service whenever they could be utilized, either in this country or abroad' " (pp. 157–158). Delano also said that she had taken up the matter with the surgeon general's office, hoping to assign Black nurses, regularly enrolled, wearing the same uniform and with all the privileges as White nurses, to the mobilization camp at Des Moines, Iowa, or wherever desired by the surgeon general. Delano claimed that she had no authority over duty or placement of these nurses, but wanted their papers so she could act without delay if assignment to duty became possible. She assured Thoms that Black nurses would receive the same pay as White nurses, along with allowances for transportation and maintenance.

The Red Cross women advised enrollment of Black nurses, but admitted that utilizing them was an uncertain proposition. One Black nurse was supplied by the Red Cross to Camp Sherman, but her services were refused. A Miss Thompson asked Catherine L. Leary, chief nurse at Camp Sherman, why the Black nurse's services were refused. Leary responded that their appeal to the Red Cross had produced so many nurses that she had to refuse several nurses, including the "intelligent young colored woman . . . [who] seemed much disappointed. I offered her a bed for the night, which she accepted and later refused. . . . I felt very sorry that she should have to go away disappointed, so I paid her fare to and from Columbus to the Camp" (p. 160). Leary assured Thompson that when quarters were ready for Black nurses, they would be glad of their services. Later, an emergency detachment of 10 Black nurses was assigned to the camp. One of the nurses, Aileen B. Cole, wrote that they were cordially received by the chief nurse, visited the Black hostess house, and attended the Black YMCA, where "'it warmed our hearts to see how thoroughly glad those boys were to have us with them and to hear them cheer!'" (p. 161). She continued: "'We are accepting conditions exactly as we find them. We have met with individual prejudice, but, generally speaking, every one so far has been exceedingly kind'" (p. 161).

Another nurse, Clara A. Rollins, said each nurse had her own room and everything was done to make them feel at home. She said, "'Our boys are in the same wards with the white soldiers'" (p. 162). Chief nurse Mary M. Roberts wrote that she would never forget Rollins' "'splendidly cooperative spirit'" (p. 162). Assigned to the surgical ward, Rollins was so loved that on a possible change of personnel, a request signed by every man on the ward begged that she not be taken away from them. Roberts added, "'As I recall that group of patients, there were very few colored men in it'" (p. 163). Roberts noted that the Black nurses did not share social activities with the White nurses, although they were welcome at all program affairs. Describing her own fear of managing the Black nurses, Roberts said she was sure she was about to meet her "Waterloo," but she found they gave valuable service to patients: "'I now find myself deeply interested in the problems of all colored nurses and believe in giving them such opportunities as they can grasp for advancement'" (p. 164).

Similar accolades came from Camp Sevier, South Carolina, where Sayres L. Milliken, chief nurse, wrote that at the peak of the influenza epidemic, about half the nurses were sick. With 3,000 patients, the idea of securing the services of Black nurses still did not meet with enthusiasm: "'fully seventy-five percent of the nurses were women of southern birth and had very positive objections to working with colored nurses'" (pp. 166–167). The need was very great, however, and twelve reported for duty in subordinate positions: "'these young women were found to be well-trained, quiet and dignified, and there was never at any time evidence of friction between the white and colored nurses'" (p. 167).

Thoms states that "no report can be made of the whole number of colored nurses who served in the Army Corps during the World War, as their records were not kept separate" (p. 167). However, Major Julia Stimson, acting superintendent of the Army Nurse Corp and acting dean of the Army School of Nursing, mentions in a 1928 letter several Black nurses who rendered valuable service.

NURSES' FIGHT FOR MILITARY RANK

Both Black and White women faced the problem of powerlessness as reflected in their lack of rank. Annabelle Petersen (1942) wrote on nurses' fight for military rank during the First World War and men's opposition to it. "'Rank for nurses! A bill to give authority to women nurses to give orders to men! Never! I will never vote for any measure that gives *any* woman the right to give any order to any man'" (p. 98). Thus spoke Samuel J. Nicholls, congressional representative from South Carolina, about a bill giving rank to members of the Army Nurse Corps. The deadly earnest fight in 1918 and 1919 culminated in success in 1920.

Without rank, the women complained, the men refused to obey them, saying, "'Oh, you don't amount to anything, you are no better than we are'" (p. 98). Orderlies would stop scrubbing a ward floor to obey a contrary command of an officer to wash windows. Orderlies went on strike when a night nurse called them to duty instead of letting them sleep. Because they were often assigned to hospitals as punishment, the orderlies' morale was bad, according to Petersen, and their training negligible. By 1918 the National Committee to Secure Rank for Nurses, with Helen Hoy Greeley as counsel, pressured for legislation and the Lewis–Raker bill was introduced. It stalled in committee, however, because "it lacked the indorsement of the War Department and . . . there was no demand from constituents" (p. 98). But the thousands of Red Cross nurses who had served at home or overseas, led by Jane Delano, exerted political pressure. Julia Stimson, representing army nurses, and Ella Phillips Crandall, representing public health nurses and chairperson of the Committee on Nursing, Council of National Defense, also provided their influential support.

Throughout World War I, the lack of nurses' status was disadvantageous, as can be seen in a 1919 letter by Mary Christy (1987), requested by Attorney Helen Hoy Greeley of the National Committee to Secure Military Rank for Nurses. Christy, a nurse from Dayton, Ohio, served in France from June 1917 to February 1919. In a trip from Neufchateau across France to the coast, their train car provided scarcely enough seating room for the officers and nurses; it had no heat, light, or lavatory. The commanding officer ordered the nurses to another train at Is-Sur-Tille, to which they had to walk, carrying their luggage half a mile. They were met by an ambulance large enough to transport only five of the nine nurses. Upon reaching the new train, they stumbled across tracks in the dark with mud up to their shoe tops, only to find the train locked and unlighted.

Deciding to return to their commanding officer and original train, they found their four companions waiting for them, unsheltered in the severe cold. When they finally returned to the unit train, they were told to go to the Is-Sur-Tille station and wait. There, they learned of hotels run by the Red Cross for officers, but with no places for nurses. There was a canteen a mile away, where, after standing in a truck, bouncing over bumps and mud, they arrived to line up with 100 enlisted men. Next, they visited Camp Hospital 41, where the chief nurse gave them supper and offered five night nurses' beds to them, the only vacant ones available. Returning to the Red Cross canteen, a phone message informed them there was no room on the new train; they would have to wait another 24 hours. Furthermore, the Red Cross hotel accommodations were not available to them because of rules prohibiting taking in nurses. They returned to Camp Hospital 41, slept two to a bed, and rose early so the tired night nurses returning from duty could sleep.

By now, some of the nurses were sick, so they went to the American dispensary for medicine where the medical officer said it was a shame the way nurses were treated: " 'many a night he had sheltered nurses, enroute to the front, who had to change trains with no place to wait, and as many as twenty to thirty had slept on the floor of the dispensary in one night' " (p. 7). Returning to the station, they found the train still unavailable. The Red Cross flatly refused to even let them sit in the hotel sitting room for the night. There was no place in the station to sit, but they received permission to stay in two passenger cars sitting on the tracks. While trying to sleep, however, a French railroad yard man persistently opened the doors to let them know they did not belong there. At six in the morning, a porter finally kicked them out, leaving them no time to even lace their shoes. Still no train for them, and this time their lieutenant told the Red Cross hotel that he was bringing the nurses to breakfast. Christy stated: " 'It surely made one's blood boil when we saw the comfortable quarters and ample room available for our officers and not for us' " (p. 8).

Finally, the train arrived, but contrary to what they had been led to expect, the nurses had to ride in dingy second-class cars with hard wooden seats and no heat, while the male officers rode in first class with a diner attached. In order to eat, the women had to wait for the train to stop, then get out and walk to the diner, and then back along the tracks to their own car. On arriving in LaBaule, their embarkation station, they walked a mile in driving rain to an unheated hotel, where they waited three weeks for transportation to New York. Such was the gratitude of men to women for their care of the wounded, sick, and dying in the First World War!

During the fight to obtain military rank for nurses, the surgeon general, himself a major general, made it clear that he would grant no higher grade than "major to the superintendent of the corps, captain to the director, assistant director and two or three assistants, and first lieutenant to head nurses, but . . . could not see the necessity for commissioning the great number of working nurses" (Petersen, 1942, p. 98). He stated they were to have authority next to the medical officers and were to be obeyed and respected, but " 'That is enough' " (p. 99). The women did not agree. They renewed their fight, and the Lewis-Jones-Raker bill was reintroduced in 1919. The secretary of war went on record as opposing the bill, which would bestow rank on army nurses, placing a considerable number of them above a large array of army officers, including medical officers; thus, the bill would serve no useful purpose. Certainly not from the male point of view! Kalisch (1976) notes that the argument for granting rank to nurses was that the efficiency of nursing service would be increased. "Rank for nurses would allow them to maintain authority against well-meaning but harmful amateurs" (p. 167).

At the 1919 hearings before the Senate subcommittee on military affairs, one senator spoke in favor of the bill because of complaints that commissioned personnel persistently treated nurses as enlisted men, who in turn refused to obey the nurses' orders. A newly appointed surgeon general declared himself the original advocate of the nurse corps. Sara E. Parsons, superintendent of the Massachusetts General Hospital School of Nursing and formerly a chief nurse at an army hospital in France, told of indignities toward nurses in matters of transportation, leave, and pay. British nurses had rank, she pointed out, Canadian and Australian nurses relative rank. An expert nurse anesthetist who served at the front finally complained after three months of no pay and was told by the quartermaster that he could pay only officers and enlisted men. Petersen notes that many women's organizations joined the battle: the Equal Suffrage Leagues, the Federation of Women's Clubs, as well as the American Nurses Association. Lawyer Greeley states final victory was claimed because every nurse to a woman sent "such thousands of telegrams to their congressmen that they were convinced of the bill's popularity, in spite of its enemies" (Petersen, 1942, pp. 99–100).

However, the enemies continued their assault. Brigadier General Lyster, assistant to the surgeon general, claimed that rank would "wean" nurses from patients. If regular army officers were trained to order other people about, nurses, if given rank, would not do nursing work but order others to do it. Evidently, rank for medical officers did not wean them from patients. Presumably, they had nurses to order about! Army officers feared the nurses " 'would go beyond bounds and become licentious' " (p. 100).

The sexist basis of the opposition to nurses receiving rank is clear in one congressman's statement: " 'The fact that a nurse is a woman is the best and strongest card she can play' " (p. 100). He claimed that a sensible woman, because she is a woman, has a great deal more power than any rank or artificial authority can possibly give her. The more sensible and womanly, the more power. This, of course, depends on the woman: " 'If she is the right sort, the men will obey her and fairly worship her' " (p. 100). Of course, if she is not, she does not need rank because " 'all the rank in the world won't supply what she lacks' " (p. 100).

In World War I women nurses were used in greater numbers than ever before. Adelaide Nutting, involved with the American army nurses, was confronted with growing evidence that women were severely handicapped in their work by the lack of military rank. Most women nurses were functioning below the grade of private. In writing to Dr. Franklin Martin of the United States Council of National Defense, Nutting sustained a spirited communication in support of female commissions. Nutting's attitude toward the army medical department became more critical as time passed. To her, the Army Nurse Corps was comprised of a group of educated and skilled professional women with well-recognized duties and responsibilities; however, they had little power to insure control of resources, agencies, and persons needed to facilitate the conduct of their work.

In the prolonged fight to grant rank to nurses in the military, Nutting was joined by Annie Goodrich, who was dean of the Army School of Nursing. Julia Stimson, who earlier opposed the Equal Rights Amendment, became the new superintendent of the Army Nurse Corps, and in her role opposed rank for nurses, rejecting the position promulgated by Nutting and Goodrich. Despite Stimson's opposition and a last-ditch effort to take away rank from staff nurses by an opponent, who under cover was "ready to save the Army," rank for nurses was finally achieved through the Army Reorganization Act of 1920 and signed into law by President Woodrow Wilson. The physicians' recommendation that nurses' ranks be inferior to their own remained, even though they lost on assigning rank to staff nurses who were appointed second lieutenants. Further, all nurses were subject to medical officers' authority since the nurses had relative standing only; they were merely appointed, and not commissioned. Thus, they had unequal employment benefits, a problem that continued to plague women.

Petersen noted that the honor of being commissioned as colonels, for the duration of World War II *only*, was conferred on the two women directing the Army Nurse Corps. Interestingly, there is no evidence in Petersen's article that she opposed relative rank. It would not be until 1947 that nurses would actually be commissioned officers. A short note on the "Etiquette of Salutes for Nurses in the Service," appended to Petersen's article, states that only since World War II have nurses, now in uniform, been saluted by any officer junior to them in rank.

THE WHITE PEACE BANNER: WORLD WAR I

Not all nurses were willing to support men in war. For many women, war was anathema, but although they detested war, they were caught up in it. Again, we see the multiple perceptions and major incongruities that nurses as women faced in such paradoxical situations. What was a nurse to do? Offer her services to the military and risk perpetuating war, or remain uninvolved while injured men were untended, sick, and dying? Many nurses struggled with these confusing and conflicting values and roles.

Robert L. Duffus (1938) described Lillian Wald and the Peace Parade of 1914 in which women of all ethnic groups moved "softly and silently down the echoing streets" (p. 146). Wald, like Jane Addams at Hull House in Chicago, realized that "war was the negation of all that she, and the army of nurses and humanitarians to which she belonged, had ever done" (p. 146). Wald saw that "women more than men can strip war of its glamour, and its out-of-date heroisms and patriotisms, and see it a demon of destruction and hideous wrong—murder devastating home and happiness" (p. 147). She believed that sending nurses to the field of battle was a way of perpetuating war and its atrocities.

Similarly, while Lavinia Dock continued her work in the cause of suffrage and as a member of the National's Women Party, she saw these activities as part of the cause of equality and peace. In 1916 she supported Wald, stating, "War is an integral part of the competitive system" (Dock, 1916, p. 58). Dock warned that the European war was a product of cut-throat industrial and commercial conflict. Taking a strong socialist and feminist position, she asserted: "We believe that cooperation is the law of life and growth; competition, of destruction and death" (p. 58). Dock believed that war is preventable through justice and regard for others, not through jealousy and hatred. She called for the saving power of the International Idea: "the world our one common country, international association and organization for world law the only hope for our future" (p. 59). Dock clearly enunciated women's values: cooperation, peace, unification, and unity. In contrast, men espoused the values of competition, war, and disunity as essential for individual enhancement. War uncompromisingly forces recognition of the different values of male and female cultures. However, all men and all women do not partake equally of these cultural values. Some men were and are pacifists; some women were and are war mongers.

The future, however, belonged to the military men. Following the war, Dock called for love, decrying Christians whose "holy duty" was to hate Germans. What, she asked, could be done for "our German sisters," nurses who were in serious distress with a so-called peace that was nothing but continued financial war, reducing even the middle class to poverty? Though German nurses had "not asked us for help, nor uttered a complaint," Dock recommended that gifts be sent to the German Nurses' Association (Dock, 1922, p. 209). Placing war on the shoulders of men, Dock said, "Whoever was to blame for the war, the nurses certainly were not" (p. 209).

The following year, Dock (1923) reported that Sister Agnes Karll wrote with "touching appreciation," telling of using every dollar to relieve the destitution of older, unemployed nurses. With the cost of living doubled, American nurses needed to support the nurses in a country that had "thrown off its imperialistic militarism; which has enfranchised women and given them seats in Parliament" (Dock, 1923, p. 493). That Dock's position was correct is sadly apparent; the economic turmoil following World War I set the conditions for the subsequent emergence of Hitler and Nazism in a Germany racked by dissension.

Although not as radically involved in antiwar activities as Dock was, Lillian Wald did make her pacifist position clear. Beatrice Siegel (1983) notes that while on vacation, Wald received a telegram asking her to lead a peace parade in New York City. In accepting the invitation, Wald found herself affiliated with women activists who opposed the war and expressed solidarity with European women. One month after the outbreak of World War I, "Fifteen hundred women silently marched down Fifth Avenue to the beat of muffled drums . . . [following] a young woman carrying the only flag, a white peace banner of a dove and olive branch" (pp. 115–116). Siegel states that 20,000 spectators lined the streets while thousands more looked on silently from crowded office buildings. The interconnections between nurses and other women from social work, labor, and reform movements is clear. Following Wald were "Mary E. Dreier, Rose Schneiderman, and Leonora O'Reilly of the Women's Trade Union League; author and leading feminist Charlotte Perkins Gilman; suffragists Anna Howard Shaw and Carrie Chapman Catt" (p. 116). They were followed by hundreds of women marching together, including some from the warring nations—Germany, England, Austria, and France.

According to Siegel, women were the first to warn that a war in Europe could drag the United States into battle. To them, war was an obsolete way to settle grievances. Enculturated as healers and nurturers, they understood pacifist women and called for international solidarity against sending husbands and sons to slaughter. By 1916 Wald was head of the American Union Against Militarism coalition, with Crystal Eastman as its executive secretary. Fighting for peace took away time and effort from gaining power for women, but, if won, could show the power of women's values. Requests for nurses from Europe met with a response from Wald similar to Dock's: " 'I think we must acknowledge that when we send relief, surgeons and nurses . . . to the fields of battle, we are to some extent perpetuating, and, in a way, glorifying war and its barbarisms' " (p. 120). Quite correctly, Wald saw that peace and social reform were cojoined; war would bring an end to the progressive and the feminist era.

In 1915, inspired by two European peace activists and suffragists, Englishwoman Emmeline Pethick-Lawrence and Hungarian Rosika Schwimmer, thousands of women met in Washington, DC to form the Woman's Peace Party. Carrie Chapman Catt, head of the National Women's Suffrage Association, chaired the first meeting and Jane Addams was elected the national chairwoman. The strong feminist influence is obvious in the preamble, which "urged women to recognize their united power . . . [as] 'custodians of the life of the ages . . . charged with the future of childhood' " (p. 121).

Dock (1915) reported to nurses that a Woman's Peace Party had been formed to protest all wars. Her article included a portion of their proclamation; Dock stated that women's patient drudgery had built the foundation of home and peaceful industry, which, after centuries of toil, could be destroyed in a matter of hours. Women would no longer endure without protest the reckless destruction of war, and men must hear and heed. Nor would women without determined opposition suffer the denial of reason and justice that war promotes. As human beings and the mothers of half of humanity, the women demanded the right to be consulted in settling questions not only about individuals, but nations as well, and demanded that women be given a share in deciding between war and peace.

Dock believed there should be a World Health Department that would ban war as the most prolific cause of diseases and pestilences. Already, as a result of the European War, ailments such as gas gangrene had reappeared that had been previously almost nonexistent. Typhus fever raged, always the "unerring sign of the presence of the most complete human misery. Prolonged and widespread starvation, exposure and wretchedness . . . [were] the soil on which typhus spreads" (Dock, 1915, p. 666). Dock demanded that war reports refrain from passive wording such as "typhus is prevalent," to the active assertion of causes: "Man's actions have produced gas-gangrene and typhus" (p. 666).

The women demanded a share in deciding between war and peace in home, school, church, industry, and state. No longer giving consent to the reckless destruction of life, gone was any facade of women tagging along behind men. In opposition to their own men, the women crossed the war lines between nations. Siegel notes that suffrage leader and pioneer physician Aletta Jacobs asked Jane Addams to preside over a peace conference at the Hague in the Netherlands. Wald could not go, but the Henry Street unofficial representative, Mabel Hyde Kittredge, did attend. After her colleagues sailed, Wald faced hostile reactions to the women contingent, characterized as silly, base, and physical cowards in Theodore Roosevelt's words. European men attacked and ridiculed the 2,000 women at the conference, but the women from war-torn countries met with their "enemies," an "act of heroism," according to Jane Addams. Her own courage was obvious when she led a group of women to belligerent countries to talk peace with the leaders. Siegel observes that this action was called "treasonable" by the press after 200 Americans were killed in the German sinking of the *Lusitania*.

The work of antiwar women was counteracted by prowar society women, who were "giving up" bridge to create the Special Relief Society in 1915. According to Siegel, the split between women prompted Lavinia Dock to state: "If war was something which fell upon the human race from the skies like hail, I could understand these ladies and think they were very prudent and wise. But as war comes about solely by and through the actions of human individuals and therefore can be avoided by them, I confess I do not understand their point of view" (Siegel, 1983, p. 125). War propaganda and preparedness increased with fifty banking and business houses agreeing to pay $2 million for the salaries of camp workers. Men's power became more evident as munitions exports rose and unemployment declined. Wald headed a delegation to President Woodrow Wilson to protest entering a war in which

2,500,000 men had been killed already, families destroyed, millions made homeless, and countries laid waste in only two and a half years. Meanwhile, suffrage efforts declined and Dock denounced Wilson, who refused to back a federal suffrage amendment.

By 1917 war seemed inevitable for the United States. Militarism dominated, says Siegel, and finally Carrie Chapman Catt offered the services of suffragists if the nation went to war. Pacifists were "traitors," who were isolated and abused in the name of patriotism. The feminist and progressive alliances were shattered, but "standing grimly opposed to the country's pitiless sweep toward war" (p. 133) were Wald, Dock, and other nurses, along with Addams and feminists such as Eastman. When the United States entered the war in 1917, Wald wrote to Yssabella Waters: " 'I have felt consecrated to the saving of human life, to promotion of happiness and the expansion of good will among people, and every expression of hatred and of the dissolution of friendly relations between people fairly paralyzes me' " (p. 135).

A ruthless brutality entered the fabric of national life, as Wilson had predicted, and militant men enacted the espionage and sedition acts, making it a crime to criticize the government and the war effort. Intelligence agencies caught not one German spy, "but many innocent people were defamed" (p. 135). Wald protested, but as Siegel notes, the Henry Street nurses eventually took part in war parades, though only as "conservers of life," carrying no flags. Wald helped the Red Cross formulate policy, but remained " 'depressed and overwhelmed with the debasement of civil liberties' " (p. 138). She opposed the drafting of nurses and urged them to remain district nurses to help her campaign to save babies. She defended men who were conscientious objectors, even visiting one man in jail. Finally, she had to resign her leadership in the American Union Against Militarism in order to save the nursing and social programs she had helped create.

The war caused many changes at Henry Street, scattering some of the original organizers such as Dock, who continued her work with Alice Paul, engaging in the militant actions of the National Woman's Party, picketing the White House while Wald met inside with Wilson. Men, "patriotic" soldiers and sailors, ripped protest banners from the women, and mass arrests of the picketers began with Dock, who, at 60 years of age, was jailed in a Virginia workhouse. When the women went on a hunger strike, the forced feedings and filthy prison conditions worried Wald. She received a report that the Virginia workhouse was a medieval institution, but that Dock was " 'taking the regimen like a veteran' " (p. 143). Publicity of the cruel treatment suffered by the women brought wider support.

In a show of public approval, the nurses at Henry Street gave a reception for Jeanette Rankin, the only woman in Congress to vote against the war. Siegel notes that in 1917 Wald addressed a dinner given by the New York State Woman Suffrage Party, the antiwar, anti-Wilson wing of the suffrage movement to which Dock belonged. Funds were withdrawn from the

Settlement house as punishment for Wald's antiwar sentiment. The staff of 170 skilled nurses had to be maintained, particularly as the tragic 1918 influenza epidemic brought demands for 40,000 nurses. In the end, the epidemic wiped out 20 million civilians and combatants. Additionally, the "Red Scare" continued after the war, finally bringing dissent and reform activities into ill-repute. The Depression followed, and, as Siegel notes, the role of women in war and of women themselves lost the strong feminist orientation of previous years.

"WHO CAN WEIGH THEIR HUMAN VALUE?"
NURSING IN WORLD WAR II

The stupidity and uselessness of World War I, nevertheless, laid the foundation for an even larger conflagration in the 1940s. Women were needed again in still another worldwide conflict, World War II. In contrast to many women who opposed war, others, such as Grace Lally (1897–1983), nicknamed "Tugboat Annie," enrolled in the Army Nurse Corps from 1918 to 1919. She had originally wanted to be a pianist, not a nurse or even a military nurse; however, her mother refused to allow her to use her scholarship to a music school. Through a chance encounter, Lally turned to nursing and shifted to the Navy Nurse Corps in 1921, where she remained until she retired as a lieutenant commander in 1946; thus, she was a woman who was a nurse in *both* World Wars. She was one of four women who wore the China ribbon for service in 1938 during the Japanese invasion of China, and held several additional honors. Her career was covered by several writers: Cooper (1946), Newcomb (1945), and Blassingame (1967).

In 1991, on the 50th anniversary of the Japanese attack on Pearl Harbor, Lally was again credited with being a "hero" by nurses Joellen Hawkins and Irene Matthews (1991). As chief nurse of the hospital ship USS *Solace*, Lally was dressing to go to church on December 7, 1941, when she heard what she first thought were American drills, but realized was an enemy attack when she saw a dive bomber hit the battleship *Arizona*, causing it to explode and sink in burning oil. The survival of the *Solace* increased the sense of unreality, but Lally and her 12 nurses immediately set up emergency wards as bombs fell all around their ship. The male mess attendants huddled together in the galley, but Lally mobilized them and by evening more than 300 casualties had been cared for.

According to Hawkins and Matthews, Lally, on the *only* ship of the 96 in the harbor equipped to provide emergency medical and surgical care, was determined that the wounded men should feel that life would go on. Therefore, the nurses smiled and joked and even raised a Christmas tree on the mast and provided gifts from the Red Cross. Subsequently, Lally and her nurses made trips to the fighting front to transfer patients to New Zealand, "caring for 7,500 casualties during the first 20 months of the war, losing only 16" (p. 185). But Lally said " 'I never get used to the first look at those stretchers. But if they [the men] can smile I guess we can and, look, they are smiling' " (p. 185). Despite her outstanding career, "few nurses know that one of our own was a key figure in the events of that day" (p. 185).

Indeed, the loss of nurses' history in wars was an issue that the Kalisches (1976) try to redress when they describe the history and founding of the Cadet Nurse Corps in 1941, during the first year of World War II. The United States was already faced with an appalling shortage of nurses and even more were needed as the war continued. At the same time that nurses were being drawn into the military, civilian hospitals were forced to close whole wards or units because of the lack of nurses. "The severe shortage of nurses caused by World War II prompted the first massive federal aid to nursing education. The program that resulted sparked improvements in nursing education" (p. 240). The nurse responsible for the program that recruited 125,000 women in two years was Lucile Petry (later Lucile Petry Leone). The Cadet Nurse Program was to prepare women to go immediately into the military and then to the war zones, where nurses were credited with saving the lives of thousands of soldiers.

In 1987 Leone published a retrospective review of her work as director of the U.S. Cadet Nurse Corps, nursing's answer to the demands of World War II. Administered through the U.S. Public Health Service, its purpose as a nonmilitary program was to increase the number of women nurses to meet both civilian and military needs, but it was supported by the War Department (now the Department of Defense—an interesting exercise in semantics). In 1940 the American Nurses Association sponsored a meeting from which emerged the Nursing Council on National Defense, later for War Service. Six national nursing organizations, the Red Cross, and federal nursing agencies collaborated to recruit more students, induce inactive women back to service, train voluntary nurses' aides, and improve the training of graduate nurses. Congresswoman Frances Payne Bolton's bill created the corps in 1943; funded with $65 million, it provided, for the first time, full scholarships for women in nursing.

Leone stresses the fact that students still provided free labor for two-thirds of the nursing services in hospitals through schools of nursing. Increasing the number of students would release registered nurses for military service. In a very short time, almost every one of the 1,300 schools of nursing was reached in a major barnstorming effort. Leone notes that nurse consultants advised reducing some clinical practice experiences, while adding others, often in psychiatry. Senior cadets often had to take their clinical training in hospitals without established schools of nursing; thus, nursing instructors had to be added to the staff. Expert nurses met in curriculum conferences, realizing that training for teaching and supervision was necessary to replace the supervisors, teachers, and public health nurses, who volunteered for service in high numbers.

As Leone states, the women from all, not just the "best" schools, were in ferment as they moved out of provincialism and into the mainstream of health and education. For the first time, the women used the War Advertising Council, which was easily persuaded that nursing was vital to the war effort. The council reached every city and small town through newspapers, magazines, posters, and billboards. The cost of the program, $160 million, established the precedent of federal aid for nursing education and research. Leone, the director of this massive effort, referring to the 150,000 women who contributed, asks, "Who can weigh their human value?" (p. 48).

What was the relationship between the Army Nurse Corps and other women in the military during World War II? As noted earlier, nurses have at times led the way for other women, but says Donald Leopard (1984), they often fail to reap the benefits of their leadership. To Leopard, the nurses led the way in the First World War, but with the Second World War, the initial rewards went to the Women's Army Auxiliary Corps (WAACs).

Edith Nourse Rogers, a Red Cross nurse during World War I and congresswoman during World War II, testified that nurses had received no compensation of any kind if they were sick or injured. Furthermore, " 'these women who gave of their service, unselfishly, patriotically, and under conditions comparable to men, should have received pay privileges for that service' " (Leopard, 1984, p. 4). The bitterness of these loyal and patriotic women, some even heart-breaking cases, was a primary issue in her proposal to establish the WAACs in 1942. Although Congress approved the legislation, Major (later Colonel) Julia Flikke, director of the Army Nurse Corps, opposed Rogers' proposal, stating that the disadvantages outweighed the advantages and that complications would arise between the organizations. And, notes Leopard, complications did arise.

Amazingly, the nurses had a more tenuous relationship with the army than did the WAACs. But far more important, many nurses enlisted in the WAACs and those over age forty, according to the Army Nurse Corps standards, were assigned as orderlies, taking orders from younger, less experienced women. Others were dismayed when they could not transfer to the U.S. Cadet Nurse Corps for civilian training. Nurses resented the more rapid promotions and greater publicity given the WAACs. Leopard concludes that the nurses' complaints were justified; the WAACs did get more media coverage, attracted strong support from political and military men in power, and were accepted so quickly that the word "auxiliary" was dropped from their title. Thus, women officers and noncommissioned officers received full military status and privileges, which, ironically, the nurses in the Army Nurse Corps did not receive until the next year. After a century or more of service, the nurses, who paved the way for other women, fell behind them, probably in large part as a result of their subordination to physicians.

Nevertheless, as Bonnie Bullough (1976) points out, World War II had a lasting impact on nursing. Health "manpower" assumed an importance to successful warfare approaching that of arms and bearers of arms. "From the beginning," states Bullough, "organized nursing supported the war effort. Not that nurses favored the war before it started, but documents suggest that they believed it was inevitable so they might as well prepare" (p. 118). It was at this time that an accurate national census of registered nurses in the United States was initiated. By the time the war ended in 1945, 100,000 nurses had volunteered and 76,000 had actually served in the Army or Navy Nurse Corps. The long-range effects of nursing's involvement in World War II included full commission for female nurses, cessation of segregation of Black nurses, and the admission of male nurses as officers.

The struggle for rank had more than symbolic significance. From Bullough's perspective it was a critical struggle for nurses to gain the professional power that was needed to plan and deliver good nursing care. "What they won when regular rank was finally achieved was the right to manage nursing care, including both the care they themselves delivered and nursing functions carried out by the enlisted corpsmen. In gaining this managerial power, military nurses set the direction for all members of the nursing profession to move toward more autonomy and more responsible managerial positions" (p. 120). The determination with which nurses struggled to achieve equity with men during this conservative period is commendable, especially since they had little support from the women's groups, since the feminist organizations had collapsed or been transformed to deal with social issues. Strong feminist groups would not be formed again until the late 1960s.

The war changed nursing from a single- to a multilevel system. Another result was to bring large members of female students into nursing schools, preparing them for nursing after graduation, to be sure, but also using their services while they were in training. To Bullough, this trend continued the earlier use of free female labor in hospital schools, since students became a major source of nursing "manpower." However, as federal funds became available to nursing schools for the preparation of nurses, educators achieved stronger bargaining positions within both hospital and university schools of nursing.

NURSES HAVE NO ENEMIES:
NURSE ACTIVISTS AND THE COLD WAR

During the Crimean War, the Civil War, the Spanish-American War, and World Wars I and II, nurses were often seen by the public as heroines, angels of mercy, lifesavers. Their public images were exalted, although treatment of them was often sexist and shabby. Many nurses also saw themselves as patriots, providing a service to their country that was important and valued.

Following the Second World War, few voices could be heard against war. But what of those women who continued to affirm peace values and reject war? At the beginning of the Cold War, Lavinia Dock again spoke out for international unity among women. Lois A. Monteiro (1978) published several of Dock's letters that detailed an episode from the International Council of Nurses' meetings in Atlantic City in 1947. Held just a few years after the end of World War II, the ICN conference was the first postwar international meeting of nurses from throughout the world. As Monteiro notes, the Truman Doctrine (1947) established a foreign policy of worldwide containment of communism. Russian nurses were "conspicuously absent from the meeting" (p. 47), but this was not reported in newspapers, nor even in the *American Journal of Nursing*.

In 1947 Dock was 89 years old. She had been a moving force in establishing international nursing; consequently, she had earlier worked with women who supported the new Russian state. Thus, says Monteiro, "when the United States government, in keeping with the Truman foreign policy, was against the invitation of Russian nurses to the Atlantic City meetings, Miss Dock was quickly brought to action" (p. 48). She wrote to the secretary of state, receiving an unsatisfactory response. She wrote again and, receiving no satisfaction, she then sent a letter to the Soviet ambassador.

In her letter to Secretary (formerly General) George Marshall, she minced no words, since "'our public men are not mincing their words'" (p. 48). Writing as a good American citizen, a taxpayer, and "'an old trained nurse of over fifty years service'" Dock stated that she had a genuine appeal and a "'*bitter* and justifiable grievance against the so-called Truman Doctrine and . . . the State Department acquiescence in it'" (p. 49). She enclosed a report of the ICN meetings and flatly stated: "We should have had the *Russian Nurses* at our meeting in Atlantic City. . . . It was an important event. There were several hundred nurses from Europe, Asia and Africa as well as at home and in the Pacific. There were altogether about 5000 nurses in attendance and we had, as you see, distinguished medical speakers" (p. 49). Again, she repeated forcefully, underlining all words: "'*The Russian Nurses should have been here*'" (p. 49).

Dock then stated that American nurses had previously met with Dr. Lebedenko, who had promised to have Russian members join the ICN. Subsequently, the ICN secretary wrote to the Russian embassy and to Moscow directly, with no result. Dock said to Marshall, "'*This is your fault*'" (p. 49). The daily insults, malice, ingratitude, and cold-blooded threats in American newspapers, radio, and numerous books were too much for the Soviets to overlook.

Writing in true feminist form, Dock stated: "'We nurses have no enemies. We do not recognize national jealousies. We care nothing for men's quarrels. We consider it an undeserved grievance that our Russian sisters have been alienated by our American Government's attitude'" (p. 50). She asked

Marshall to reply to her as a founding member of ICN, and said curtly, " 'I can only sign my name' " (p. 50). On receiving a bulletin containing the opinions of Congress, Dock sarcastically wrote her thanks for the Bulletin of the State Department, which " 'courteous gesture . . . does not in any way amend or alter the cleavage in the International Council of Nurses' " (p. 50). What, she asked Marshall, can be done in " 'our Sisterhood of trained nurses?' " (p. 50). From the world's perspective, the Russians were ignored: "No delegates were here, no report could be made, as to why there was no response from their country; no mention even was made of their absence, for this would have necessitated giving a reason . . . [which] would have necessitated laying the blame flatly on our own country" (p. 50).

Given the heightened fear of communism at the time, Dock claimed (her judgment later to be borne out in the McCarthy hearings) that the ICN women, being more ethical than the government, were unwilling to refer to the political hysteria, but, she stated, " 'I personally, as one of the oldest founders, *am not* so ethical' " (p. 51). She then asked Marshall to write a statement of the nurses' grievance to the Russian ambassador and offer regret at the impasse, noting that nurses worldwide had been called to work with the World Health Organization: " 'And the Russian Nurses, who served through the War, who suffered everything—devastation, ruin, even imprisonment—starvation, torture and outrage, are to be left out, as if Russia had been an enemy instead of our strongest ally' " (p. 51).

Dock threatened to write an apology to the Russian ambassador, which she did! Introducing herself as belonging to no political party, Dock surmised that her name was on the black list of the Thomas–Rankin committee. As one of the early founders of organization among nurses, she had helped form the International Council of Nurses, which now had over thirty countries represented in its membership. Dock recounted the unsuccessful efforts made to include Russian women in the ICN, sadly noting the nurses met without the women from the Soviet Union: " 'This was a grievous thing to us elders, perhaps more so than to the younger generation who have less awareness of history in the making' " (p. 52). She blamed America's political leaders for the volley of abuse, slander, threats, and warnings, for which she apologized. She then informed the Soviet ambassador of her letter to Marshall, quoting herself on nurses knowing no boundary lines and having no enemies and no part in men's quarrels. She told the ambassador that she had asked Marshall to send an apology. Since he did not do this, she was sending her own. As an old nurse, she declared she had " 'a right to complain of the slight to nurses, all of whom, and Russians conspicuously, have given service in men's horrible wars' " (p. 53).

Monteiro is to be thanked for bringing these letters to light. As she states, they show Dock's refusal to be silent, even in the face of considerable personal risk. Monteiro concludes that these letters show Dock not simply as an "early nursing leader," but as a person whose courage is timely for "current professional and women's rights advocacy" (p. 54).

THE INVISIBLE VETERANS: NURSES AND MODERN WARFARE

Public images and beliefs about the heroism and courage of men and women in battle were sustained throughout the Korean War but underwent a significant change during the Vietnam War. The horrors of the battlefield and the consequences of modern warfare were brought as never before to the public's awareness. The unpopularity of America's involvement in the Vietnam War, coupled with the appalling physical casualties, created severe and long-lasting psychological problems for the men and women who participated in that conflict; many of these problems are still unresolved. As Pete Earley stated in 1982, nurses were still haunted by memories of service in Vietnam. Although 6,250 nurses served in Vietnam, much was written about the problems of the 2.8 million male Vietnam veterans; but at the time Earley wrote, no study of the female veterans had been conducted: "Even the eight-year Veterans Administration-sponsored study of the war's multiple impacts on 1,340 veterans released failed to include a single woman" (p. 8). One army psychologist, who served in Vietnam, said that the women were forgotten, and " 'We are only now beginning to see the war through their eyes' " (p. 8). Most researchers assumed that since women and men lived through the war, their reactions to it had been the same. But woman's role was unique in Vietnam and still is an inadequately explored issue to this day. The nurses, predominantly women, again saw the worst of the war, "an endless procession of mangled bodies across the operating table" (p. 8). This was one war where the image of the nurse was not publicized. No one saw her as a heroine and she did not necessarily see herself as a patriot. Furthermore, the breakdown of the mythology of protection of women by men was evident. Women nurses were uncompromisingly placed in dangerous situations in Vietnam, exposed to unfamiliar infectious diseases, enemy attack, and chemical warfare. The contradictions between men in war and women in a profession devoted to sustaining life were most glaring in the Vietnamese conflict.

Sara J. McVicker (1985) calls the women who served in Vietnam the "Invisible Veterans." By 1985 only one study of women in military health care in Vietnam existed, despite numerous articles, books, and studies on post-traumatic stress disorders in male veterans. From interviews with women veterans, McVicker found loneliness was a major difficulty: some women described "being virtually confined to quarters . . . with guards outside to 'protect' them from male servicemen" (p. 14). Sometimes essential equipment, medicine, and blood samples were not available.

War injuries were severe, with amputations 300% higher than those in World War II and 70% higher than in Korea; paraplegia was 1,000% higher than in World War II and 50% higher than in Korea. The use of helicopters for fast transport from the battlefield brought in men who would have died in previous wars. Nurses sometimes had to decide "who would receive immediate care, who could wait, and who had to be set aside to die" (p. 14). Furthermore, Vietnamese military personnel, civilians, and prisoners as patients created communication problems and forced nurses to deal with diseases such as cholera, plague, and leprosy. Women worked 12 hours a day, 6 days a week, sometimes going for days without sleep. There was no safety since any base could be attacked.

McVicker discovered that many women veterans denied their feelings, while those who sought help were belittled, forcing them to avoid Veterans Administration facilities, where sexist attitudes from male counselors or veterans negated the women's status as veterans. With little help, feelings of anger or depression were common. Romantic or sexual relations were often bittersweet. About half the women in one study reported reluctance to have children because of war atrocities or exposure to chemicals. The negative effects of war on women can be very different from the effects on men: "One nurse freezes when startled by loud noises" because she never learned to hit the floor since she was always "going for the patients" (p. 19).

As in previous wars, the invisibility of these women nurses is obvious. The theme emerges again of underrating and undervaluing women who made life-and-death decisions; trivializing the efforts of war nurses who worked incredibly long hours protecting the men rather than themselves. There was little feminist analysis of the nurse veterans; therefore, there was no way for them to understand their plight as women. They were simply excluded from the research, many of the health services, and even from the concern extended to some of their military counterparts upon return to the United States. Indeed, the late appearance of the few articles on Vietnam nurses shows the impact of feminism in uncovering their experiences. The general public probably is still largely unaware of the heroic services performed by these women, even with the recent efforts and publicity given to the monument constructed in Washington, DC which finally memorializes and honors the nurses who served and died in Vietnam.

Equally concerned with these forgotten veterans, Marilyn L. Steffel and Margaret G. Kaczmarek (1987) present a historical perspective on women in the military, noting that during the Revolutionary War, 10 nurses and one matron were authorized for every 100 sick or wounded soldiers. In the Civil War, 6,000 women served the Union and Confederate soldiers. In the Spanish-American War, nurses established themselves as essential. In World War I, more than 20,000 nurses, half stationed overseas, served; 200 died from pneumonia and influenza. In World War II, 57,000 army nurses and 11,000 navy nurses were on active duty: 217 died from enemy action and 78 were prisoners of the Japanese in the Philippines. In Korea, 500 nurses served, often in combat areas. (These statistics will vary according to time periods surveyed and adequacy of records of the different branches of the armed forces.)

As noted previously, most of these women served without rank, officer status, or equal pay or benefits, such as retirement and veterans rights. Steffel and Kaczmarek state: "Without rank, nurses did not officially exist within the military social system and hence had no power or influence . . . they received no recognition of consequence from the structural hierarchy" (p. 34). Even the top leaders were not fully acceptable: it was not until 1971 that an army nurse became a brigadier general. The superintendent of the Army Nurse Corps was, until 1984, "not a 'person' in the sense of the law under which she was promoted" (p. 35). It is clear that there is an invisible barrier, and beyond "the lace curtain," women cannot go. Even if women do more than men, they usually rise only to middle management positions and there they may stagnate.

Women nurses in the military have also been denied their usual female roles; in 1951 they were forbidden to be parents, and until 1973 women who were married were deprived of military entitlements. As late as 1974 nurses who were pregnant or had children were discharged from the military. These restrictions meant that women could not remain in rank or move up to positions of power. Males were excluded from the Army Nurse Corps until 1955 and, when admitted, it was not until 1970 that they lost their special privileges, not granted to the female nurses. Slander and sexual harassment have continued, and changes have been forced only by litigation initiated by women nurses.

Linda Spoonster Schwartz (1987) also draws attention to women and the Vietnam experience: "One of the best kept secrets of the war is that more than 263,000 women served in the military between 1964 and 1975" (p. 168). Amazingly, the records are still insufficient (as they have been for over two centuries) to determine how many women were in the Orient, or more specifically, Vietnam. Although a few articles have appeared, Schwartz notes the inadequacy of research and presents her own informal research on the military experience. She begins with the falsity of recruiting advertisements that glamorized the role of the military nurse, showing her caring for children, socializing at parties, or tending for the wounded in air flight. Actually, flight missions were exclusively reserved for men.

As many as 45% of the women serving in Vietnam had no prior service experience. The women had to maintain decorum and deal with an "extremely authoritarian system" that often extended to off-duty social activities, which, if refused, led to "transfers to more dangerous locations, denial of 'R and R' or changes in duty schedule" (p. 169). Thus, when women are placed in male authority systems, the clear message is that they must be professionally *and* socially available.

Experiences of sexual harassment, ranging from sexist remarks about lesbianism to rape, often went unreported and unpunished because of fears of reprisal. The incongruence of values was sharply drawn: the women's values of helping, healing, and serving humanity were incompatible with the male war values of death, destruction, and devastation. Unprepared for the personal danger they faced, many nurses felt that nothing could prepare them for the violence. They withdrew into health care for the Vietnamese, submerged themselves in work that glossed over the reality of war, or engaged in substance abuse or partying. Conflicting and multiple role expectations of being mother, nurse, sister, girl-next-door, and girlfriend created impossible situations for them.

A terrible rage at enemies, whom they could not confront, led to disillusionment, cynicism, and mistrust. There was no place for them to vent their anger. Whether the nurses were actually in Vietnam, the care of war casualties was very distressing because of the severity of the multiple mutilating wounds and injuries. Napalm caused massive, smoldering burns. Paraplegia and multiple amputations were, as noted previously, much more common than in previous wars.

As Lillian Wald had recognized decades ago, the most tragic fatalities of war were the women and children. The tragedies of these innocent by-standers appalled the nurses. In one instance, nurses faced 1,500 dead and wounded civilians; not one of these had seen a hospital or morgue for six days. One nurse took out shrapnel and removed sheets of skin and fingers and toes while constantly under mortar fire.

Schwartz states that a normal duty was 11 to 12 hours a day for 6 days each week. Sometimes duty required around-the-clock contact with mass casualties, the worst receiving least treatment, reversing the women's usual approach. Hospitals were often under attack, and the nurses were themselves wounded, injured, and disabled. These heroic actions were carried out by women who were not supposed to do anything without authorization from military and medical men! One of the most difficult adjustments for these nurses was to accept the imposed, restricted sphere of activity upon their return to the United States. They were not allowed to carry out the complex medical procedures that they had performed so effectively in Vietnam.

The role confusion and dissonance bewildered feminists as well. How should they deal with these military nurses? How should they deal with nurses in general? Women in uniform on return to the United States reported "being spat on, having eggs thrown at them" (p. 172), and being called "baby killers." Feminist groups, mostly antiwar, did not welcome the self-reliance and egalitarian attitude of women veterans, who were, ironically, also excluded from veterans' organizations. In civilian hospitals, they were forced to return to restricted roles, not even allowed to "hang a pint of blood." Although a majority stayed, many simply left nursing. About 80% used VA benefits to get more education, and although 22% to 53% were estimated to suffer aspects of post-traumatic stress syndrome, few received the help they needed.

Both the editors of *IMAGE* and author Linda Schwartz received considerable correspondence in response to her article. One military man recalled nurses living in tents, showering outside, and hiding between sandbags when under rocket fire: "A statue of a woman, unarmed, on foot, needs to be added to all those around the country of male generals on horseback armed to the teeth" (*IMAGE*, 1988, p. 176). Army nurse Gail Russell said the war "impacted my life in a mixture of ways that is so hard to articulate!" (p. 176). Russell had worked for the VA, but was never involved in veterans' groups: "Your article brings me out of the closet" (p. 176). A younger nurse, still in elementary school when the war was over, urged a statue of a nurse to honor and recognize the duty these women performed: "I only regret that it has taken so long for it to come about" (p. 176). Willa Adelstein, an Air National Guard Reserve nurse who accompanied casualties back to California, stated: "This experience was by far the most unrewarding, depressing hours I have ever spent in nursing . . . there was no time to think about anything but getting the jobs done. . . . I vividly remember, even now, looking at all those young faces of severely mentally and physically injured and wondering what their lives would be when we got them 'home'. Now we all know" (p. 176). Adelstein said she did not know how the regular air force nurses, fatigued and overburdened, did their job.

Colonel Doris S. Frazier praised Schwartz for the finest and most honest exposition of women's experiences in Vietnam and claimed the scars, particularly on the younger women, remained and that their experiences exacted a terrible toll. Timothy A. Jacob, an army nurse, recalled: "Half way into my tour of duty, an enemy rifle's sharp staccato cracks—one, then two, three burning rounds—suddenly piercing the fading afternoon light, and just as quickly, a life and a career was forever changed . . . years after countless surgeries, nearly two years of lonely hospitalization and painful rehabilitation, I am, as they say, 'disabled'—a damaged disfigured arm and hand, never to be the same again" (p. 177). Theresa M. Stephany said, "I am one of many who had no idea of what went on over there. . . . I am joyously (and somberly) sending a copy to every feminist I know" (p. 177).

Many women outside of nursing also know little of nurses' work in the Vietnam War, or for that matter in any of the previous ones. Since the impact on women, for better or worse, is integral to the history of women, it is vital that feminists incorporate nurses' experiences into feminist understanding. This, particularly for the Vietnamese conflict, has rarely been done. In one attempt, a complete issue of the feminist journal, *Women and Therapy* (1986), was given over to 12 responses from feminist therapists and activists, each from a different theoretical position, to "A Woman's Recovery from the Trauma of War."

The case of "Ruth" (a fictional name), a nurse who lived in her family home until she entered the navy at age 23, was presented by editors Esther D. Rothblum and Ellen Cole. In 1968 Ruth began treating severely wounded men who had been flown to New York after the Tet offensive. Many were horribly burned, with severe infections and often missing limbs. Ruth was transferred to Da Nang in 1969, where she was under constant threat of attack; the hospital received regular, often daily, mortar shelling; off-base sniper, grenade, and terrorist attacks were common. Her patients, with whole body burns, traumatic amputations, or terminal malaria, either died or were evacuated. Not only was Ruth exposed daily to maimed or dead bodies at work, but often off-duty as well: "she once witnessed the surfacing of the drowned bodies of three airmen who had crashed into the bay, while she sat having lunch with a friend at a cafe that overlooked the water" (p. 8).

Ruth's first sexual experience was in Vietnam, with a married physician in a relationship that was abusive. Her belief in religion crumbled because she could no longer believe in a caring deity. On her return to California, she complained of pain, chills, and fevers, all diagnosed by physicians as psychosomatic, leading her to spend nine months as an inpatient in a neuropsychiatric hospital. She was finally correctly diagnosed as having pulmonary tuberculosis with a lesion at the site of her pain. Her psychiatrist diagnosed her as having conversion symptoms and prescribed Valium for four years, despite his knowledge that she was drinking alcohol to deal with her pain. This continued, even after she was correctly diagnosed as tubercular. She dropped out of nursing, became a salesperson for a window cleaning company, withdrew from her family, and continued drinking, which did not over time succeed in blocking her distress. Ruth experienced "frequent visual hallucinations and nightmares of dead, maimed, and bleeding bodies, and a recurrent olfactory hallucination of the smell of pseudomonas, a common infection of burn victims" (p. 10). In addition, feeling chronically anxious, Ruth was hyperalert to sounds resembling explosions and to overhead helicopters. In a recurring nightmare, she was being sought out and hurt by the badly wounded men she had cared for. Eventually suicidal and self-mutilating, feeling numb and cut-off, then tearful, she entered therapeutic groups to deal with her alcoholism.

Feminist activists and professors Joy A. Livingston and Joanna M. Rankin (1986), both members of the Women's International League for Peace and Freedom, the current version of the earlier organization fostered by Wald, Dock, and other feminists, responded to Ruth's case. Referring to Cynthia Enloe's (1983) work on the militarization of women's lives, they believe that the armed forces may be nervous if nurses tell their stories because they "reveal so much about the nature of war itself" (p. 107). To Enloe, the military gender structure and its basic legitimacy are protected by nurses' silence. Beginning with this premise, Livingston and Rankin develop a feminist analysis of militarism, as an institution of patriarchy, which defines power as control of and dominance over others with the goal to win, not negotiate conflict. The authors contrast this model with a feminist one, which defines power as a choice from within, to express cooperation to achieve a high quality of life, "not death in the pursuit of winning" (p. 108). To these feminists, Ruth, like all women who are coerced or persuaded to collaborate, was caught in militarism that justifies patriarchal power, "a system for domestic control as much as a protection against external threats" (p. 108). In short, the military is the ultimate expression of men's control of society. The more power the military has, the greater the power of patriarchy and the less the power of women to protest it or live outside of it in alternative structures.

Livingston and Rankin recognize that military nurses are essential to war, but military ideology sees women as irrelevant; thus, Ruth's abilities were used but also marginalized and devalued. This paradox is obvious—first, in the psychiatric evaluation of her real physical disorder as an imagined one; and second, in being actively discouraged from discussing her wartime experiences with her psychiatrist, leading her to question the reality of her symptoms. Since many men deny that women have anything to do with combat, that they are in the military for romance or adventure, that they have nothing to do with the "real thing" at the front (where women in nursing actually often are), it is never admitted that Ruth or other women experience real trauma.

Actually, claim Livingston and Rankin, war is not an atypical response to particular circumstances, but an integral part of patriarchal structure. Although denied, "Women are essential to warfare. Given that at least 10 support people are required for every actual soldier, it is women who make the military possible" (p. 109). As mothers of sons, military wives, workers in military industries, military service workers, recreation workers, military nurses, even prostitutes, and as a reserve work force to replace men even as combatants, women make the military possible. This fact cannot be admitted because it challenges the "masculinity men earn by having combat experience" (p. 109). Such experiences cannot be shared with women; thus, the "conspiracy of silence" invalidating Ruth's intimate experience of death and destruction cannot be acknowledged.

Furthermore, women's presence may interfere with male bonding to produce the obedience necessary to validate killing through a chain of command. But women are always present; thus, this paradox must be denied—Ruth's experience must be invalidated. To these analysts, Ruth was coopted into thinking hierarchically in her early Roman Catholic and later naval nurse's training. Rather than threaten these structures, and thus the fundamental patriarchy, she isolated herself rather than bonding with other women who had been to the front, seen unspeakable horrors, and been used and abused. Ruth, they agree, was marginalized and coped with it alone—all alone.

What amazes Livingston is that "we treat all these forms of violence (wars, abuse, rape) as if they are abnormal . . . violence is hardly abnormal, but very normal . . . vital to maintaining patriarchal structures" (p. 111). Under these circumstances, notes Rankin, Vietnam nurses have struggled to be recognized as suffering from post-traumatic syndrome. They were not in combat but actually saw the worst of war, an unending flow of mutilated and dead bodies. If women spoke out loudly enough about the realities of warfare, as Clara Barton, Lavinia Dock, and others tried to do, they would undermine militarism, the basis of the patriarchal structure that keeps men, the dominants, believing that everything is right and good for both them and their subordinates, women. But Ruth and other nurses, more than most women, are particularly threatening because they can uncover the myth; thus, they are even more severely abused and silenced. This makes Ruth's tragedy so intense; acting competently and humanely, she is subsequently rewarded by being denied, trivialized, and marginalized.

Rankin notes that Vietnam nurse Lynda Van Devanter (1983) claimed that there has always been a fine line between a prostitute and a military nurse in men's historical accounts. Nurses have had to fight this stigma in order to bond together, to reveal the enormity of war, to be seen as professional military nurses. Further, military depersonalization must affect many nurses, who often do not see wounded men recover; they either die or are evacuated. If soldiers or nurses take things too personally, the pain is too great. Soldiers may distance themselves, but nurses, as caring women, and supposedly peripheral to war, may personalize and blame themselves for not being able to save the victims. The military forces men not to have feelings, but nurses cannot disconnect. If they did, few wounded men would survive.

How do women bond with other women? If they share feelings in any deep relationship, they can be broken up by simply labeling the nurses, not as prostitutes, but as lesbians, women who love women. Homophobia, states Rankin, isolates women: "Given the small number of women and the proscriptions against meaningful relationships, it is frightening to think how isolated were women in the Vietnam war" (p. 114). How then can nurses organize to tell the truth of war, to shatter the myth that war does not have terrible, long-lasting, negative consequences? If men do not talk of combat, then women as nurses are some of the few who can. But Ruth's psychiatrist, seemingly in collusion, actively discouraged her from talking about her war experiences. To Livingston and Rankin, a substantial number of men are not able to function in combat, some being so terrified that they are unable to fire their weapons. They wonder if the taboo against talking about combat is because it would expose the fear and other reactions that would not support the masculine image. On the other hand, it may also expose the sheer barbarism that makes military masculinity unacceptable.

In language reminiscent of Wald and Dock, Livingston and Rankin question whether in fact military nurses prop up the warrior mythology. To them, war is about killing people so it is farcical to have medical services at the front, where nurses, who patch up people, help perpetuate the idea that war is not primarily about killing. For nurses, war is the killing and destruction of their feelings, the validity of their own experiences. From this perspective, not cooperating is the affirmation of life. Caught as victim in a system of death, the nurse herself becomes suicidal, attempting to kill literally the remembrance of war as it really is. To help Ruth, these feminists recommend support groups of women who also served in Vietnam, helping her put her experiences in a political context so she can actively resist the militarism of herself, others, and society. She must be helped to learn her own power by telling her stories, avoiding "endless repetitions of this distress for future generations" (p. 118). To break silence, to identify with others in pain, rather than suffering silently in isolation—to break the "shame of the oppressed"—this, the authors believe, can change the militarism, the patriarchy, itself. More than any other women, nurses have the power to destroy the myths surrounding war.

This radical feminist analysis collides with simple civil libertarian actions; to open not only nursing but the entire military structure to women, even abolishing laws that exclude women from combat. Clearly, the conflict over women and war continues. Once women are allowed in military structures they cannot move for advancement and promotion unless all avenues are open to them. Commander Barry J. Coyle (1989) tells how women represented as much as 28% of VQ-3, part of the navy nuclear strike forces, in the early 1980s. The squadron won several awards and commendations, proving that women could potentially function well in a combat environment as part of integrated male-female teams, serving as mission commanders, aircraft commanders, instructor pilots, division officers, flight surgeons, and intelligence officers, as well as in many enlisted positions.

Sexist attitudes were the major barriers to high performance in mixed units. Many military men think women cannot fight, fly, lead, or do heavy work—that they would be "freaks" leading men into combat. Coyle states that even with daily proof of the absurdity of these attitudes, men still deny that women can perform traditionally male tasks. Women, he claims, expect men to change their behavior, but this is a "bad" approach. According to Coyle, one cannot change the "basic nature" of men or women, but one can get them to work together. He sets, however, an upper limit of 30% women! This, of course, assures that they are always in a minority.

Not pregnancy itself, but the navy's restrictive rules concerning allowable activities for pregnant women caused problems. Occupational and sports injuries, drug and alcohol abuse, and unexcused absences were rated higher than pregnancy as reasons for loss of time from work. Fraternization, a strange, male-defined word for sexual relations, occurred, but the couples were not allowed to work or fly together. Sexual harassment, Coyle thinks, is infrequent. Clearly, many military nurses would not agree.

Indeed, the perceptions and stereotypes about women nurses are still prevalent today, particularly among physicians. Debbie Tipton Winters (1985) hypothesized that nurses and physicians, both commissioned army officers, would perceive themselves as having similar occupational status. However, physicians ascribed a higher occupational rank to the physician than nurses ascribed to the nurse. Although the nurses were more likely to see the nurse's status as similar to the physician's, the latter refused to see the same degree of status similarity. Thus, even the achievement of officer's rank and status has not overcome the gendered battle between nurses, predominantly women, and physicians, predominantly men. This finding was sustained regardless of any background variables, including level of education, amount of direct contact with nurses, or pursuit of specialty training or advanced degree. As Winters states, this finding is consistent also with those of several other studies in which physicians overvalue medicine and undervalue nursing. Further, Winters concludes that this is consistent with the stereotypes of physician educational preparation and control over patients, and with the erroneous public perception that nursing requires no advanced academic training and has no input into decision making. Perhaps, Winters says, greater collegiality will change perceptions. But if Livingston and Rankin are right, nothing, including comparable rank, will substantially change these perceptions, because they are necessary to maintain the militaristic structure basic to both hospitals and the armed forces. In their view, only by changing sexist social structures will genuine equality be achieved.

If physicians refuse to credit women in the military, and if they become invisible to the public, the only recourse nurses have is to fight for recognition. Thus, the efforts of Donna Marie Boulay, nurse and lawyer, who spearheaded the Vietnam Women's Memorial Project, have received widespread attention and acclaim. Rejecting the invisibility of military women, Boulay, as reported by Marlene Jezierski (1987), toured the Smithsonian and found to her surprise information about the civilian female pilots who had ferried planes across the Atlantic Ocean during World War II. Why did she not know about these women before she was 40 years old? To her, their invisibility was similar to her own experiences when she talked in social situations about her tour of duty as a nurse in Vietnam. To set the record right, former army nurse and Vietnam veteran, Diane Carlson-Evans, and Gerald C. Bender, attorney and a veteran wounded in Vietnam, joined with Boulay in 1984 to consider how to fill in history's gaps. Initially, they considered a statue, created by veteran Roger Brodin, of a slightly gaunt young woman in fatigues, stethoscope around her neck, scissors in her pocket, helmet in her hand, and "searching eyes reaching far away" (Jezierski, 1987, p. 122). The statue would represent nurses' military history. Later, sculptor Glenna Goodacre's depiction of three women and a wounded soldier was chosen as the preferred memorial.

Boulay spent 20 hours a week on the project on top of her full-time legal work. A labor of love, she remembered that when she volunteered as a nurse for Vietnam, she had no idea whether nurses were there or what their roles were. Her Vietnam experience still looms large in her life with memories, for example, of a young man she nursed three times, who returned to combat, only to come back and die in her arms. On her return to the United States she had nightmares for six months, married another veteran, and seven years later went to law school. To her, the deeds of over 11,000 women who served as nurses, Red Cross workers, and in other capacities had to be documented and made visible.

The proposed site for the statue was at the opposite end of the Vietnam Memorial in Washington, DC and is meant to recognize not only the women who served, but the women who sent their family members in the military to Vietnam. To Jezierski: "This is much more than a noble cause. This is the only way we can have honest history and thus build our futures. It is imperative that an attempt be made to do justice not only to the women who served and to the women who sent their loved ones, but to the future generations of women who will be making choices" (p. 124).

By 1985 the Vietnam Veterans Memorial was supporting the project of Boulay and her colleagues, and in 1986 the design was also approved by the secretary of the interior, but J. Carter Brown of the Fine Arts Commission rejected the monument, "expressing the opinion that if a monument of a woman were allowed, other statues, such as one for the Canine Corps, would be needed" (*AD Nurse*, 1988, p. 8). To be equated with dogs was and is an interesting expression of sexism. (Perhaps, however, it is time to honor animals as well!) Brown's denial contradicted public law #96-297, which authorizes a memorial for military men *and* women. His rejection should have been, but was not, based on artistic merits. Now special legislation was required—a serious setback despite the overwhelming support of nursing and veteran organizations. The American public needs to know about all the women Vietnam veterans, but finding them is a challenge, since "There are no accurate records of the numbers of women who served in Vietnam. Finding them will promote a healing process" (p. 8).

Four years later, Leslie C. Blum (1989–1990) reported that the national memorial to nurses, a legacy of healing and hope, was finally becoming a reality. After a six-year effort, President George Bush signed legislation authorizing the memorial, subject to review by the National Capital Memorial Commission, the National Capital Planning Commission, and, once again, the Fine Arts Commission. The time to completion would be between 31 and 37 months.

To Diane Evans (1989–1990) of the Memorial Project, the images of war and men were common in history and the media, and she acknowledged their needs for psychological and physical healing. But no such healing had been provided to women: "After years of invisibility, silence, isolation, and denial, women veterans are very gradually stepping forward to acknowledge their veteran status, share their experience, and find the help they need. Before the inception of the Vietnam Women's Memorial Project there were no networks established, women's contributions were not covered by the media, and there was no tangible symbol for their recognition" (p. 2). Finally the monument was erected and dedicated on November 11, 1993. Perhaps partial healing for so many women veterans will now occur through some public recognition.

THE PARADOX CONTINUES

The feminist view of women and war is still divided, reflecting both a negation of militarism and an affirmation of the rights of women in the military. In the war with Iraq, the influence of feminism in opening up the military at all ranks and in all aspects, even combat, was clearly apparent. Ironically, once again, the spotlight was directed, not on military nurses, but on the women who were in the front lines. With some amazement, the nation and the world watched televised coverage of women helicopter pilots, female prisoners of war, and women officers and enlisted personnel, both Black and White, who were involved in support and front line jobs. Their presence, as Clara Barton predicted, further eroded the one remaining excuse for male dominance: the presumed "protection" of women and children.

In modern warfare, as Lillian Wald said, the civilians, mostly women, children, and the aged, are not protected from the effects of war, as can be seen in the hundreds of Iraqi civilian deaths. And, as Barton said in the 19th century, women and children experience war at its worst, subjected to injury, rape, and death, with no weapons to defend themselves. What the aftermath of this latest armed struggle will be for American, allied, Kuwaiti, and Iraqi nurses is still unclear. What is clear is that the sex discrimination against women in the Middle East affected Western military women as well as local women. Once again the war between the sexes was being played out within the confines of the larger war primarily created and conducted by men. And, once again, women in the peace movement took to the streets to protest the brutality of war and to assert women's protest against militarism in any form. And, again, women in nursing were caught between the militant and the peaceful, but went to war to take care of the wounded and dying.

Once again, nurses received little attention from the media and the public for their humanitarian work during the Iraq war. Given military censorship of the media during the war, this could be expected since focusing on the number of "surgical" strikes, of tanks and other nonhuman objects "taken out," riveted all attention on the technological wonders of warfare, not on the human beings damaged or destroyed. Since it is the wounded and dying that nurses care for, it is not surprising that their work was unreported. Images of women caring for maimed and mutilated men, women, and children did not fit with those of the technological precision of Patriot missiles or of pilots of F16s.

Nurse Meta Seltzer (1991) did publish some of the letters she had written from "Operation Desert Storm" to other nurses at home. A member of the

U.S. Army Reserves, in Combat Hospital Support, she served in Saudi Arabia. Writing home on January 27, 1991, she reported that she and 11 other nurses were huddled in the hallway of their apartment building, listening to the roar and explosions almost over their heads of the first Patriot missile used to intercept the first SCUD missile. Expecting germ or chemical warfare, the nurses carried their masks and other equipment with them even to meals. Seltzer was assigned to a field station, but en route observed fighter planes taking off every minute, exclaiming, "It was a beautiful sight at night with the red flame from the jet propulsion very visible. My heart went out to those brave men in the jets. I prayed for their safe return" (p. 372). She did not comment on the destruction of both Iraqi military personnel and civilians that the pilots would cause.

Caught in a rainstorm in tents, the nurses dealt with water running through like a river out of control. Setting up for their field station, all supplies had to be located, unpacked, and repacked. Trying to sleep in their tents, the nurses listened to bombs dropping near the border, making the ground shake all during the cold nights. The physicians gave emergency treatment classes on chest traumas, cervical spine, and facial injuries. Two orthopedic physicians argued about how to pin or stabilize extremities.

By March 23, 1991, the tone of Seltzer's letters had substantially changed: "As the days pass it becomes more difficult for me to write about the war" (p. 373). Located in a field hospital 16 miles from the Iraqi border, the nurses were all praying that peace talks would be fruitful, but by February 24, continuous bombing, with no pause between bombs, preceded the start of the ground war. The next day the wounded started to arrive, including three Iraqi soldiers, who had not eaten for five to seven days, had been drinking water from vehicle radiators, and were suffering fractures of the humerus and femur, missile wounds to chest, lacerations to the liver, fractured wrists, and tuberculosis.

Over time, the nurses treated about 60 Iraqis and 40 American and British soldiers. The American injuries were often related to tanks or land mines. The Bradley tanks seemed very dangerous: one young man's face was burned, hair scorched, and eyes swollen; both his legs were fractured; he had open wounds on both tibiae and both feet had flesh missing. When he asked Seltzer if his legs could be saved, she said yes, but did not tell him there was a significant amount of missing bone and it would be many operations and a long time before he could walk again. Indeed, the only minor injury she encountered was a tank driver's fractured arm.

Seltzer found that the Iraqi injuries were more severe and their physical conditions were poorer; often they were caked with dirt. All these factors complicated their recovery. However, the elite Republican Guard soldiers were neither starved nor dirty, but well fed, clean, mean looking, and suspicious of everything. One feared anesthesia because he had been told Americans would cut off his legs and arms. However, when the Iraqis left "they all thanked us, and some even kissed our hands!" (p. 374). Two even wanted to get to California. However, cultural and gender differences did cause problems, particularly with catheters and urination. Indeed, the Arab men who came to sell souvenirs ogled the women, even peering into the female showers, a practice that persisted despite warnings from officers to stop this harassment.

Seltzer constantly feared for her son who was in another military unit, holding her breath when she scrutinized the admittance list of the wounded during the night shift. Eventually, they were united and Seltzer said, "Thank God the war only lasted for 100 hours, because I don't think I could have endured much more stress" (p. 375). She concluded, "I will never forget the injured—on both sides—and continue to question the righteousness of war" (p. 375). Nevertheless, she was proud to be an American and to serve and care.

What would Seltzer and other nurses have said if they had served, as Barton did, for *years* in the Civil War, or as Lally had for years in *both* World Wars? Thankfully, the Gulf War was over too soon to know. But even in the few months of carnage, Seltzer, although still patriotic, had come to question the rightness of war. Whether she and other nurses would, over time, become as invisible as thousands of previous nurses in the military is unclear. There is no doubt, however, that the effects of war are long-lasting; as Rankin notes, there have been more veteran deaths from suicide than from combat in Vietnam. Men, who come back from war in pieces and not "safely" dead, are supposed to remain quiet and be brave. Nurses, too, are constrained to silence; those who tell the truth expose the reality of war, of militarism, the basis of patriarchal dominance, the reality of the violence normal to such a structure. Certainly, the strongest way "to not cooperate with patriarchy is to affirm life and live it fully and completely" (Livingston & Rankin, 1986, p. 117).

The fundamental problem pertains to women's life-giving and sustaining values and men's war-making and death-bringing values. Even for strong feminists the issue of women in the military is difficult. However, it is clear, as Clara Barton knew, that if women cannot engage in self-protection, this will be used as the ultimate reason for men's assumption of leadership, not only in the military, but in all other social institutions. As Lillian Wald reasoned, the problem is to make men's war obsolete and to so diminish the importance of aggression and war to a society that boys and men will not be attracted to destruction as a "glorified" way of asserting manhood. Until that time, nurses, more than any other women, are subject to direct involvement with male warriors. As such, they are the "test case" for the gendered conflict over life and death cultural themes.

Chapter 4

The Lively Debate: Nurses and Suffrage, the Equal Rights Amendment, and Social Reform

Nurses' involvement during times of war certainly exemplifies one form of public duty or social consciousness and activism. To what extent, however, have nurses reflected a greater social consciousness? Over time, how actively have they worked for change and social reform? In this chapter we take a closer look at the social issues of deepest concern to several of the nurse activists discussed in Chapter 2: the Equal Rights Amendment, the political enfranchisement of women, and other women's rights issues. To what extent did organized nursing, the professional associations, support the efforts of its activist members? Who were the leaders and who were the followers? How committed was the profession to social reforms and feminist goals?

Organized feminism in the United States took root in 1848 at Seneca Falls, NY, where the Declaration of Sentiments was signed, expressing the revolt of American women against patriarchal dominance. From that time until 1900, little is to be found in the published nursing literature on the status of women in relation to the status of nursing. This is partially because few periodicals had been founded in the 19th century by nurses in the newly emerging profession. Although a few earlier historical accounts by nurses do provide some information, previously unpublished materials, such as letters, diaries, minutes from meetings, government documents, and other sources, have only recently been uncovered and analyzed. When more thorough analyses of original sources are available, a different picture may emerge, but at present it appears that, for many nurses, the development of the profession in the 19th century took precedence over a concerted struggle for women's rights. If the creation of a public, paid occupation for women is considered a feminist activity, then many nurses have historically been a part of the women's movement. And if the first two decades of this century are examined, some nurses were actively involved in the debate over the Equal Rights Amendment (ERA). Several nursing leaders, particularly those in the urban Northeast about whom more is known, pursued nursing as well as social and feminist goals. As noted in Chapter 2, Lavinia Dock interconnected the relationships between the status of nursing and women, focusing attention on suffrage and on the ERA, among other issues important to women. The lack of attention given to Dock as a feminist indicates the extent to which nurses, until the 1970s, had lost touch with the problems of nursing as a woman's profession in societies that subordinate women. And the extent to which Dock and other nurse activists have been ignored by women's studies scholars is further evidence of modern feminists' lack of attention to nursing.

"UNTIL WE POSSESS THE BALLOT": WOMEN'S ISSUES, NURSES' ISSUES

A true pioneer of her time, Lavinia Dock urged nurses to be involved in women's issues and social issues. She deplored nurses' conservatism, their reluctance to consider political issues, and their lack of analysis of male-dominated power structures. In 1907 the *American Journal of Nursing* (*AJN*) published a paper delivered by Dock to the National Association of Nursing Alumnae (the American Nurses Association as of 1911). In her article on "Some Urgent Social Claims," Dock affirmed that the political enfranchisement of women had a direct bearing on the profession of nursing and on the lives of nurses as women. She recognized that to the majority of nurses the issue of women's political enfranchisement was a remote, far off, uninteresting idea to be avoided with disapproval or indifference. But Dock said: "I am ardently convinced that our national association will fail of its highest opportunities and fall short of its best mission if it restricts itself to the narrow path of purely professional questions and withholds its interest and sympathy and its moral support from the great, urgent, throbbing, pressing social claims of our day and generation" (p. 895). She urged the members of the association to look beyond the bounds of their professional organization, to emphasize and encompass the social movements and needs of the day: "Women who are indifferent to the movement for political emancipation are often amazed when they are confronted with the facts of the actual advance of this social change" (p. 899).

Dock admonished the National Association of Nurse Alumnae (NANA) to rise to a broader consideration of larger social issues than it had done before, leaving smaller concerns to the local regional bodies of the association. Imploring the group to widen the scope of its interests, she believed the day had come when the NANA "might here decide on our place, our share, and our policy toward the great social claims of education and educational reforms—industry and the industrial situation—especially as it relates to women-child-labor, its iniquities and dangers . . . prostitution and the white slave traffic" (p. 899). She did not think that many nurses could individually take any active or direct part in extending themselves to solve many of these problems, but she said, "to all of such movements we could give at least intelligent sympathy and moral support—perhaps occasionally some useful service" (p. 899). Finally, she stated:

> I would like to have our journals not afraid to mention the words political equality for women. I would like to see our local groups give more time to a consideration of their relation to other bodies of workers, for it has been said by a wise person that those who only know their own specialty do not even know that one. . . . Until we possess the ballot we shall not know when we may get up in the morning to find that all we had gained has been taken from us. (p. 901)

Lavinia Dock's words at this meeting had little immediate impact. One year later, the NANA by a large majority voted against "the reasonable and temperately expressed suffrage resolution" (Dock, 1908a, p. 925). This was a great shock to Dock, who said: "I have never been disappointed in the actions of that body [the association] . . . until this year, when I read, with humiliation . . . that a negative vote 'by a large majority' was recorded at San Francisco" (p. 925). She ended her distressed letter to the editor with the statement: "I hope that at a future meeting our members will reconsider their hasty snapshot verdict" (p. 926).

Dock's letter to the editor was followed by several other letters and responses throughout the months of 1908 and 1909. For example, in September 1908 Sophia Palmer, then editor-in-chief of the *AJN*, published an editorial on neutrality, explaining the editorial board's policy on the suffrage question. That editorial prompted a letter in October 1908 by Mary Bartlett Dixon, in which she criticized the editor for remaining neutral on "broad questions" such as the women's suffrage issue. Dixon believed that the editorial policy was to avoid important issues: "If you continue to remain neutral on the woman suffrage movement, may I suggest to you that your logical attitude must be that a 'nurse's place is inside *the* sickroom, not mixing up in affairs outside of her sphere'" (p. 49).

In the same issue of the *AJN*, Palmer responded to Dixon's criticism, saying that until such time as the NANA was ready to endorse suffrage, the editorial policy must remain neutral. Palmer personally regretted the action of the association's delegates, and stated that if she had been present, "I should have thrown the weight of my voice in favor of suffrage" (Palmer, 1908, p. 50). However, she believed that her support would not have influenced the result of the vote "as I understand the subject was ably argued by members who support the suffrage movement" (p. 50). Palmer believed that the vote of the delegates at the San Francisco meeting represented either the sentiment of their home associations or doubt as to what their sentiments really were: "In my judgment those nurses who were instrumental in turning the vote against the suffrage movement should give their reasons through this department of the magazine" (p. 50).

In an August 1908 letter to the *Nurses' Journal of the Pacific Coast* (*NJPC*), Dock said that she "felt so chagrined and pained over the surprising incident relating to equal suffrage that occurred at the San Francisco meeting. . . . Where were our Western sisters when this unfortunate vote came about? How did it happen?" (p. 366). In response to that letter, the *NJPC* editor stated: "Not guilty!" Dixon also sent her thoughts to the *NJPC*, asking the West Coast nurses if they had ever really thought about this question of votes for women. Dixon stated that she was told by a delegate who attended the San Francisco meeting: "It was the consensus of opinion 'that nurses had affairs enough of their own to attend to without getting mixed up in politics'" (Dixon, 1908b, p. 442). Dixon countered: "I claim that we were 'mixed up in politics' before we were born, and that it is impossible to attend to the smallest part of our own affairs without taking politics into consideration" (p. 442).

The debate continued with a letter from Adelaide Nutting to the editor of the *AJN* in November 1908. Nutting had been vacationing and her magazines had not reached her for two months. On learning from her friends, Lavinia Dock and Florence Kelly, of the failure of the NANA to support the resolution of the Women's Suffrage League, she wrote: "in thinking the matter over, I am rather inclined to conclude that their action was due more to a lack of knowledge of what woman suffrage really means and involves, than to any deep-seated conviction that it is an undesirable and unworthy cause to support, for otherwise it hardly seems credible that such action could be taken by working women (such as we nurses are) who are also thinking women" (p. 134). It is hard to believe that these nurses were ignorant of suffrage issues since they had been publicly debated since at least 1848. Why did they not know about them? It is difficult to accept a "lack of knowledge" and to assume that over half a century of debate on the issue, the pros and cons of suffrage, had not been transmitted to nurses. Perhaps Nutting was simply trying to be tactful, giving them an excuse for their "hardly credible" behavior.

In the same issue of the *AJN* another view was presented by Louie Croft Boyd (1908), who believed that the refusal to support the suffrage resolution was right because it was "in no sense vital to the nursing profession. Equal suffrage, although a matter of justice, should not be an issue with the nurses of the country because their issue is a uniform training throughout the United States, and this can only be accomplished through the registration laws which in time should be made uniform" (p. 136). In contrast, Nora Holman (1908), in her letter to the editor in the same issue, supported Nutting and Dock:

When nurses, as citizens, are entitled to vote for legislation in furtherance of their interests, for efficient men and women in government, and for health measures, far-reaching in results, will the *Journal*, editorially, still remain neutral and uninterested? . . . Those of us who were impressed recently by the vigorous support of suffrage shown by the English nurses, cannot but feel that the nurses of America, though spirited in *individual* matters, still lack the true spirit of the times, an awakening *social* responsibility. (p. 135)

Holman clearly realized the inevitable movement toward not only national but also *international* women's rights. It is unclear how many nurses at this time embraced such a world view and how many ignored the broader implications of the struggle for enfranchisement.

The debate continued into 1909 as the editor of the *NJPC* wrote, "Again the 'Woman Question,'" hoping that the next time the convention met they would have a better understanding of the suffrage question and vote in favor of it. In the same year, Ada M. Safford (1909) added her voice: "It is well that the endorsement did not carry at the San Francisco convention, for it would not have truly represented the nurses. I do not say that we should pass it at the next meeting, but the question has come up and I make a plea for information that shall help us to know why we do or why we do not" (p. 360). Safford insisted that nurses as business and professional women "need to recognize the debt we owe to the women who have *done things* before us, making it possible for us to hold the positions that we do today" (p. 360). It is a sad commentary, she asserted, that the demand for nurses and their technical training could not be met at the present time. However, directly following Ada Safford's letter, is one by Bessie Louise Dickson (1909), who expressed satisfaction with the neutral editorial stance of the *AJN*. She believed that the subject of suffrage or political equality should have no place in a magazine devoted to nursing, and commended the action of the convention. It is hard to imagine that women would vote against their own self-interests, but one might assume that early nurses like Dickson were inured to their subordinate status, reacting in an oppressed group manner, not realizing the damage they were causing to the full professionalization of nursing. This short-sighted behavior would make itself felt in decades to come.

Lavinia Dock (1909, May) again presented her opinions on the relation of the nursing profession to the woman's movement in a speech at a mass meeting of nurses in Philadelphia:

It is not at all that I think you could, or should, take an active part in the woman's movement; I know that your nursing duties make that, for the largest number of you, impossible. The foremost reason I have for wishing to present this subject to nurses is that we owe the existence of our profession to the woman movement; we owe it all that we are, all that we have of opportunity and advancement; we owe it our social and educational and economic *status*; and, all this being true, we surely owe it our gratitude and our recognition; we owe it our loyal allegiance and our moral support. (p. 197)

Once more, Dock pleaded for nurses to understand that their position as nurses was integrally related to their position as women in society.

Finally, in 1909, under the weight of opinion and the continuing barrage of letters to the editor, the editorial board of the *AJN* decided to consider broader social issues, not just narrow topics pertaining to the profession itself. Thus, in April 1909 Julia Ward Howe wrote to the *AJN* presenting "The Case for Women Suffrage." In this article, Howe claimed that suffrage is fundamentally simple justice and if there were no other reason, this one would be enough. Fortunately, there were other powerful arguments to be made. Suffrage would open positions of increased dignity and influence to women; broaden their minds; lead to improvements in the laws and to the defeat of dishonest candidates; bring women's direct and quick influence on legislation; make elections and political meetings more orderly; and raise the political honesty of voters. Note how Julia Ward Howe's reasons for supporting the suffrage movement emanate from one of the prevailing ideological constructs of the time: that women were perceived as the moral force of the nation. While men engaged in intellectual, analytical, and business activities, women's nature was to provide moral and spiritual guidance for the family and community. Because of their "inner goodness," women would supposedly influence the political process by raising its moral and ethical stature.

In the same *AJN* issue, and immediately following Julia Ward Howe's articulate article, is one by Lyman Abbott (1909), who protested: "I am an advocate of woman's rights: her right to an open door to every vocation, her right to a fair opportunity for the highest and broadest education, her right to do whatever she can do and be whatever she can become" (p. 566). However, Abbott believed that the movement for the emancipation of women had been accompanied by extravagances that constituted nothing less than an assault on womanhood: "this assault is the more dangerous to society not only because it is always veiled behind fine phrases, but also because it has among its leaders women prompted by noble motives" (p. 568). He deplored the fact that "the opening of all vocations to women has been followed by an inrush of women into industrial competition with men; [resulting in] the real and serious increase in the death rate among women" (p. 569). He denied the economic independence of women or of men: "Economic independence is the hazy dream of an unintelligent doctrinaire. . . . The question of woman suffrage is therefore really one for the women themselves to determine. Whenever they wish the suffrage they will have the suffrage. At present they do not wish it. . . . The hysterical appeals of the suffragettes, the unfeminine appeals of the masculine women who wish that God had made them men, we may wisely disregard" (p. 571). Abbott's supercilious and condescending statements are little more than thinly veiled attacks on women's rights to compete with men, particularly in the economic sphere. "Industrial competition" equals monetary competition. Abbott's fears are easily recognized as he differentiates "freedom" from economic freedom. Further, Abbott negates women activists and feminists, simultaneously calling them hysterical *and* masculine; in doing this he negates women's rights in totality, even if illogically.

Although some nurses were by now engaging in feminist activities and were perceived as radicals by some of their colleagues, the involvement of the rank and file in these social concerns may have been somewhat tardy. The organized women's movement emerged in the mid-19th century, and women external to nursing had debated the suffrage question and related economic issues for decades. Thus, nurses were restating what had already been explicated by earlier feminists; nevertheless, the debate on the suffrage question continued in nursing throughout the early 20th century. In 1911 a letter to the *AJN* editor by Mary Johnston explained the reason why she believed in votes for women. According to her, 25 million women in the United States were wage earning, a number larger than all the men, women, and children in the thirteen colonies when the fundamental statements of freedom were written in 1776. "Women," she asserted, "because they are women, are taxed without representation" (p. 77).

In 1911 the National Association of Nursing Alumnae had changed its name to the American Nurses Association; by 1913 it had also changed its neutral or negative position and had finally voted in favor of suffrage. An editorial comment in the *AJN*, published in April 1913, includes a description by nurse Isabel McIsaac of the experience of the nursing section of a suffrage parade, which took place on March 3, 1913, in Washington, DC:

As we waited for over an hour beyond the appointed time for starting we had not the remotest idea that the head of the procession was being hemmed in and buffeted by a seething, restless, jeering multitude, upon which an indifferent, incompetent police had as much effect as a broom against the tides of Fundy.

It would seem that on the whole the nursing section fared much better than many others, perhaps because even the worst of men can recall having been nursed by someone. But mingled with the chaff was a sinister slime which . . . is ever ready to burst its bondage and only needed a word of hostility or a jostle to have aroused its malignant fury and to have made an appalling disaster.

Never did we appreciate training as much as at that moment we ducked our heads under the necks of those fine [trooper] horses as they shoved the intruders out of our path. What happened to us after we were freed and among the respectable element is an indistinct blur—we only realized that we had sight of depths which will never be closed until women help to do it . . . . we came away astounded at what had been revealed, but more than ever determined to be working parts of the great struggle—world without end. (p. 491)

In 1915, as the United States prepared for its entry into World War I, Lillian Wald added her voice to those of Dock, Dixon, Nutting, and Kelly. In an article called the "Business of Being a Woman," Wald is emphatic about the importance of women to general societal issues and trends during the second decade of the 20th century: "Feminist, that word so newly coined . . . is nothing at all but the age old desire that women express in a new way, holding on to the things that are theirs, and ever have been and shall be" (p. 16). She points out that in the previous two decades, coinciding with social unrest, "the nurse has emerged into public movements, and the appeal to her mind is the appeal of the community" (p. 16). The nurse, she states, is beginning to realize her place in society, not only her place in the profession of nursing. Wald refers to a major theme that was clearly apparent in the late 19th century and early 20th century: the relationship between an understanding of the critical social issues of the time and the development and expansion of public health in which increasing numbers of nurses were involved.

While this debate on the question of votes for women in the United States continued, women in nursing were being observed carefully by their colleagues in Britain. Even during World War I, in 1917, Ethel Gordon Fenwick in the *British Journal of Nursing* sent "Congratulations to our American Cousins." British nurses applauded the fact that, finally, New York State and New York City had at last both voted for the enfranchisement of women, "a glorious triumph for right and justice, after a struggle for seventy years" (p. 342). They recognized that the great champion of full citizenship for American nurses and, indeed, for nurses all over the world, was Lavinia L. Dock. Fenwick extended "warmest congratulations to our American cousins, coupled with the name of our dear Miss Dock" (p. 342).

The women of Britain, of course, were also fighting for the right to vote and in 1918 another editorial by Fenwick expressed hope for the women of Britain because the first paragraph in the king's speech before Parliament dealt with the representation of the People's Act of 1918: "The Act which has removed the disability to exercise the Parliamentary Franchise placed upon women, and so has expunged the blot which has disgraced the English Constitution" (p. 107). The writer noted that it was a good omen for the preservation of national unity, because women would have an important share in reconstruction after the war. "To members of the nursing profession the prospect of political freedom for six millions of women brings the hope that the end of their struggle for the effective organization of their profession will speedily receive statutory authority" (p. 107). Fenwick continued that nurses have no doubt that Mr. Lloyd George "will soon add to his laurels by providing for the professional enfranchisement on 'self-determination' lines, of trained nurses, a status their work for the community has earned, and the public interest demands" (p. 107). It is apparent that early on, Fenwick rightly connected the issue of women's right to vote to the necessity of registration for nurses. Whether this interrelationship was obliquely or directly recognized by the majority of British or American nurses in the 19th century is not known.

THE ACTIONS OF THE MAJORITY:
VOTES AND RESOLUTIONS OF THE FOUR NATIONAL
NURSES ASSOCIATIONS BETWEEN 1895 AND 1920

More detailed research on the involvement of the newly founded American nursing organizations and the suffrage movement was published by Sandra B. Lewenson (1990), who rejects the idea that nurses, as historian Jo Ann Ashley (1975) says, were conservative on feminist issues, or as historian Susan Reverby (1987b) claims, that nurses' sense of duty, altruism, and social hierarchy had compromised their support for gender equality. However, Lewenson's time frame for her study was limited to 1893 through 1920; thus, excluding at least a half century of prior feminist activity from her analysis. Certainly there is strong evidence that individual nurse leaders, such as Clara Barton, were deeply involved in feminist work during the earlier time period, but there are inadequate data to establish the broad spectrum of nurses' involvement. Indeed, in the half century of struggle preceding the early 1900s, much of the pioneering work in feminism had been conducted, narrowing to suffrage issues only later and losing some of the more radical approaches and emphases in the early 1900s in order to create national coalitions with less feminist women's organizations. Since the time frame of Lewenson's work is limited to this later period, it is still unclear whether nurses were previously involved in any large numbers in pioneering feminism in either the United States or other countries.

While admitting that as late as 1908 nurses voted to reject suffrage at their national convention, Lewenson's research on the four national organizations indicates that suffrage was repeatedly debated and that nurses voted on organizational support seven different times, five of which were in favor of suffrage—during 1912, 1915, 1918, and 1919—but all of these had been obliterated from memory, except the 1915 vote when the resolution was passed. As important as these votes were, it is necessary to remember that many women's organizations by this time were in favor of suffrage. The national coalition on the narrower, less radical issue of the vote had largely succeeded in bringing together women's organizations on this one issue. Thus, the votes by organized nurses could be seen as similar to those expressed by women in other organizations reflecting the prevailing sentiment, but hardly similar to the pioneering feminists in the 19th century, who for 50 or more years had worked to create the climate of opinion and the coalition of groups that expressed it. Only more research on nurses' degree of involvement during the pioneering, earlier phase of feminism can resolve the issue of nurses' conservatism or nonfeminism on issues external to the professional development of nursing.

Nevertheless, Lewenson's research on the later period is important because it establishes the involvement of organized nursing in suffrage. She examines, first, the American Society of Superintendents of Training Schools for Nurses, founded in 1893 and renamed the National League of Nursing Education in 1912 and the National League for Nursing in 1952. At their sixth annual convention in 1899, Maud Banfield expressed concern that nurses were denied positions on boards of health, which were filled as political favors. Without the vote, women nurses were outside the political process. An organizational motion passed that a committee be formed to support nurses' placement on health boards. At the ninth annual convention, Sophia Palmer said that Susan B. Anthony had "'contributed as much to the advancement of nurses as any other woman, improving our legal status, and all those things we enjoy'" (p. 125). President Annie Daimer wanted members to support the Susan B. Anthony Memorial. In 1908 Dr. Margaret Bigelow from the National Suffrage Association spoke to the nurses, who were enthusiastic, according to a newspaper report. Helen Parker Criswell, president of the California Nurses Association, asked in 1908 how the largest organized body of professional women in existence would affect the status of 20th-century women. To her, professional problems could not be solved without addressing women's status. Nevertheless, at the 11th annual national convention, the suffrage resolution was defeated. As noted, there followed efforts to educate and enlist nurses' support and assuage their fears that supporting suffrage would negatively affect registration. The Superintendents Society and the National Association of Nursing Alumnae of the United States and Canada planned jointly to send a delegation to the International Council of Nurses convention. A resolution for the delegation to support women's suffrage was again defeated in 1909. According to Lewenson, nurses' attitudes toward suffrage then began to change. This change was expressed by Annie Daimer, who noted a feeling of unrest in all the meetings. In some, nurses were openly demanding the vote. At the 12th annual convention of the NANA, Annie Goodrich said "'eighteen years of this struggle has made a woman's suffragist of me'" (p. 128). By 1912 the American Nurses Association (ANA) had approved sending a delegation to the next International Congress of Nursing (ICN) meeting to support suffrage. Both Jane Delano and Isabel McIsaac supported the resolution, not wanting future delegates to go again to the ICN meetings with a negative position. McIsaac exclaimed: "'How in the world will we ever face Miss Dock if we do?'" (p. 129). Subsequently, the ICN in the same year voted to endorse woman suffrage.

Lewenson's data on the National Association of Colored Graduate Nurses, founded in 1908, are weaker, including one reference to indirect support, presumably derived from their delegation's attendance at the 1912 International Council meeting when suffrage was supported. However, by 1915 the Susan B. Anthony bill was voted on and supported by all three nursing associations, as well as a fourth, the National Organization for Public Health Nursing, founded in 1912. Speaking for all but the Association of Colored Graduate Nurses, D. Elva Mills Stanley wrote in the 1915 *AJN*, " 'Unanimously these associations stand for the enfranchisement of women'" (cited in Lewenson, 1990, p. 129).

In 1918 the executive board of the National League of Nursing Education passed another resolution and an endorsement to be sent to the Senate. According to Lewenson, in 1918 a joint resolution of the American Nurses Association, the National League of Nursing Education, and the National Organization of Public Health Nursing agreed to advocate publicly for passage and for a message to the president to support suffrage in the deliberations in Congress. Lewenson notes that the Association of Colored Graduate Nurses never recorded an official vote of endorsement, but President Adah Thoms, at their 12th annual convention, urged the women to consider the ballot as important to their goal since " 'education, registration, health, and racial prejudice could be addressed via the vote'" (p. 130).

In her research, Lewenson found 200 statements on nursing and suffrage, signifying to her the active role of nurses in the 20th-century women's movement and the significance of suffrage to the autonomy of nursing practice. Indeed, Lewenson asks why nursing's contribution to the women's movement has been so ignored and misrepresented. To her, there is an underlying societal prejudice toward nursing. She uses the term "nursism" to express a prejudice toward the field reflecting a devalued and subordinate view of nursing. By jarring the recollections of nurses' actual contributions to the women's movement, perhaps the struggle to be seen as valued, educated, and autonomous may sustain "the image of nursing that our pioneer leaders have intended" (p. 132).

THE VOTE WON, THE ERA LOST

Women won the right to vote in America in 1920, and in November 1922 the National Women's Party adopted "The Declaration of Principles." This declaration was presented as a federal constitutional amendment and introduced into Congress in December 1923. It stated: "Men and women shall have equal rights throughout the United States and in every place subject to its jurisdiction" (*Public Health Nurse*, 1924, p. 135). The declaration was named for a famous feminist and was often referred to as the Lucretia Mott Amendment. The *Public Health Nurse* published the substance of this amendment so that the nursing community could understand the importance of the ERA and the issues surrounding it. This amendment was strongly supported by Lavinia Dock. It is difficult to assess the support of individual nurses, but at least the nursing journals were presenting the issue to their readers.

After the editorial on the Lucretia Mott Amendment appeared, letters to the editor again were sent to the *AJN*, many of them appearing in 1924. Julia Stimson (1924), for example, presented arguments against ratifying the ERA and gave a list of national organizations that were opposed to the National Women's Party Amendment, or the ERA. Organizations opposed to the amendment included: the National League of Women Voters, National Women's Trade Union League, American Federation of Teachers, National Council of Jewish Women, National Council of Catholic Women, National Council of Women, the YWCA, United Textiles Workers, Republican National Committee, Democratic National Committee, and American Association of University Women. Clearly, many women were afraid that newly won labor "protection" laws for women and children would be lost. Ironically, much of this "protective" legislation was used subsequently in a discriminatory manner, which continued the subjugation of women in succeeding decades.

In the next issue of the *AJN*, July 1924, there appeared another letter to the editor by Lavinia Dock, who continued her fight for women's rights. In her letter, Dock explained that social reforms, such as mothers' or widows' pensions and maternity aid would not be destroyed; thus, the opponents of the amendment had misinterpreted it. Dock believed that passage of the ERA would provide first, ample protection for boys and girls; second, equal conditions of protection for young workers of both sexes; and third, equal rights and opportunities for adult women and men without restriction or exclusion based on sex alone. Dock and other women lost on the ERA and in consequence, so did all nurses and women in general. Even when the ERA was defeated and after the First World War, Dock still credited the women's movement with influencing the international movement of nurses toward feminism. In 1929 she wrote: "looking back. . . . I realize afresh how much our profession has owed to the Woman Movement and its leaders, and how greatly the earliest international experiments in organization were both indirectly made easier by the influence of feminism . . . and directly aided by the counsel and sisterly help of eminent suffragists" (Dock, 1929, p. 14).

LESSONS FROM THE PAST: STILL IGNORED?

In 1985 Charlene Eldridge Wheeler analyzed the editorial position and content of each issue of the first twenty years of the *AJN*, finding three themes: professional issues, socialization of nurses, and influences of major social and political movements. According to Wheeler, her study contradicts prevalent popular views about the history of nursing. To Wheeler, it is common for nursing students to graduate without learning about early nursing leaders or the nature of their contributions: "When reference is made to a nurse from a bygone era, the nurse is often overtly or covertly degraded and represented as somewhat of an oddity, a crock, or abnormal" (p. 21). This treatment of women nurses parallels the exclusion of women from history or the trivialization of women's history, which are both well documented in the women's studies literature (see Spender, 1983).

Wheeler further asserts that current problems in professional socialization can be traced to the failure to learn lessons from the past. Even nursing history texts create a lack of interest in early leaders. For example, Wheeler takes issue with the Bulloughs' (1978) history text in which, from her perspective, selective obliteration distorts early women leaders' contributions. According to Wheeler, the unspoken assumption, for instance, that early nurses wanted to be subordinate and that subordination in the larger cultural paradigm was normal, distorts and prevents an accurate professional image.

Wheeler also claims that the Bulloughs' presentation of Lavinia Dock is distorted. For example, to state that Dock permitted no mention of World War I in her column in the *AJN* and then to omit her rationale for this decision produces a view of Dock as a "dyspeptic individual who performed her editorial role irresponsibly" (p. 22). Wheeler claims that Dock was not alone in her disapproval of the war and was consistent in her views with those of editor Sophia Palmer, who deplored the "'slaughter of thousands, the desolation of homes, the retardation of industry'" (p. 23). Both Palmer and Dock expressed solidarity with nurses in foreign countries by their refusal to report "successes" of those promoting war, justifying this stance on the ground that *all* nurses were devoted to alleviation of the suffering caused by war. Clearly, Wheeler insists on seeing nursing history as a part of women's history.

In the first decade of the 20th century, the *AJN* was involved in establishing the foundations for nursing's autonomy. Sophia Palmer, editor-in-chief from 1900 to her death in 1920, claimed that previous journals had not been owned or controlled by nurses, and that the *AJN* would be a channel of communication, managed and edited by recognized women supervisors and educators who were both conscientious and thorough. To Wheeler, there is strong evidence that nursing leaders were concerned about nurses' education, registration, and service. They were clearly aware that organization and legislation were needed to obtain professional status: "Nurses were urged to become familiar with parliamentary law so they could have a more powerful voice in public meetings, and the Associated Alumnae openly allied themselves with the National Council of Women" (p. 25).

By 1901 a column on medical facts in condensed form openly acknowledged that nurses could learn from medical literature, but this did not suggest subservience since nursing leaders were "determined to have nursing under the direction of women in nursing" (p. 26). They believed that when state registration became a reality, education comparable to other professions would follow and from this would come appropriate recognition. Sophia

Palmer stated, " 'the trained nurse will rank, not as a subordinate of the medical man, but as his associate' " (p. 26). Furthermore, though nursing was seen as an occupation for women, nurses were not isolated from the broader community of women since, as one writer stated, they were " 'part of the great woman's movement of the age' " (p. 27); women in other lines of work needed nurses, just as they needed other women to prevent one-sided narrowness. As Wheeler notes, an *AJN* tribute to Susan B. Anthony on her death in 1906 recognized her indefatigable efforts in behalf of women.

As the second decade began, tributes to Florence Nightingale and Isabel Hampton Robb on their deaths demonstrate to Wheeler that nursing leaders were "revered, deeply loved, and respected for their diversity and non-conformity" (p. 28). In addition, increased emphasis on membership in the professional organizations and on moral social institutions was evident, for example, in Palmer's outrage over the blatant disregard of the treatment of women confined for venereal disease. Nurses were urged to teach and distribute information on the spread and prevention of gonorrhea and syphilis through a series of *AJN* articles on sex hygiene.

Early nurses took successful political action in declaring as unconstitutional a portion of the Page bill, which "allowed any woman to be arrested for suspicion of prostitution, held in jail at least 24 hours or until her bacteriology results were available . . . and publicly charged with the crime of being infected with a social disease" (p. 29). The neglect of real health problems for the poor, such as malnutrition and tuberculosis, made the issue of medical treatment of prostitutes not one of aiding poor women, but of protecting the upper classes of men who used them. Nurses themselves did not always agree on these issues, one arguing that a "clean journal" should not deal with moral and professional shortcomings of nurses and physicians, nor with prophylactic measures of specific diseases, nor with the pros and cons of duties of, for example, the catheterization of male patients. Sophia Palmer responded: "The whole world has, in the last few years, wakened to a recognition of the fact that it is what has been called 'the conspiracy of silence' more than any other factor which has brought about the shocking prevalence of social diseases, the white slave traffic, and all the ills that follow in their wake" (pp. 29–30). To her, nurses needed knowledge to protect themselves and to act as properly informed teachers of the public.

Wheeler contends that nursing leaders were *not* isolated and *were* actively involved in the women's movement, even though she admits that the official organizational policy on suffrage was originally one of neutrality. Since 1848 marks the beginning of *organized* feminist action, as reflected in the Declaration of Sentiments at Seneca Falls, it is again debatable whether early nurses were leaders in the women's movement, at least on the issue of suffrage. Again, it is clear that some individual nurses in the latter 19th century were involved, but national nursing organizations were largely nonexistent and could hardly be credited as early leaders on key political issues. However, we should again state that the creation of a woman's occupation, led by women, represented a major struggle against the prevailing social constructs and norms.

The negative position toward war softened, according to Wheeler, as the United States entered World War I, which placed heavy pressure on nurses to volunteer for war service. Caught between traditional women's and men's values and activities, nurses who subsequently supported the war became disillusioned with the Red Cross, which was willing to accept nonregistered nurses for war service. Wheeler concludes that the movement to recognize nursing as a self-controlled body occurred against "incredible odds and intense opposition" (p. 32). The nurses eventually expressed "solidarity with and great loyalty to the cause of women's progress . . . a guiding principle for the majority of the first two decades" (p. 33). Tragically, it was the war, Wheeler claims, and nurses' immersion in it that subsumed their energies and eventually destroyed nurses' solidarity, their radical critiques of social ills, and the effects of these on women and children. Nevertheless, Wheeler urges nurses today to see early nursing leaders as "courageous women who dared to dream, to have visions, and to struggle" (p. 33), whose work demands respect and admiration, not derision and judgment based on myths of subservience and ignorance. The continual erasure or distortion of the past must, according to Wheeler, be superseded by reclaiming these strong, decisive women in order to restore nursing to its rightful place.

"THESE WOMEN CARE": NURSES PARADING, CANVASSING, AND LOBBYING

What were these nursing leaders actually doing? The importance of nursing leaders located in New York was obvious to suffrage leaders, since a victory in this large and influential state would be critical to their national campaign. As Doris Daniels (1976) notes, suffrage legislation had been rejected by the men in the New York State legislature every year since 1854. This continuous rejection of female political rights caused the women to be influenced by the more militant women's movement in Great Britain, leading to the creation of the Women's Political Union organized in New York City. Carrie Chapman Catt, former president of the National American Woman's Suffrage Association, consolidated many organizations into the Woman Suffrage Party, which led two referenda campaigns, the second of which succeeded in 1917. The feminists asked Lillian Wald to be a candidate for the women in the city, but Wald refused. Later, however, she agreed to be honorary vice chair of the planned Woman's City Convention, organized around assembly districts. Lavinia Dock represented at least three districts, in which she worked with nurses Helen McDowell, Yssabella Waters, and Beula Weldon. Parading, canvassing, and lobbying, these and many other women forced the legislators to submit a referendum to the voters.

The feminists conducted an impressive campaign and Wald, as R. L. Duffus (1938) said, " 'could no more keep out of the suffrage movement than a fish could keep out of water' " (p. 214). Duffus claimed that Wald was "hot" on the suffrage issue, throwing the resources of the Henry Street Settlement into the struggle. But, as Daniels points out, Wald was often not involved formally in women's groups; instead she pressured politicians, published articles, and gave speeches, often getting through to groups that were impervious to other feminists. In addition, Wald was used as "a model of what women could do if they had the power. . . . Ironically, even the anti-suffragists used Wald as an example, for she showed what women managed to do without the vote" (p. 215). In contrast to Dock, Wald eschewed militant tactics, preferring the many good arguments for suffrage; yet, as Daniels notes, Wald marshaled support for the Pankhursts in Britain and for Dock, even though they disagreed on tactics and strategies.

It is Lavinia Dock, active in the Congressional Union (later the National Woman's Party), with its adaptation of the Pankhursts' methods in Britain, who put her life on the line. For example, she went to the polls and insisted, as Susan B. Anthony had earlier, on her right to vote, hoping to be arrested and thus force the issue legally. As indicated previously, she was "one of the first pickets of the White House to be jailed . . . [serving] a total of forty-three days including twenty-five days in Occoquan prison where she claimed conditions were so bad that she had 'hard work choking down enough food to keep the life in me' " (pp. 216–217). Wald protested to the White House over the jailing of the pickets and pleaded with Dock not to go to jail again because Wald could not bear the thought. As Daniels notes, Wald thought militant tactics unnecessary because in a democracy everyone has the right to be represented and the force of this right would naturally evolve into a reality. Women, carrying the world's burdens on their shoulders, were obviously capable of voting wisely.

The nurses of Henry Street were particularly valuable in countering prejudice toward immigrants. The suffragists needed the support of ethnic and religious minorities and the poor. Foreign-born males in other referenda had voted against suffrage, yet native-born women still could not vote at all. Daniels acknowledges that suffragists espoused views that violated traditions and religious teachings of the new immigrants. Given these facts, how were the feminists going to get the immigrants' vote *for* women's suffrage? They turned to the nurses, who had worked hard in and knew the immigrant neighborhoods; in 1910, for example, 47 nurses had made 50,000 home visits; by 1917, 100 had made 250,000 home visits. Daily, the immigrants could see liberated women nurses, who were concerned about "womanly" issues. Thus, Wald and the nurses became interpreters of feminism, explaining suffrage to immigrants and, in turn, explaining the immigrants to the suffragists.

Believing that working women needed the vote to gain protective laws, Wald claimed she was a suffragist because she wanted to dignify the home and mothers, the fundamental source of society; mothers would vote to preserve that which was "valuable and important to them" (p. 222). Wald defended foreign-born women who, she said, were earnestly concerned about making life happier and safer: "They knew from bitter experience about labor conditions. 'And these women care. It would be extraordinary if they did not care'" (p. 223). Furthermore, the vote was important to them. Wald noted that one could see working-class women and mothers on soap boxes, exhorting their audience to give women equality. Wald also brought the suffrage issue to Jewish voters, asking the men to vote for women because it was just. With education, women would, she said, perform their full duties in a democracy.

According to Daniels, the effects of the work done by the Henry Street Settlement nurses were obvious in the polls and the referenda results in their districts. The first referendum was lost and some women blamed the immigrant men, but the Lower East Side vote was more favorable than in any other district in New York City. The Russian and Austrian immigrant voters were positive toward suffrage, while the German, Irish, and Italian were more negative. By 1917 the enfranchisement issue would be tested again, but with World War I creating patriotic fervor, would the pacifism of the women leaders negatively affect the issue? The momentum was still strong, however, and even President Woodrow Wilson had by then agreed to a federal amendment. Lillian Wald again served as a symbolic leader, and the Henry Street nurses "duplicated their massive effort of 1915" (p. 229). This time Wald was in disagreement with some of the suffrage leaders who had offered their services to the government during the war crisis. She agreed to serve only if the Woman's Suffrage Party would commit the women to relieving "'suffering or distress in any form'" (p. 229), but even that, she feared, might increase the "war spirit."

The testimony to the dogged, determined, hard work of the nurses was that the urban centers did give women the victory. According to Daniels, the nurses' districts carried 69% of the favorable votes in Manhattan. In contrast, in the same year (1917), Ohio rejected suffrage, demonstrating that the war did not influence positively the national suffrage trends. After so many years of work, Wald wrote to Jane Addams, "We are nearly bursting over our citizenship. . . . I had no idea that I could thrill over the right to vote. . . . The carrying of New York State is the greatest single victory that the suffrage cause . . . has yet won. It breaks the backbone of the opposition [and] forces the blindest reactionary to see the handwriting on the wall; it insures the speedy passage through Congress of the nation-wide suffrage amendment" (p. 231).

Wald and her nurses immediately moved to educate women in the mechanics of government in order to make the city safer and better. She urged women to remain independent; instead of being absorbed in men's political machines, women could demand definite programs from both parties—indeed, this was the model for the League of Women Voters, the reorganized National American Woman's Suffrage Association. Daniels claims that Wald did not believe suffrage was a panacea, but she did make her audiences believe that women were interested primarily in social reform. Interestingly, Daniels and other feminist scholars blame the suffragists for *not* becoming attached to the male political machinery, for espousing independent action and concentrating on individual issues and social concerns. Rather, states Daniels, "The new voters should have been urged to enter political parties, to gain a constituency, to wield influence by choosing candidates and to develop reputations for achievement and ability. To claim 'power,' women had to reach places where they made final decisions for the political process" (pp. 232–233).

The war had taken attention away from women's concerns and in the postwar society of the 1920s, successes were less frequent. As money went to the war effort, the nurses were hard pressed to obtain funds to sustain their work. Daniels claims: "Youth took advantage of the benefits won by the older generation, but it may be that the easier access to education and the professions thwarted the development of a feminist consciousness" (p. 279). Increased opportunities for women, gained by enfranchisement, now created new challenges, but Wald found the new generation did not believe strenuous effort was required to meet them. The younger generation was disinterested, "even hostile to those things which Wald believed to be most important" (p. 280). Novelists, even Nobel Prize winner Sinclair Lewis, "satirized liberal 'uplifters'" (p. 281), settlement house women, alluding to lesbianism, and giving one reforming woman, in his novel *Ann Vickers*, "five lovers, one abortion and one illegitimate child" (p. 281). Thus, powerful men were actively attacking women leaders and trivializing their persons and work. The conservative shift following the war was apparent in the apathy of the young, but at least, Wald said, they were more frank, with less "'hypocrisy and surreptitious experiment'" (p. 282) in sexuality. Further, some began to think they could have both marriage and career.

By the 1930s the Depression dealt a severe blow to feminism; married women were fired, regardless of their abilities or economic status, and women lost many of their rights—ironically, a situation that was accepted if it meant that men could be employed. Other thinkers, however, claimed that social feminism slowed, but was not destroyed. Wald continued to battle for women's rights to serve on juries, for laws against women's loss of citizenship on marrying a foreigner, and for passage of the Sheppard–Towner bill in 1921, which provided federal funds to promote maternal and infant health care. Male politicians refused to renew the bill in 1930, claiming it was fundamentally a "woman's measure" that forced states to take responsibility for welfare and increased public health nurses' responsibilities for educating the public about maternal and child care. As with many social issues, nurses were pitted against physicians who, along with politicians, saw the bill as a "feminist-socialist-communist conspiracy" (p. 286). By 1930 "red-baiting" had become fashionable, and President Hoover and the Republicans allowed the bill to lapse.

A new Woman's Party was formed in 1921 and its first convention was attended by nurse delegates, including Wald and Dock. Unfortunately, notes Daniels, "radical" issues, Black women's participation, birth control, disarmament, and marriage and divorce laws were pushed aside. The ERA took precedence, but this also split the group, particularly offending women who had fought previously for protective legislation. Other women claimed these laws should extend to all instead of segregating women and children in a separate caste. Nurses were also divided: Dock and Goodrich supported the ERA, while Wald did not, believing the amendment would destroy the unity of women established during the prewar decades. Daniels notes that Dock regretted these divisions and tried to persuade Wald to see another point of view, urging her to see the protective laws as deceptive, used to exercise exclusion and segregation. In retrospect, Dock was right and Wald was wrong. Finally, in 1938 Wald wrote to a congressional body that was holding a hearing on the amendment. She spoke against the amendment, emphasizing her 40-year support of protective measures; later, she corresponded with several nurses, urging them to reject the amendment. Still, even these divisions among the women did not stop them from working together on social legislation.

As the early leaders grew old and died, many younger nurses did not emulate their foremothers. World War I and then the Depression put the independent nursing organizations in great financial jeopardy, eventually leading to their demise or incorporation. Daniels concludes Wald was a propagandist, and needed to popularize "suffrage, unions for women, professionalization of nursing, the women's peace movement and almost every other campaign to effect sexual equality" (p. 297). To Daniels, Wald was "instinctively a feminist"; she violated the stereotype of a woman's place in society by becoming a nurse; she became a model of what women could do in public life. Her power was grounded in the nurses of the Henry Street Settlement and the Visiting Nurse Service, and from this base she could make sisterhood a reality.

Given the mixed pattern of support that the professional nursing associations gave to the suffrage issue and the ERA during this period, it is interesting to read a 1976 historical summary of the record of the ANA on numerous social issues. Written by Ann Zimmerman for the *AJN*, a passing comment notes that "the organization itself was not among the avant-garde defenders of women's right to vote" (p. 589). Zimmerman emphasizes those issues that the association supported strongly throughout the 1900s: between 1910 and 1930, legislation affecting mothers and children, such as child labor laws; in the 1930s, disability and old age insurance programs as well as governmental funding for mental and public health services; in 1946, removal of barriers preventing full "professional development" of minority nurses; civil rights bills affecting health, education, and equal employment opportunities; in 1950, inclusion of nursing service in medical insurance plans; and finally, in 1971, support of the ERA. Though some of these issues directly affected women, the article is limited in presenting important women's issues, such as the right to vote or the right to constitutional coverage for women.

Certainly, nursing, often in opposition to medicine, has taken important stands on social issues directly affecting women, children, and families. On political issues directly concerned with women's rights, however, nursing's support was somewhat tardy, given the data currently available. It is difficult to determine how many nurses actually understood the many important linkages between women's issues and what the nursing profession could achieve if women's equality became embedded in societal norms and in constitutional law. Until more historical research on this issue is conducted, we can only conclude that during the latter half of the 19th century, it seems that feminists outside of nursing took the brunt of the derision, social ostracism, and even imprisonment. Nevertheless, on issues of women and war, a few early nurse pioneers experienced the full force of sexist attacks. And certainly, some nurses in the early 20th century were directly involved in the struggle for women's rights, experiencing along with non-nurses the negative societal reactions to their acts of courage and commitment. Furthermore, if we conceive of the development of organized nursing itself as a movement of women outside the home and into the public world controlled by men, then nurses have been continuously involved in feminist activity, even during times when other women were quiescent. In 1971 the ANA did approve the most recent version of the ERA, but, again, organized nursing was not a pioneer in the reemergence of feminism. Fortunately, there are individual avant garde nurses whom we can thank for speaking up on the linkages between nursing and female subordination, both in the previous century and in this century as well.

Chapter 5

"What We May Become": The Sounds of Transition

The collapse of militant feminism or the transmutation of it into generalized social activism from the 1930s on left nurses without activists to protest women's subordination or to provide an overarching social analysis of women's status. The voices of the leaders of the early 20th century were muted by the derision toward "suffragists" of the earlier period. After women achieved the vote, the Equal Rights Amendment was brought before Congress in 1923, and in every succeeding year, and defeated each year until 1972 when it was passed, only to fail to be ratified by a sufficient number of states. The roaring twenties collapsed into the grinding Depression of the 1930s. Although the unjust system of sex discrimination remained, few women in nursing published any systematic statements on the issues involved.

Some major nursing reports alluded to the effects of gender on, for example, employment and salaries, but there were few sustained analyses of sexism in the nursing journals. World War II led nurses into renewed demands for equal treatment, but these demands were presented as professional rights and seldom overtly and systematically related to women's status in general. Women's voices in the postwar period from the late 1940s to the middle 1960s, were even more muted and many previous gains in independence were temporarily lost for all women. On the other hand, there is no doubt that many women pressed for some social reform action during the 1960s—the war on poverty, passage of the 1964 Civil Rights Act, including Title VII, and the 1963 Equal Pay Act—all of which had direct, beneficial outcomes for women's status. Some nurses gave their support to these issues, but much of their involvement was not reflected in the nursing literature. Nevertheless, during the postwar decades, nurses, as noted in Chapter 3, did take advantage of their military experience to press for improvements in the profession. A few nurses, in quiet voices, kept some other feminist issues alive.

THE IMAGE OF HOPE

In the 1950s and 1960s some women began to publish their concerns about the status of women and of nursing as a predominantly woman's profession. Most lacked the fiery assurance of earlier women. Byrne Hope Sanders (1956), for example, tentatively asked, "Are We Equal to Our Future?" Codirector of the Canadian Institute of Public Opinion, Sanders addressed nurses, asking them to set aside their roles as nurses and concentrate on their roles as women: "Will you think of yourselves, for a little, just as women? As women, let us think of ourselves, what we are and what we may become. Let us set the image of our hope before us" (p. 782). On the need to achieve a nation-wide awareness of being Canadian, she said, "as women we are half that national consciousness" (p.783). She asked nurses to give thought to what being Canadian means: "we women have to develop our opinions on national and international matters more definitively" (p. 783). Based on her work on national surveys, Sanders claimed there is only one major difference between women and men: "On many important questions one finds a far greater proportion of women than men who say 'I have no opinion'" (p. 783).

Sanders emphasized that nurses have a commitment to society to become involved as women in professional associations external to nursing. From surveys, she found that nursing was the most popular profession for women in Canada. When asked what occupation, outside of marriage, offers most for the young girl, she said, "nursing leads the list far above any others, such as secretarial work or teaching" (p. 783). Those who say nursing offers the least do so because the work is viewed as too hard. Sanders told the nurses that a key problem is the dedicated nature of their work, which might make their world of ideas narrow down to only the fields of nursing and medicine. In a faint echo of Lavinia Dock, Sanders encouraged nurses to involve themselves in social issues, and to extend their lives as women beyond the narrow confines of the nursing profession.

Although no longer espousing the belief that there is a *woman's point of view*, Sanders, nevertheless, urged nurses to "learn of women's problems in other lines of work than your own. Quite frankly, I wish more nurses would enter community or public life" (p. 783). Admitting how busy nurses are, still she advised them not to become too introverted in their professional lives. Sanders stated the main purpose of her message: "As a woman, will you think seriously about the importance of *supporting other women?* Believe in women, help them, like them—as intelligences, as workers, as citizens" (p. 784). She cautioned against belittling women in ways unrecognized. Sanders shared the story of one woman in politics who asked her to join a crusade, requesting her to say, when she hears of a man who has been particularly brilliant, "'He thinks just like a woman!' or 'He's got a brain like a woman!'" (p. 784). To this, Sanders responded, "I am not an ardent feminist" (p. 784), believing women no better, nor worse, no kinder, no more cruel than men.

Nevertheless, as "intelligences," Sanders claimed that women must exercise their minds, forcing themselves to look beyond their own life habits. She leaves the nurses with three words—intelligence, courage, sensitivity—to hang onto in the rough and tumble of life.

THE TEMPO QUICKENS

By the early 1960s the first evidence for the reemergence of feminism appeared with the establishment and report of President John F. Kennedy's Commission on the Status of Women (1963) and the publication of Betty Friedan's *The Feminine Mystique* (1963). Dorothy Kelly (1963), editor of the *Catholic Nurse*, wrote an editorial prompted by the work of the commission, which was established at women's insistence. Many members were older women such as Eleanor Roosevelt who had been committed to feminism in the earlier part of the century. Contrary to popular opinion, at least some women had continued their concern for and commitment to women's equality and, when the time was right, they acted. In fact, Wilma Scott Heide (1983) recalled in a personal communication to Joan Roberts that as a nursing student in the 1940s, she had asked Eleanor Roosevelt, who was then addressing issues of human rights to a group of nurses, when President Roosevelt would deal with issues of women's subordinate status. To this, Eleanor replied that the time was not ripe, but that she would notify Heide when it was politically advisable to act. Heide recalled her astonishment when she received a communication in the early 1960s from Eleanor Roosevelt that indicated the time for women had come once again. Heide exclaimed about a woman who, with such great responsibilities, still, after 20 years had elapsed, remembered and responded to Heide's inquiry as a young nursing student in the 1940s.

Responding to the work of such women, Kelly found the commission report interesting and not strident in tone. She believed that the Report of the President's Commission on the Status of Women proved that "Particular groups of women are in a sad plight, indeed, beset by color prejudice on one hand and by sex discrimination on the other" (p. 16). She stressed that women themselves were not using their rights, opportunities, and talents: "nor have they pushed very hard for the elimination of discriminatory practices" (p. 16). Of particular importance to Kelly was the report's assertion that war had brought women great economic opportunities, but thereafter they were treated as a marginal group. Kelly found nothing in the report with which she could disagree, but warned against those who say a woman's place is in the home, recommending they look at the statistics, consider the pressures on women, and remember that "the home just isn't what it used to be!" (p. 16). Kelly noted that every third worker was a woman and of these workers, three of five were married. Given the increased life span of women, "it ill befits us to maintain an outmoded social climate which relegates women either to certain traditional fields (poorly remunerated because they are 'womanly' tasks) or to lower grades in occupations followed by both men and women" (p. 16).

The report, an invitation to action, called for changes in education; Kelly claimed too little is expected of girls educationally and thus, individuals, family, and all of society suffer alike, adding the church to her list of sufferers. The distance between women now and those earlier, who had to fight for the vote, was so great that earlier feminists would "find their present-day sisters' indifference both to the ballot box and to political office downright incomprehensible" (p. 17). Given the report's conclusion that the desire of young women to excel in intellectual fields has weakened, Kelly asked what ideal do we hold out to them. "The movie version of marriage? the career that pays off through beauty and sex appeal rather than through intellectual endeavor? Or does it have to do with defective attitudes on the part of American males?" (p. 17).

In a related article, Gretchen Gerds (1963) interviewed Esther Peterson, executive vice chairwoman of the President's Commission, about the commission's report and its significance to nursing. Peterson considered the most important message in the entire report to be that "there is a new pattern to women's lives and our social thinking has not caught up with this reality as yet" (p. 70). She stressed the importance of education to women, particularly given the increased number of women managing the combined roles of single mothers, homemakers, and employed workers: "in 1900 the average age of employed women was 26; as of 1960, the average age was 41, and, in 1963, more than half of all women in the age group from 45 to 54 were in paid employment" (p. 70).

When asked to identify areas of the report relevant to nurses, Peterson responded that the idea of women working as a normal, expected event may encourage them to choose a nursing career. In addition, there could be greater preparation of women for new kinds of technical jobs and increased attention to economic issues affecting women, both nurses and non-nurses. "The Commission believes that we must upgrade, both financially and in working conditions, those areas where large numbers of women are employed" (p. 70). Furthermore, women should be covered by basic protections enjoyed by other workers. For example, nurses and many women were not covered under the Federal Fair Labor Standards Act and could not use their right to bargain collectively. The report recommended coverage of workers at nonprofit institutions, including hospitals, and state laws that would protect the right of all workers to join unions and bargain collectively. At that time, only 3 million of 24 million women were covered by collective bargaining agreements.

Peterson emphasized the lower economic status of women based on the depressed salary statistics in the 1960s, and on the need for continuing education to retool women for the job market. But, asked Gerds, how did

Peterson respond to the charge that the commission wants to take women away from the home? Peterson responded, "Very simply. Women are already away from the home. . . . Then, too, many of the Commission's recommendations are really aimed at strengthening home and community life" (p. 72). Homemaker services in times of emergency, services for ill, disabled, or convalescing women, easily accessible maternal and child health services—these and many other recommendations that would involve nurses were enumerated by Peterson. Extensive child care services were particularly stressed as important supportive services for women working outside the home: "licensed day care is available to only some 185,000 children. But in nearly half a million families with children under six, the mother is frequently the sole support" (p. 72).

The report, claimed Peterson, was the first attempt in many years to bring to nurses once again the magnitude of the discriminatory social structure. She expected women's associations to select certain recommendations and work for them and the newly created state women's commissions to carry on the work. To her, nursing was vitally affected by the whole report, particularly in economic areas, but even she could not predict the explosion of women's energies and political actions that followed in subsequent years, which went far beyond existing women's organizations of the early 1960s.

Few in nursing were writing on women's issues at this time. Non-nurse and free-lance writer, Opal D. David (1962), director of the Commission on the Education of Women, American Council of Education from 1958 to 1961, noted that concepts about women were changing and, to anticipate the future for students and teachers in nursing, these changes must be understood and predicted. David stressed that women urgently needed opportunities to update their education, so that they might prepare themselves to return to the job market after having spent several years in childbearing and homemaking activities. Note that David, writing during the early 1960s, still seemed to assume that most women were married, bearing children, and staying at home.

David thought that women may have emancipated themselves into a new slavery of complex and multiple demands. She stated that women wanted higher education and from "four brash young females who matriculated at Oberlin College in 1837 . . . [has come a] 1961 contingent of a million and a half" (p. 82). Women wanted the vote, which has not created perfection, but in specific instances in education, welfare, and consumer interests, "the influence of women's votes has been decisive" (p. 82). Women, said David, did not want wars or the technological economy, so they could not be completely saddled with responsibility for the idea that women "can combine family responsibilities with work outside the home. . . . Whoever is to blame, there has been a disconcerting blurring between the masculine and feminine roles in our culture" (p. 82). Women were moving into men's occupations, but there was no threat to the child-bearing role, the one unchanging woman's role to which all else must be related. It is clear that David simply assumed that all women are, will or should be in this role.

David believed that people assumed that when a woman moves into areas previously reserved to men, her performance must equal his, but women's and men's life patterns are different. A young woman may marry at 20, and if she is intelligent and ambitious may obtain a bachelor's degree, but her probabilities of getting an MA is less, and a PhD, extremely slight. Although not wishing to discourage a girl for postponing or even foregoing marriage, David nevertheless stated, "it does not seem wise, or even desirable" for a girl who is committed to be a homemaker for 10 to 20 years "to invest large amounts of time in specialized training" (p. 83). With continuing education, however, perhaps marriage is not a foreclosure but a postponement of a professional career. Again, it is very obvious that the 1960s thinking on women's education assumed marriage and children and that all women's lives are based first on this expectation.

David did point to experimental programs that enabled older, returning women to obtain education. Still, she claimed, there are few women who expected to be free to work immediately after graduation. She noted that rapid technological changes and increases in knowledge required easier access for women to update their education without going through regular degree programs. But even with refresher and retraining courses, women had "to come to terms with the facts of [their] continuing role in the home. This means that, just as women probably always will earn fewer PhD's than men, so also fewer women are going to reach positions of top eminence in the professions or in business and industry" (p. 84).

A fortunate few, richly endowed with talent and energy, might be teachers. Quite clearly, the conservative nature of this expert's advice to nurses as women continued to limit them in both personal and professional roles. In addition, David's article made no sense to nurses whose leaders were women, nor to married nurses who were already working full-time in large numbers. Here is a woman, in charge of women's education for the nation's most prestigious organization in higher education, who restated and perpetuated the limitations on women's lives and work. Nevertheless, nurses continued to accept and print articles on women by non-nurses. The initial response by nurses to the reemerging feminist movement seems minimal. For many nurses, interest and involvement with feminist issues did not become a dominant motif in the profession until the 1970s.

The emerging concern for women's rights in the 1960s was not limited to the United States. In 1965 Claire Kirkland-Casgrain, Quebec minister of transportation and communications, provided an interesting portrayal of what was happening to women in Canada because of Bill 16. She claimed that the Quebec code was a "synthesis of two great traditions in western law—the Napoleonic Code and English statute law . . . [upholding the] law laid down by that rabid anti-feminist, Napoleon Bonaparte" (p. 527). The complete subjugation of women was avoided by applying some minor points of the old Anglo-Saxon tradition. After correctly condemning Napoleon, Kirkland-Casgrain satirically let him off the hook: "Was it for the faithlessness of Josephine that we have paid so dearly?" (p. 527).

To change the code, clear-thinking Canadian women had to elect representatives, but the struggle for the vote in Quebec stretched from 1922 to 1940, when the franchise was finally achieved. But for 25 years, "the Quebec wife remained, as before, under the domination of her husband . . . she enjoyed fewer privileges than a mentally retarded individual" (p. 527). Bill 16 provided that a married woman, in relation to property, was finally free to act as an individual and was restrained only when property was held in common. The minister said that future court decisions would be based on the presumption of the equality of two human beings, not on the notion of the servitude of wife to husband. But, asked Kirkland-Casgrain, how many women know of their freedom? Very few, she said, have used legal channels to change their status. Instead of blaming the male-controlled system, Kirkland-Casgrain believed women themselves had failed to break away from their preconceived ideas and their passivity regarding customs that still did not grant equality: "It seems to me that this is our own fault" (p. 528).

Some 25 years after franchise, there was only one woman in the 95-member Canadian Legislative Assembly. Quoting another woman (Menie Gregoire), Kirkland-Casgrain claimed, " 'The age of mature womanhood has started. Feminism is outdated' " (p. 528). Previously, women had struggled for the right to work or vote. This was now outmoded; women must simply *do* these things: "They must be worthy of their freedom" (p. 528). Again, instead of focusing on a male-defined system of justice that had, for centuries, denied women their property rights, nurses were told they had to be worthy of what should have been theirs all along! One wonders what men must be worthy of—since it is their system that forced Quebec women in marriage to forfeit all rights to property and even to their own children.

In 1965 Dorothy Kelly wrote another editorial on women, stating that her main reason for writing about women "is that women are such underdogs and, by and large, they don't even know they are. Why not, then, leave them in peace? Because we are not convinced that peace at any price is a suitable attitude for a human being" (p. 16). Kelly pointed to a Swiss Catholic woman, who had recently recommended that the priesthood be opened to women: "We were properly shocked, we must admit . . . the clergy either dismissed the Swiss woman as a crackpot or reiterated the usual male nonsense about the proper place of women which is you know where" (p. 16). Other women, said Kelly, were now tracing the history of the "forgotten sex" and she recommended that women do more than organize church suppers and raise piddly sums. Kelly took no position on women as priests. However, she did say, "We wish, for instance, that the women who blithely repeat that canard *All Women Were Made to be Mothers* would think about this instead of swallowing it whole and passing it on to other benighted individuals" (p. 17). Before relegating women to passive roles, Kelly wished women would use their brains to reflect on some of the ideas that were "afloat"; she could not believe that "God made two kinds of brains—male and female" (p. 17).

CLAIMING NORMALITY AND REPUDIATING OLD STEREOTYPES OF WOMEN LEADERS

Who would lead nurses to examine the new ideas "afloat"? In 1965 Mary Ann C. Iafolla wrote on the dilemma of nursing leaders, saying, "Women today have attained neither the amount nor the quality of leadership that the pioneers of the feminist movement anticipated they would, once the legal framework of women's rights was provided" (p. 54). Floundering in roughly the same three situations identified decades ago, women leaders, said Iafolla, had to deny their sex and rise above it, or compensate in leadership for inabilities to function as women, or try to combine both housewife and career roles.

Looking back to feminist leaders Lucretia Mott, Susan B. Anthony, and Elizabeth Cady Stanton, Iafolla said such women provided proof from the 19th century on that women can be powerful leaders. By the 1960s *The Feminine Mystique* had again empowered women and denied any innate female inferiority. Reviewing the evidence on stereotyped socialization and focusing on the emotional stress of career versus marriage, Iafolla asserted that women, whether single or married, were still likely to find gender "a handicap in the achievement of leadership status in a business or profession" (p. 58). The refrain, "I wouldn't work for a woman!" still indicated the subordination expected of women. What traits, asked Iafolla, evoke such a reaction? Gender-stereotyped responses to one survey portrayed female leaders as inconsistent, narrow, and dogmatic; or as autocrats and sticklers for ethical behavior, unfeeling, insecure, and selfish. To Iafolla, the reality was different: "Well organized occupations have usually been able to prevent the entry of women . . . discontinuity of employment [so common among women] is fatal to the development of occupational solidarity. The same attitudes and prejudices which keep women out of supervisory positions also limit their ability to develop strong leadership" (p. 59). Furthermore, male perceptions of female leaders may be shared by women, who may also stereotype female authority: "Women have traditionally been taught to think of men as managers, and in scrutinizing female leaders to see how they compare, they may be captious and unsympathetic in picking flaws" (p. 60).

To Iafolla, a degree of consensus did seem to substantiate some of the charges against women leaders, at least to a limited degree. Perhaps American women as a subordinated group reflected a conception of their status, and maybe "the female stereotype provides the images which the professional woman has of herself" (p. 60). The woman may assume characteristics of the dominant group as members of other subordinate groups have done. Her insecurity may also be exacerbated by the hostility expressed by work associates of both sexes; thus, a vicious circle is established.

In agreement with French feminist Simone de Beauvoir, Iafolla believed that subordination engendered a lack of self-assurance, causing the woman leader to be unable to forget herself, placing "too much emphasis upon her successes and failures" (p. 62). What does this mean for women who are nurses? To Iafolla, an effective nurse must be a leader; yet she, like other women leaders, encounters the same responses, particularly from male physicians who treat her as their handmaiden; by women physicians, who assert their superiority in order to achieve recognition; by male nurses, who automatically get leadership positions; and by female staff nurses, who may react with competition or jealousy.

To achieve a synthesis of status and functional leadership, the nurse must recognize that she is assigned contradictory roles. Even within herself, conflicting gender roles of wife and mother may make her feel abnormal. Therefore, the leader nurse must *claim normality* and *repudiate the old image*, refusing to identify with demeaning stereotypes. Qualities of leadership must be learned during education in which nurses and physicians are jointly conditioned through common experience in the same university settings. If the nurse wishes to be judged on merit, not gender, she must seek the answer inside herself.

Thus, in the mid-1960s the approach to power recognized societal causes, but focused on individual solutions and analyses. Still, Iafolla was hopeful: "As she becomes more dissatisfied with her lot in life and recognizes the need to change and then desires to change, she will change. Someday—not today, tomorrow, or the next day, but someday—enlightened by the examples of even greater women leaders, society's attitudes will also change" (p. 66).

THE PROPER PLACE OF WOMEN

With few exceptions, nurses as women were not writing on gender and sexist issues. Although some were expressing strong concern about economic inequities, others were still engaged in "blaming the victim," behavior typical of oppressed groups. In 1968 the *Catholic Nurse* reprinted a speech by Lillian O'Connor, presented to the Congress of the World Union of Catholic Women's Organizations. In her speech, O'Connor claimed that throughout history and in every corner of the globe, women have been revered and honored as very special creatures, but, at the same time, their ideas have been scorned and their activities outside the home have been denied and belittled. Women themselves have tended to support the "myth of angelic sweetness in home as a haven" (p. 26). Relying on feminist Simone de Beauvoir, O'Connor stated that women realize what they would lose, but not what they might gain from changes in this ideology.

That women have not counted for much in the public world is, to O'Connor, a state of affairs for which "women share as much blame as our fathers and brothers—if not more" (p. 27). Thought of as special, women are not aware of their part in fostering discrimination against themselves: "What has brought us to this third quarter of the 20th century still arranged in the swaddling clothes of earlier times? Still unsure of our own identity as persons, insecure, full of self-distrust, unable to exult in being what we are?" (p. 27). Despite great achievements of individual women, nowhere are freedom, equality, and full participation complete, and, in fact, said O'Connor, there are even instances of retrogressions during the past few decades. It is fascinating that O'Connor does not name those who were rejecting women's ideas; who were turning them, discouraged and apathetic, back to their familiar corners to seek "security" in familiar routines. Indeed, it is women, not men, who must change before the "World of Tomorrow" obliterates the whole human race. Just who or what controls this world is, again, not stated. Nevertheless, O'Connor did realize that women have forcibly espoused change, but have "never expressed ideas that would destroy the race, every member of which she has, at the risk of her own life, brought into being" (p. 27).

By the 1960s women's history had again become obliterated, forcing O'Connor to insist that women must seek out the records of those "courageous women who wrote and spoke out for humanity" (p. 27). Trying to maintain her Christian roots, O'Connor turned to Eve, who was blamed for the first disobedience, but whose own ideas on this issue went unrecorded. "Perhaps," said O'Connor, "she was too insecure and thus left Adam to do all the talking!" (p. 28). Realizing that she was not going to get anywhere with such biblical stories, O'Connor leaped forward to the Industrial Revolution and the gradual recognition of the "rights of the weak." O'Connor, in agreement with novelist Pearl Buck, said this marked a tremendous evolutionary step forward.

To once again give back to women their obliterated history, O'Connor asserted that, with the printing press, ideas were more widely spread and women could quietly read men's thoughts. Some women even began to write and speak, but were "reviled, heaped with abuse, and sometimes physically attacked . . . [other women] joined in the contumely heaped upon their outspoken sisters even more vigorously than did their fathers and mothers" (p. 28). Thus, the more outspoken and vigorous women presumably were blamed most by other women. Although O'Connor was reticent about naming men as the aggressors, she was eloquent in her tribute to feminists Mary Wollstonecraft, Frances Wright, and Lucy Stone, who were often only mentioned in footnotes to history, but were all significant motivating forces for the rights of the weak.

Wollstonecraft's 1792 book, *Vindication of the Rights of Woman*, was little known by the 1960s and when mentioned at all, as in encyclopedias, O'Connor found the focus was not on Wollstonecraft's ideas, but on the storm of opposition created against her in England. O'Connor next resurrected Frances Wright, a Scotswoman who advocated universal education, political equality, abolition of slavery, and better working conditions for women. But, said O'Connor, Lafayette regarded Wright as a woman, who with ruthless violence, had broken loose from the restraints of decorum and, with contemptuous disregard, leaped the boundary of feminine modesty, exhibiting herself as a female lecturer; nevertheless, he admitted she had a lofty philanthropy, sincerity, purity of heart, brilliance, and power of mind. Despite less laudatory male critics, women, claimed O'Connor, were Wright's harshest critics.

O'Connor noted that American Lucy Stone had to work nine years before she could enter Oberlin College because her father would not help her financially. At Oberlin, only a few courses were open to her, provided that she would sit in silence. Stone persisted, however; she spoke against slavery, recognized women's lack of freedom, and worked for their rights. Again, O'Connor blames the great majority of women from whom came the most bitter criticism of Stone. O'Connor says that Stone merits "only a sarcastic comment or two in the historical records of the day" (p. 30). That most, if not all, historians in the 19th century were male is a fact left unstated.

That these three women were from the industrialized Western world was, to O'Connor, accidental, since their situations were common to women everywhere—women who live in a prescribed circle of activity, suffer rejection of their ideas, experience difficulty obtaining education, and hear the "monotonous reiteration of prejudice" (p. 31). Again, O'Connor blamed the majority of women who, less courageous and daring, are "bowed into a passivity they themselves do not recognize" (p. 31).

Indeed, O'Connor claimed that women enjoy all the advances of the world, "having barely lifted a finger to bring them about" (p. 32). It is particularly ironic that this article, published by nurses, specifically denies women's central role in controlling epidemics, improving sanitation, and instituting health measures. It is women who were largely responsible for changes in public health, but this O'Connor did not know or recognize. To her, women are derelict in following through on the humanitarian ideas of our foremothers, losing sight of their leadership, now buried, she said, in a few footnotes to history. The processes of that burial, how it was accomplished (predominantly by men in control of publishing and education), remains unrecognized by O'Connor.

Are we afraid of recognizing our foremothers' accomplishments? Are we ashamed of our female pioneers because we fear being accused of neglecting wife and mother roles? O'Connor turned for an answer to psychology, but, despite finding volumes of work in the social sciences, concluded that few of the experts encouraged women to do any thinking and advised women, who defied the men's expertise, to keep to their own sphere. To O'Connor, the psychological and psychoanalytic writing had not reduced, but added to the mountains of prejudice. Freud's "anatomy is destiny" was, for example, derived from his own wishes and needs, which were uppermost; for example, when he became irritated with the noise from his sister's piano playing, her piano was simply removed from the house.

Although it is obvious that Freud was only one of many "scholarly" men who defined woman by keeping her in her place, O'Connor continued to focus on the women, the conformists, driven to acceptance of passivity, who bring up their children by reinforcing the so-called inferiority of daughters. Furthermore, O'Connor claimed that women thoughtlessly accepted scientific and technological changes, except if they made chores a little less dreary. They did not comprehend that each change altered their whole situation and that of "mankind." Ironically, nurses republished these sentiments even though they themselves had actively participated in scientific advances—to the extent they could force medical, hospital, and university men to admit them to scientific knowledge in formal education in institutions of higher learning.

O'Connor asserted that anatomy includes the brain, so it is women's destiny to think and use their mental powers, which have been stunted and warped away from the essential to the trivial. This has been done, not by men, said O'Connor, but by the "very women who have suffered most under the dictates of society" (p. 35). Indeed, O'Connor said that women should not find fault with fathers and brothers until women themselves can recognize their own worth: "The human race cannot continue with half of its members refusing to function at the level required in the 20th century" (p. 69). O'Connor urged women to help each other recognize their own worth so they could focus on the larger picture of humanity. Clearly, she still blamed the victim, not the victimizer. Nevertheless, she believed that women must develop their own scholars who could delve into original documents and winnow out the essentials; that women must reject totally the thought that "the brain that comes with a little girl baby is somehow inferior" (p. 69). Speaking to Catholic women from all over the world, she told them that women must teach their children, "all of them, boys and girls alike, that insecurity is the fate of MAN and is not the peculiar prerogative of women" (p. 69).

A FAIRER, SQUARER DEAL

By the end of the decade, the focus had shifted. In a 1969 article, Catherine East, executive secretary of the Citizens Advisory Council on the Status of Women, U.S. Department of Labor, concluded: "Most men have been unabashedly 'masculinists' since Adam. [Women] shall have to be unabashedly 'feminists,' working with the protective mantle of our organizations, until we all become full members of the human race" (p. 60). East's paper, given before the Women's Joint Congressional Committee in Washington, DC, and reprinted for a nursing audience, began with a rationale for the issue of what women really want. East feared that the topic might sound selfish, grasping, and unfeminine since women are trained to be unselfish, thinking always of others, expected to be kind, gracious, sympathetic, cooperative—in other words, tractable. East asserted that a better world for women will also be a better world for men and children, "but our first hurdle is the need to recognize openly and honestly that we want a fairer, squarer deal for ourselves, our daughters, and our granddaughters—simply because we are human beings, entitled to the same rights, respect, and dignity accorded other human beings" (p. 38).

There is, stated East, nothing wrong or unfeminine in seeking to be considered fully human. As a *Ladies Home Journal* poll found, many women felt their husbands treated them as not too bright children. In contrast to O'Connor, East emphasized organized action. To her it was unproductive for individual women to talk in general of sexism or specifically of personal experiences with discrimination unless they banded together with other women to take action.

Women in poverty, said East, particularly needed help: by the end of the 1960s two-thirds of all poor adults were women—11.2 million, compared to 6.9 million men. Children in women-headed families, because of lower earnings of women, were more likely to grow up in poverty. The gender differences were so severe that, according to East, women of all races, who had finished high school, earned less than White men with only eight years of education. Clearly, feminist foremothers had won some battles, but there were many still ahead. East briefly summarized the salient facts. She condemned the high unemployment rates and the programs to alleviate poverty, since most of these ignored women and girls. This was particularly damaging to teenage girls, among whom the pregnancy rate was increasing. Women's jails and prisons, especially those for delinquents, were inadequate, providing gender stereotyped training or none at all. In addition, longer jail sentences were given to women than to men for the same offenses. Girls were not admitted to schools or universities under the same standards as boys. Newspapers were unwilling to abandon segregated employment ads, even opposing new civil rights legislation.

East recommended a drastic revision of marital property laws. Women must have both public and private discussions *with men* and insist that all decision-making bodies include women, particularly on issues affecting them. By what means feminists would force men and resistant women to face these problems was left unclear. Indeed, East asserted that sex discrimination was still a matter of laughter and ridicule.

With women's issues largely ignored in the media, how could women keep informed about their rights? Major federal court decisions went unnoticed in the press—even the important *Weeks v. Southern Bell* case, which established

employment access for women and equity of opportunity. Most women knew
nothing of this, and not one in a thousand women understood discriminatory
marital property laws or court cases pending about them. East credited
women's sections in newspapers for beginning to publicize feminist issues and
newly emerging organizations that were dedicated to equity. Even some men,
whose help should be acknowledged, were beginning to write articles and lend
their support.

These few messages to nurses on gender roles and feminism were often
written by non-nurses and were interspersed among the more familiar
exhortations for women to sustain their traditional societal roles. These mixed
messages were no doubt confusing to nurses. For example, Mary Hoffman
(1970), a physician, advised the traditional role for women in the *Occupational
Health Nursing Journal*: "We should develop our feminine traits and use them
to their best advantage. Men are to be respected as the head of the home and
business, and be admired for their male aggressiveness and mechanical minds;
but in these traits, women should not try to imitate them. Women should be
the heart instead of the head. They should be subtle with true empathy and
unemotional sympathy, and should rule with kindness" (pp. 16–17).

Hoffman warned nurses that no one likes a domineering woman; thus, they
should be realistic, shifting from "blind obedience to prudence" (p. 17).
Furthermore, nurses should make people like them by being genuinely
interested in others, by smiling, being good listeners, talking in terms of
others. To win others over, nurses should avoid arguments, never telling a
man he is wrong, letting him talk a great deal and making him feel the idea
is his: "As women, we must remember not to nag, not to try to make people
over, or to criticize them" (p. 17), giving instead courteous attention and
appreciation. After all these traditional injunctions, Hoffman claimed that "we
must never underestimate the power of a woman . . . no one will be known
as a great heroine but each woman, as she does her share of work—and a little
more, will be able to see and bring out the best in her fellow man" (p. 17).
The nurse's skills are outdated, said Hoffman, so she must change not only
these but her role as a woman as well: "She must not fear these changes or
refuse to accept them, but rather see them as a challenge to increase her skill
in the art of nursing" (p. 17).

It is astonishing that such an article would appear in a nursing journal at
a time when so many women were becoming assertive, using their *heads* as
well as hearts to analyze women's problems and rights. Indeed, it is clear that
the majority of women who wrote on gender issues during the 1960s were
non-nurses. President Kennedy's Commission on the Status of Women and
Friedan's *Feminist Mystique* served as catalysts for women such as Sanders,
Peterson, David, and East to write about gender inequities. Articles by nurses
such as Kelly, Iafolla, and O'Connor were few and far between. Fortunately,
the 1970s marked a period of increasing activism, an explosion of very

different articles by nurses on women's rights—quite unlike Hoffman's restatement of the old sexist mythology.

Chapter 6

The Turning Point:
Nurses Connect with the
Women's Movement

The few lone voices in the 1950s and 1960s, mostly those of non-nurses, had become, by the early 1970s, radicalized by the second wave of feminism. Women in nursing began speaking out more and more about sex discrimination, becoming more assertive in their published analyses, urging empowerment through role changes, and calling for political, social, and economic action to right the wrongs experienced by women. A clear feminist construction of nursing history was advocated by several nurse scholars and, increasingly, attention was given to the negative effects of media and public stereotyped images of nurses. Nurses' consciousness of their subordinated and oppressed group status became heightened, propelling some nurses to advocate radical role-breaking, risk-taking behaviors. A strong movement emerged calling for unity among all women, but professional unity in particular. Nurses began to work to improve their economic conditions, some even advocating union membership to gain pay equity. In their many professional journals, women in nursing began to reflect and expand on the earlier themes of their feminist foremothers. As noted previously, reemerging feminist activities in the broader society can be traced to the early 1960s; however, it was not until 1970 that one of the first clearly activist articles was again published by a nursing leader.

RESURRECTING THE POWER MOTIF

Sixty-two years after Lavinia Dock made her impassioned pleas for nurses to vote for suffrage, Mary Kelly Mullane (1970) acknowledged that a "women's liberation movement" was visible in the media. Although she placed these words in quotes, as if the reality of reemerging feminism was not quite real, Mullane, nevertheless, recognized that nurses could grapple with their situation only if they understood the past history of women. To her, men's history, an unending progression of battles, peace treaties, and conflicts, leading to more battles and peace treaties, had excluded women as unimportant to the cycles of war, peace, and again war. Further, Judeo-Christian religious history depicted women "as helpers to the clergy, unworthy to be admitted, except as observers" (p. 7) to church rites. Indeed, orthodox Jews daily thanked God they were not created women, a view presumably established by Paul and passed on to subsequent generations of Christian male authorities.

Mullane claimed that a woman's life was traditionally the life of the family at home; and, until a century ago, most everyone was at home. When men migrated so did women. Indeed, Alexis de Tocqueville, noted Mullane, claimed in the early 1830s that the strength of the American people could be mainly attributed to the superiority of their women. Although Mullane claimed that gender interdependence existed in the 19th century, this assertion blurs the reality of women's legal subjugation. She was correct, however, in observing the increased separation of private and public lives. Indeed, society had changed faster than had men's and women's adjustment to change.

Mullane asserted that women's future role in shaping society was up to them. In agreement with Catherine East (1969), Mullane said that what women needed were the same rights, respect, and dignity accorded to all human beings. Relying on East's data, Mullane emphasized that two-thirds of adults in poverty were women; earnings revealed gross discrimination and injustice; courts supported different laws for women and different prison sentences for the same offense. However, she questioned whether women would break their lethargy, ambiguity, and escapism from the world's interests to regain control, even though this was a real possibility given the fact that women had on average almost forty years of life left after their children were in school.

Mullane urged women, especially nurses, to shape future policy through the use of their political franchise won by feminists of an earlier era. Observing that women of voting age outnumber men, she encouraged nurses to establish their rights through political processes. Further, she strongly believed that the division of occupational roles between men and women was artificial, stating, "Women can turn this world of ours around. Whether or not they will remains to be seen. There is no question of their intelligence or ability" (p. 9). Thus, like Dock, Wald, and other nurses before her, Mullane resurrected the power motif and urged nurses to recognize their own group identity as women.

Mullane cited research conducted by Gass (1967), who studied college juniors and seniors and found they planned marriage, a comfortable living, full-time care of two or three children, and possible part-time work; however, there was no evidence of a strong drive toward occupational mastery or success. Gass concluded that the students' rosy picture was a failure in the transmission of life's realities. In a second study, Gass found that middle-aged women had a dim perception of what they were or could be; believing they had much to give, they remained unsure of *how* to give. Intellectually impoverished, they felt little respect or attention was paid to what they said. Even volunteer work was dissatisfying to them. They urgently needed to move into the world beyond home. Gass's third study focused on women doing graduate work; committed to both profession and family, they experienced difficulties finding child care and negative attitudes toward them as working women who presumably needed no intellectual development.

Mullane foresaw continuous rapid social change and asserted: "I am convinced that mankind has so debased our planet and created such efficient means of its destruction that a drastic reordering of our social goals and ethical standards is imperative" (p. 9). Instead of economic territorial goals, vital human needs must take priority; and women, because of centuries of socialization to deal with essential needs, had the talent to create new priorities. But would women devote the necessary discipline, thought, and work to shape policy? Mullane warned, "Unless enough women are found to do just that our world may not survive" (p. 9).

As noted earlier, women in Canada, both nurses and non-nurses, were engaged in a reassessment of their roles and status, similar to the efforts of American women. Articles began to appear in the *Canadian Nurse* on women's status. For example, Sister M. Thomas More (1971), still using the stereotyped idea that women nag, turned the injunction against such behavior into a "right to nag," which to her was both inalienable and essential. She dismissed the definition of "nag" as an aged, inferior, or unsound horse and reconstituted the original dictionary meaning: "to affect with recurrent awareness, to make recurrently conscious of something (as a problem, issue, or concern)" (p. 38). More felt no need to teach nurses how to do this since women were all-time pros in making others recurrently conscious of something! Since women were already stereotyped as naggers, the only question remaining was, "What are fit subjects for nagging?" (p. 38).

According to Margaret Mead, many women had a cave-women mentality, concerned only with the interior decoration of their caves and with their children and husbands. More connected Mead's assertion to Friedan's comment in a seminar that there must be something better than getting the kitchen sink whiter than white. More concluded that too few women have interests that are really significant for the rest of humanity.

That human society needed renewal was not debatable. Nor was the fact that women, individually, could restore meaning to their lives. In More's life, the crises in religious orders, with "girls . . . going over the walls like flies" (p. 39), had forced her to reconsider the concept of "calling." Was it a state in life? A way of making a living? A service to the common good, involving acts to create change? For what function did women's groups exist? "Now if I were to judge the purpose of most women's organizations, I would say they exist to collect old clothes and to eat . . . and men's organizations exist to wear old clothes and to drink" (p. 39). She asked women to check out the purposes of their organizations and to seek leadership focused on vision, which is often killed when idea-women are labeled too impractical or idealistic. Because they are fearful of new ideas, More claimed, women develop cerebral contraceptive devices to prevent the birth of brain children. However, she never presented the feminist visions that would change the cave-woman mentality, except to suggest that women's organizations focus on important societal issues.

What the important issues are becomes more apparent in an editorial by Virginia A. Lindabury (1971), who reviewed the *Report of the Royal Commission on the Status of Women in Canada*, chaired by Anne Francis, and usually referred to as the *Francis Report*. Comparable to the earlier American report by President Kennedy's Commission, the well-documented and carefully compiled account of discrimination against Canadian women could, according to Lindabury, lead to radical changes if both sexes were prepared to study and react to it objectively, putting pressure for action on all levels of government. To her, equal pay for equal work remained only a principle until there was legislation to enforce it.

Lindabury deplored the discrepancies between male orderlies, with no formal training but higher wages, and female nursing assistants, with 10-month training but lower incomes. Furthermore, male orderlies were automatically promoted to specialist orderlies, but the women were not. Such inequities were not condoned in the report, which condemned women's lower earnings in predominantly female occupations and professions. According to her, the Canadian Nurses Association asserted that "the cause of the shortage of available nurses is not so much an inadequate number of trained nurses as the fact that nurses are entering other occupations with better pay and working conditions" (p. 26). But why have women stayed in traditional occupations? They simply do not have that many other options.

Gender segregation could be changed by the government in its pay scales, based on comparisons of women's professions with pay rates in other professions, rather than by prevailing market values, since these are notoriously sexist and sustain the problem. But the Canadian government did not lead the way. For example, only 6.3% of those appointed to boards of directors were women. The issue of poverty was raised in the report, which noted that thousands of elderly women were living lives of loneliness and deprivation and advised adjustments in government benefits. But, said Lindabury, the voice of the government is the voice of men; even a change in the abortion law was decided by 263 men and one woman. The political reality in Canada was succinctly stated: "Nowhere else in Canadian life is the persistent distinction between male and female roles of more consequence. No country can make a claim to having equal status for its women so long as its government lies entirely in the hands of men" (p. 26).

THE UNIVERSAL MORAL IMPERATIVE

The year 1971 represents a turning point. From this time onward, a rush of articles by nurses, and occasionally by other scholars, appeared in nursing journals. Many of these writers shared their anger, discouragement, optimism, and ideas during a decade marked by intense debate and sometimes enthusiastic support for female liberation. During this decade, some nurses began to realize that the women's movement could help them and that improvements in the status of nursing were inextricably related to the goals expressed by those in the women's movement. Thus, we find strong feminist nurses such as Wilma Scott Heide (1971), then chairwoman of the National Organization for Women, making a clear set of connections between the liberation of women and of the nursing profession. Heide pulled no punches, producing the best feminist nurse statement since Lavinia Dock's earlier uncompromising words. To Heide, in all social institutions and even in the language, men are viewed as human and women as the "other," "the deviant, the body, the reproducer, the subservient, the secondary class of people" (p. 4). Even now, said Heide, some have "the gross insensitivity to wonder why there's a women's rights/liberation movement" (p. 4). Referring to Kate Millett's (1970) book, *Sexual Politics*, Heide observed that women are conditioned to act out their "female nature." To survive, nurses do this by playing the male doctor-female nurse game. To seek fulfillment outside of marriage and family is to want to be a man or like a man. To this assumption, Heide said, what arrogance! Human wet nurse, incubator, or sperm donor are the only exceptions to the rule that "*all* interests, roles, and jobs are potentially human interests, roles, and jobs" (p. 4).

Heide believed that physicians were overtrained for cure and undereducated for care and nurturance, usually provided by nurses who, as an oppressed group, identify with and accommodate to their oppressors for survival, economic support, and career advancement. Thus, nurses become mired in the doctor-nurse game, the transactional neurosis that allows the physician to appear to be in complete authority. As noted in Chapter 2, Heide was actively involved in the civil rights movement, and claimed that we have only recently stopped training Black people to "know their place." We continue, however, to teach women that they have a predetermined place in society. At least, said Heide, Black people are aware of the racist system, which is now in the national conscience, but similar damage is caused by gender stereotyping, though many people were not aware of it, nor had it yet reached the national conscience.

Indeed, most "women's concerns," which are actually human concerns, are decided by men. Abortion, a failure of birth control, is governed by outdated laws made by men, who continue to expect women to bear and rear children as their primary role in life, regardless of the mental illness, family stress, and even violence that correlate with uncontrolled births. Peace, another issue associated with women, is one over which they have little actual control. Indeed, the sanction for violence in toys, games, and competition socialize boys for war, not peace. It is clear by the beginning of the 1970s that the hope for peace expressed by some earlier nursing leaders had not been achieved.

According to Heide, "Women's liberation is a universal moral imperative. . . . Economic and social independence . . . allows love, . . . unencumbered by duty, fear, or oppression" (p. 16). There should be no higher priority than the liberation of half the population; this, to Heide, is the fundamental human oppression out of which other social problems emerge. For example, in the health-care delivery system, many problems actually are caused by the low status and subservience of nurses, which strikingly parallel the status and subservience of all women. But, said Heide, "The Nurse Practice and Medical Practice Acts are not eternal imperatives. They've been changed before and we'll change them again" (p. 16). Indeed, Heide believed that nurses, who are committed to care, human development, and survival, must lead in developing new paradigms of the human family and society. Heide believed that women *can* create change and when people see this, women and nurses will move to a new level of self-confidence. Heide saw this emerging in the young women to whom she spoke at the National Student Nurses' Association; she invited them to join in the "most profound social movement the world has ever known!" (p. 16).

EQUALITY OF RIGHTS: AGAIN, THE ERA

Feminists in the latter 1960s had brought the Equal Rights Amendment (ERA) back to the public's consciousness. Attorney Toby Golick explained the ERA to nurses in 1971, asking, do women need it? Golick stated: "Every year since 1923, a women's rights amendment has been introduced in Congress with little publicity and less success" (p. 285). This simple statement of historical fact was, at the same time, a shocking indictment of the intransigence of political men; of women who had turned their backs on their feminist foremothers and did not even know that a few women had sustained their earlier work; and of a society that had trivialized the history of women to such a degree that it was once again invisible. Indeed, Golick even had to restate the actual words of the amendment: "Equality of rights under the law shall not be denied or abridged by the United States or any state on account of sex. Congress and the several states shall have the power, within their respective jurisdictions, to enforce this article of appropriate legislation" (p. 285). Golick further explained the process of adoption by a two-thirds majority of Congress and the ratification by legislatures in three-fourths of the states.

In 1970 the ERA passed the House, but died in the Senate; it "stirred considerable controversy, much of it ill-informed and some of it silly" (p. 285).

As in the 1920s serious debate focused on "protective" legislation for women whose "physical, emotional, psychological, and social differences," said Democrat Emanuel Celler of New York, have existed "ever since Adam gave up his rib to make a woman" (p. 285). This reversal of who actually gives birth to whom was still alive in the mythology expressed even in Congress! As in the past, women from labor unions, such as Myra K. Wolfgang, testified that the amendment would invalidate women's protection from working longer hours, which may be fine for professionals but not for women in laundries, hotels, restaurants, and assembly lines. Feminists argued that *all people* should receive the best working conditions, but that the experience of the past half century proved that men in power had used women's "protections" as ways to exclude them or to pay them less money. Certainly, nurses had seldom been protected, often working, for example, ten to sixteen hours daily, or even double shifts. In addition, nurses' absence from union coverage was often ignored by organized workers.

As Golick noted, other women unionists, such as Dorothy Haener, claimed that women were "protected" by being prevented from competing for high-paying jobs and lucrative overtime pay. Furthermore, chairs for rest periods should be provided not just for women, but also for men. More important, the absence of job security following maternity leaves in 45 states made the provision of chairs for women a comparative triviality. What Lillian Wald and other early nurse activists wanted was not what eventuated; instead "a pattern of inconsistency and irrationality" existed in the legislation on the books. For example, women could work as barmaids in all but 10 states; night work was illegal in 18 states, but phone operators and domestics continued to do such work.

To those who believed the issues should be dealt with specifically one at a time, lawyer Eleanor Norton pointed out that legislation is irregular and time consuming, and can be rescinded whenever men in legislatures decide to act. To feminists, making women a part of the Constitution, in one stroke, would force a national attack on the pervasive discrimination. The opposition centered, as Golick said, "around the rather silly issue of whether the amendment would allow separate toilets for men and women . . . [but] even the most enthusiastic supporters of women's liberation are glad to leave the men their urinals" (p. 286).

To Golick, the amendment implied that there is no rational basis for treating the sexes differently. Thus, it would eliminate blatant discrimination in laws that barred women from certain occupations; favored men in estate distribution when their deaths occurred without wills; limited or excluded women from juries; restricted wives' control of their own earnings or from going into business; allowed husbands, but not wives, to sue for divorce if women, but not men, were "unchaste" before marriage; and set different ages for marriage for men and women. All these and many other inequitable laws would be ruled unconstitutional.

Perhaps the most controversial issue was, and still is, the draft laws. Once again, as in the past, women's role in war created confusion. Feminists supporting peace said no one should be drafted. And the protest against the Vietnam War eventually led to debates on an all-volunteer army. Certainly, it was not until this century that all men would be registered and many drafted for training as warriors. Of course, military conscription could, as Golick stated, be revived, but exemptions for both women and men could be enacted, as they were for men in previous wars in this century. Surprisingly, Golick did not address the issue of nursing and the draft. As noted in Chapter 3, women in nursing have been consistently involved in wars, volunteering to serve their country and nearly being drafted toward the end of the Second World War. Thus, nurses have always been involved in men's wars, even though they have been divided on the rightness of this involvement. Should they or other women be involved in actual combat? Golick thought they would probably be exempted on the basis of strength or problems in housing both sexes, but would weaker men also be excluded? Golick concluded that the ERA might make women eligible for combat duty. Over time, it is increasingly clear that women in the armed forces have been trained for combat and have been involved in preparation for certain kinds of combat situations. For nurses, the problem of combat is peculiarly problematic, but Golick did not address this aspect of the issue.

Instead, Golick turned to other issues, such as the law on husbands' support of wives, and concluded that changes in the law would in this matter and all others probably extend women's privileges to men. In the case of racism, courts have usually extended White persons' privileges to others. Golick's position has been subsequently supported in court decisions on sexism, but women are still not full citizens under the Constitution.

No one, said Golick, expected the worst discrimination in private practice and social custom to be completely erased by the constitutional amendment, but it would commit the nation "irrevocably and absolutely to providing equality to all regardless of sex . . . [and] women will know they are supported by no less august an authority than the United States Constitution, and this will be no small achievement" (p. 287). Indeed, this achievement is yet to be accomplished. But the American Nurses Association (ANA) did reverse its position from the 1920s, as noted in Chapter 4, and voted to back the amendment; thus, Lavinia Dock's position, not Wald's, was eventually supported.

Individual nurses, such as Ruth Greenberg Edelstein (1971), urged nurses to fight for the ERA, because equal rights for women meant equal rights for nurses. However, she cautioned: "Ardent feminists have been advising women not to become nurses because by doing so they will perpetuate their inferior status as women. Rather than admonishing women to stay out of nursing, feminists would be well advised to encourage creative and talented people to enter the field, for the status of the pervasively female nursing profession with its massive membership has a major impact on the status of women" (p. 294).

Edelstein resurrected historical images of nurses and reinterpreted them as women in revolt. She defended nursing, saying that it required highly specialized functions, extensive knowledge, skill, and innovative talent. To her, nursing had functioned as a social force for women's liberation since ancient times. History, however, does not support the idea that nursing is "natural" only to women, since women and men have distinguished themselves equally. Nor, claimed Edelstein, does history support the feminine characteristics of passivity, masochism, and subservience. Midwifery, for example, had for centuries been controlled and monopolized by women as independent practitioners. Not only midwives, but nurses in general rose up in the twelfth and thirteenth centuries, organizing secular orders, such as the Beguines of Leige, who fought male church authority, which dissipated but did not entirely destroy a movement that continues to the present. Furthermore, said Edelstein, at the Hôtel Dieu in Paris in 1487, when the nursing superintendent was convicted and discharged, nurses and patients revolted against her unjust conviction; her replacement could not function, the clerical ruling body was forced from the hospital, and outside nurses were harassed into leaving. At the Hôtel Dieu in Lyons in 1801, an open struggle occurred over a wide number of issues, such as whether a lay head could place and replace nurses. Forty nurses walked out, refusing to take orders from a layman. The nurses did not give in without a fight.

In agreement with early nursing leader Isabel Stewart, Edelstein stated that the sexist stratification system, which assigned slaves and women to household manual labor, is consistent with the separation of intellectual medical functions from manual labor. In 1945 Stewart claimed that liberal education was based on the Greek distinction between free leisure and subservient working classes. Men received liberal education to develop intellect; women's training focused on developing manual skills and instilling habits of obedience and industry. Medicine, eventually subsumed in the liberal arts, was intellectual study for gentlemen scholars, while surgery, nursing, midwifery, and anatomical dissection were manual tasks for the "uneducated." Out of the class distinctions emerged a master-servant prototype based on the assumption that it is inevitable and positively functional. Edelstein, however, claimed some theorists see a rigidly stratified society, with decision making and power concentrated in a few, as unable to adapt or use the full range of intelligence and talent in the society.

Through Nightingale's work, stated Edelstein, modern nursing encouraged women to emancipate themselves to take on the real work of the world. This is probably one of the first reworkings of Nightingale as feminist to emerge in this latter period: "Nightingale did as much for the liberation of women as those who later struggled for woman suffrage" (p. 296). Edelstein relied on the Nutting and Dock (1907) history of nursing to resurrect Dorothea Dix and

Elizabeth Blackwell, quoting them on the Civil War, which " 'washed away the petty anchors which had kept the majority of women carefully moored in the quiet remote little bays of domestic seclusion, and they floated out upon the stream of public duties' " (p. 296). It is interesting that Edelstein had to return to a history of nursing from the early feminist period to obtain this view, since many subsequent nursing histories did not include these feminist perspectives. (For a more thorough discussion of this issue, see Roberts & Group, *Nursing, Physician Control, and Medical Monopoly*.)

During the past 25 years, nurses had established economic security programs, endorsing state groups of the ANA to act as bargaining agents. From these predominantly women's organizations had emerged the precedent of combining both professionalism and unionism in the same body. On the other hand, some nurses, seemingly Freudian adherents, had assisted in the construction of antifeminist nursing models that perpetuated female inferiority. Edelstein warned that when theorists equate nurse and physician to mother and father, stereotypes cannot be broken. With the feminist critique, Freudian conceptions of women and family are anachronisms, and so are the false sociological dichotomies between women and nurses as expressive and men and physicians as instrumental. Edelstein advocated a unified model in which the ratio of these behaviors would alter according to specific conditions in any situation.

Edelstein believed that nursing education in universities could change the "functional freeze" that maintains male supremacy; but "without school curriculums and policies which deliberately emphasized unlimited potential for both sexes and freedom from sex-typing roles, rigid role enactments will change slowly" (p. 297). Sociologist Amatai Etzioni had previously designated nursing, social work, and teaching—all female professions—as semiprofessions, but Edelstein said it would be more appropriate to call them "half-human" because his criteria were based on the relative lack of autonomy. To her, it is no accident that men's fields are "professional" and women's "semi." However, she cautioned nurses, in their attempts to become a profession, to not rigidify and simply become more like male groups.

Edelstein believed that role confusion was exacerbated by the newest category (in 1971) of health-care provider, the physician's assistant, foisted on nurses by physicians. What is required is open and free communication to create nursing as a science. In fact, said Edelstein, when "nursing finally emerges as a science, the rights and status of women in general will advance a thousandfold" (p. 298). She asserted again that nursing's proud history in behalf of women's emancipation qualifies it as one of the greatest of women's professions. Any helping profession can be conceived of as "maternal," stated Edelstein, who rejected feminist Caroline Bird's (1968) assertion that nurses were "old masculists," who believe that woman's place is in the home and that women are mentally and physically incapable of doing men's work. Though Edelstein claimed that current nursing leaders and young nurses will be the "new feminists" who think sex roles are obsolete, her prediction is yet to be fully realized.

Joining Edelstein in resurrecting and reinterpreting history was Betty Clemons (1971), who focused on feminist leaders, bringing alive in a brief chronology the women's movement from the mid-19th century and the early 1900s. Describing the work of pioneering feminists, such as Elizabeth Cady Stanton and Lucretia Mott, Clemons interconnected the early women's movement with the nursing profession. She advised nurses to look at woman's "lib," not simply from a woman's perspective, but from a nurse's as well. Most nurses do not associate the two turbulent movements simultaneously, but Clemons invited nurses to step back a century and see a woman, defined as inferior by Divine intention, incapable of man's education or work. Forced into prostitution or marriage for security, the wife became civilly dead, her property, land, and even sentimental trinkets became her husband's to keep, squander, or sell. When he died, the son inherited everything and could leave a mother destitute. Most women accepted their total dependency on men for life, but a few, such as Mott and Stanton, did not. Both attended the 1840 World Slavery Convention in London, but were denied seats and herded behind heavy curtains, where they determined to revolt against their own subjugation.

Clemons also asked nurses to go back to 1854, to Scutari and Nightingale, who went there to prove that female nurses would not faint, could withstand hard work and effectively nurse men. Clemons saw Nightingale as a born liberated woman, who used the Crimean adventure, as she herself said, as "a fulcrum with which to move the world" (p. 74). She provided living proof to other women of what a woman could do. To Clemons, the interaction between nurses and feminists was clear: nursing offered a new and honorable vocation at the same time that feminism challenged women and girls to break with tradition. Nursing cleansed hospitals, making them safe for humanity, but feminists gave women human status.

The historic interplay was obvious at a meeting in the Woman's Building at the Columbian Exposition in Chicago in 1893. From England, Ethel Gordon Fenwick brought a nursing exhibit and asked for space for American nurses to meet. Here, noted Clemons, women, both inside and outside of nursing, organized and the professional bodies later known as the American Nurses Association (1911) and the National League for Nursing (1952) emerged from the nurses in attendance. In 1869 two women's suffrage groups had formed; in 1890 the two consolidated into the American Woman's Suffrage Association. From 1878 to 1920 the 14th Amendment was proposed to Congress every year. The vote was finally achieved, as were property rights for married women, changes in divorce laws, entrance into colleges and universities, inroads into several occupations and professions, and improved wages and working conditions for women. Suffrage led to a new social consciousness, and feminists such as Carrie Chapman Catt urged women to put an end to war. Nurses, however, had gone to war and returned to focus on public health and higher education, broadening women's horizons. Today, nurses are still trying to humanize health care and "we hear—faintly hear—Women's Lib in the air, calling—asking for *full* equality with man" (p. 78). For nurses, the sounds echo those of Fenwick, who saw the future of nursing as dependent upon the evolution of woman herself. In this century, concluded Clemons, nurses had gained a choice. Now she urged them to articulate their convictions.

SEXISM: NURSING'S FUNDAMENTAL PROBLEM

Nursing scholars, such as Virginia S. Cleland (1971), did proclaim their convictions. Cleland realized that sex discrimination was nursing's most pervasive problem. Indeed, sexism is the most *fundamental problem* in nursing, as a women's occupation in a male-dominated culture. From previous research in which Cleland had studied inducements for and consequences of married nurses reactivating their careers, she concluded that nurses could successfully combine career and marriage. At that time, she simply *assumed* that employment was secondary to family and that male employment models need not be used for women. However, the women's movement intervened in Cleland's life, and she acted initially to support faculty colleagues in fields where sexism was frankly overt. After reading the *Feminine Mystique, Born Female, Sexual Politics*, and numerous reports, articles, and news reports, Cleland "began to recognize how closely the entire social issue of equal rights for women actually relates to nursing" (p. 1542).

Sexual politics, power-structured relations in which men control through consent or force, is inherent in all social systems. At one time, said Cleland, she thought nursing had an advantage over other women's occupations because women controlled all power positions, but now she saw nursing in utter "isolation from all vestiges of power except within its own group . . . [but] the majority of nurses, like the majority of Southern blacks, have not been vocally or obviously concerned about their lack of power . . . dominance is most complete when it is not even recognized" (p. 1543). Like segregated school systems that allowed only internal upward mobility, nursing has allowed internal power for women when other routes were closed. Nursing administrators, like Black principals, were still available only within male medical systems in medicine, hospital administration, and higher education. Younger nurses, said Cleland, have not seen the "acquiescing behavior of the Aunt Janes . . . who really have no power except over the hapless and are only female Uncle Toms" (p. 1544). She further asserted that nursing had suffered, from the 1940s to 1960s, three decades of weak and unimaginative leadership, which paralleled "the growth of the cult of women as sex symbols" (p. 1544).

To her, this trend was influenced by Freudianism, which espoused for women the route to fulfillment by way of the uterus.

In contrast to early women leaders, more recent nursing leaders had been socialized to believe that women who envied men, tried to be like men—rejecting sexual passivity, nurturing maternal love, and male domination—could only feel "less than adequate when comparing themselves against the social standard of the woman-as-sex symbol" (p. 1545). Assuming leadership in a game whose rules are set by men, nursing leaders were in double jeopardy, risking double failure. This double bind has produced a generation of acquiescent, conservative leaders who can win individual plays, but learn that the game itself must be won by the male. The woman taught to acquiesce and fail also learns self-hatred for her "successful" gender socialization.

Cleland further condemned the general lack of leadership in decision making, in communicating needs, in obtaining resources, and in establishing and maintaining professional standards. More particularly, Cleland was dismayed by the lack of power in the economic system: "I am appalled every time I am forced to recognize that the vast majority of directors of nursing do not control their departmental budgets" (p. 1545). She could not imagine a man accepting such a title with no corresponding authority, particularly when 80% to 85% of the personnel budget is allocated to nursing service. Cleland saw faculty failing to formulate educational policy and practitioners negating rather than setting policies of practice, both turning for direction to administrative authority. This was the result of early female socialization, which trains nurses to support male administrators, fight against collective bargaining efforts, written contracts, and grievance procedures, and even to risk "the lives of patients rather than take forceful, public stands to insist on the closing of improperly staffed areas. I personally have known of only one director of nursing who has had sufficient courage and conviction to use her power to close units" (p. 1545).

Cleland noted that the *American Journal of Nursing* had perpetuated the confusion between gender and professional roles by publishing ads for job recruitment that did not offer money for professional services, but rather implied sexual fulfillment or marital success. Nursing leaders, who permit sexually motivated advertisements, warned Cleland, were enticing nurses by cheap sexual inducement, rather than paying honest salaries: "Could this common practice be called 'procuring'?" (p. 1545).

To Cleland, sex discrimination could be attacked, first, by ignoring marital status as a personal relationship that has no professional significance. "It should not make any difference professionally whether a nurse lives alone, lives with another female, lives with a male, or is married" (p. 1546). These are personal decisions, not evidence of social success or failure. Instead, Cleland recommended altering the usual male-defined work patterns, allowing for part-time work and relying on the 1964 civil rights legislation under Title VII, Executive Order No. 11246, to force decent salaries. Cleland herself was part of a group that had filed a complaint on wage discrimination, forcing her own university to deal with the lower salaries of women and those in nursing who were paid less than their male colleagues. Discriminatory practices in admissions to graduate schools, scholarships and fellowships, fringe benefits for staff and faculty—these and other issues, then being urged by feminists, were also being pushed by a few nurses such as Cleland. Still, she concluded, "I am very pessimistic about nursing. I do not believe nursing leaders see the need for the drastic change in nursing I believe is necessary" (p. 1547). Whether one agrees that assimilating more male nurses will break the profession's isolation, it is easy to concur that first-rate nurse clinicians could not be prepared using the traditional preparation, which created "a trained dependency characterized by high predictability of behavior" (p. 1547). Instead, Cleland called for nurses who could take calculated risks, not ones who strive to never make a mistake. However, she noted, "many women do not want this type of freedom and responsibility" (p. 1547). To her, "a nurse is a nurse is a nurse" must be changed to acknowledge those who will accept freedom and responsibility. Cleland feared, however, that the desire for protection would win over bolder plans and that nursing would "continue to be consumed by more aggressive groups" (p. 1547).

The conflicting definitions of "femininity" in nursing were central to Cleland's concerns. Victoria Wilson (1971), on the other hand, emphasized the need to dissolve stereotyped dichotomies, such as female intuition versus male intellect, women's dependence versus male independence. If the profession of nursing is to emerge once again with dignity and self-reliance, Wilson believed that it must discover its identity, just as each woman must discover her own. By eliminating stereotyped concepts of femininity, the nursing profession might begin to believe in and restructure itself. Wilson admitted that nurses have functioned passively under terms laid down by physicians who, with male hospital administrators and paraprofessionals, have left the nurse floundering without definite roles.

Historically, Wilson claimed that men have always tried to understand women, but on men's terms, using themselves as the standards of measurement. Christian teaching dichotomized women as madonna or prostitute; blamed women for leading the species into sin; and did not recognize Mary until her sexuality was denied by making her into an impregnated virgin. In philosophical thought, women were not better off. Aristotle, for example, claimed women to be only "matter," while the male principle was divine. Nor has psychoanalytic thought improved the perceptions of women; indeed, Freud's ideas have produced the view of women as passive masochists and mutilated "men," who envy and castrate the active, objective males when, as women, they deny their passive, intuitive, subjective natures. These ideas, said Wilson, have been sustained in a number of studies that have supported female subordination as an appropriate adjustment for women.

Wilson claimed, "The problems of the profession of nursing are the problems of women" (p. 215). Nurses as mother surrogates, presumably possessed of instinctual mothering, need no intellect. Since they actually *do* possess intellect, they must deny it; thus, they are caught in the bind described by feminist Matina Horner (1969), who found in her research on women both fear of failure and fear of success. To Wilson, nursing schools have perpetuated these problems by discouraging individualism and personal initiative, teaching the young woman to stay in her place, thus allowing physicians full intellectual reign. In social life, nurses are segregated from other young people and from men, often seen as outsiders and threats to the group's integrity, which is fostered by "pseudo-professionalism"—uniforms and school rules governing even hair and fingernail length.

Similarly, nurses hold on to nurturance rather than embracing productivity. Returning to the sacred icon, Wilson emphasized Nightingale's Crimean ventures as bold, dramatic rebellions against the stupidity and boredom of Victorian demands on women. It is, nevertheless, strange to hear this brilliant woman typified by Wilson as merely "quite intelligent." Still, she uses Nightingale as a bold icon, leaving behind the nurturing image. To enlarge nursing roles, a new self-identity is necessary—first, as human beings, and then as nurses, who are no longer extensions of physicians. This requires, however, that dependency, or more precisely, seeming passivity, be denied.

THE RISING CONSCIOUSNESS OF NURSES

As concern about the status of women increased in the early 1970s, more nurses began to realize that their socialization as women was compromising them as nurses; discrimination in the workforce was a part of a system of gender stratification; their consciousness-raising refocused their analysis and activities from individual to group concerns. Does identity as a woman come first, or identity as a nurse? How does a nurse deal with the reality that her profession has never had full autonomy? That subjugation to medicine produces only contingent, internal power?

These questions were at least partly considered in a 1972 panel on the "Liberation Movement: Impact on Nursing," which was presented at the Congress of the Association of Operating Room Nurses. One panelist, Teresa Christy, claimed: "The impression that many of the Women Liberationists have is that if you have some brains you would really like to be a doctor, but because you can't get into medical school you become a nurse, and you don't think of nursing as being a truly challenging or in any way intellectual type of career" (Christy, Stein, & Wolf, 1972, p. 71). She correctly predicted: "if nursing doesn't join this bandwagon [feminism], we are going to lose some of the best people for nursing and nursing is going to suffer as a result" (p. 71).

Christy's view represents a fairly common reaction by nurses to the women's movement: dismay toward feminists because of their assumed devaluation of the nursing profession. (In searching the literature, we could find few *published* attacks on nurses by feminists; however, their emphasis on entering male occupations certainly *implied* a devaluation of traditional nursing.) There was simultaneously an affirmation of feminism by some nurses and an awareness that nursing would have to achieve greater power and autonomy if it were to survive. Christy provided the historical perspective needed for an evaluation of feminism. She defended the current women's movement, admitting it was unpopular with the media today, but it had been equally unpopular with male reporters over a century ago when the 1848 Seneca Falls Convention was reported to be organized by " 'divorced wives, childless women, and sour old maids' " (p. 67). In actuality, Christy noted that Elizabeth Cady Stanton, for example, was married and had several children. Some reporters in the 19th century used "flattery" instead of sarcasm, saying, for instance, that women are nothing, but wives are everything, having enough influence without being politicians. If a " 'pretty girl is equal to 10,000 men and a mother is next to God' " (p. 67), then ladies should maintain " 'their rights as wives, belles, virgins and mothers and not as women' " (p. 68). Other journalists, said Christy, resorted to "reason," but their rationale required no logical response since " 'Every true hearted woman will instantly feel that this [feminism] is unwomanly' " (p. 68). Women at the convention were accused of being against " 'the order of things established at the creation of mankind, and continued 6,000 years' " (p. 68). Evidently, this continuity would be completely shattered, according to the journalists, and demoralized women would be degraded, losing their high sphere and noble destiny.

Even some women, said Christy, did not support feminism, being taught, as Emily Collins asserted, that being unknown was women's highest praise; that dependence was their protection and weakness their sweetest charm. Ridicule from both men and women was then, as now, focused on feminists' presumed sexlessness: lacking personal attraction, the thin maiden ladies or women were incapable of inducing any man, young or old, into marriage. These women "ravaged" themselves on the male sex. And, of course, homophobia also was implied. Susan B. Anthony was called repulsive, supposedly having strong hatred toward men. Sometimes, said Christy, marriage was acknowledged, but confined by the media to antiquated, homely females with henpecked husbands who could not say no to strong-minded women.

Although such allegations were denied by the actions of earlier feminists, Christy claimed that the views of the male-dominated press had not changed much, merely becoming a little more subtle toward current feminists: "inferences that she is probably sexually perverted, at the least a bra burner, or a man hater, and at the extreme the possibility that she is homosexual are common" (p. 69). Seeming to assume that earlier feminists primarily wanted the vote, Christy, nevertheless, did prove that early nursing leaders could not make headway with male legislators, because as women, nurses without the franchise had little political clout. Even when suffrage was won, Christy correctly noted that feminist nurses, such as Lavinia Dock, knew it was insufficient. As noted previously, Dock vigorously supported the ERA, which, said Christy, most nurses did not support until 1971 when the ANA finally voted to approve it (see discussion in Chapter 4).

Christy placed feminism in historical perspective, taking the sting out of identification of nurses as feminists; nevertheless, she noted nurses' tardy support of feminist efforts. Christy also examined current sexism in nursing, referring to Cleland's article (1971) and affirming her conclusions as true. Christy connected Cleland's work with Helen Creighton's (1971) discussion of legal cases pertaining to sex discrimination. One, for example, involved higher pay for male orderlies, which was sustained because they lifted patients and, according to the court, provided the psychological effect of security that female nursing aides could not give. What nurse, asked Christy, has not lifted patients? And what so-called psychological security is really given by the male presence? Discrimination in pay and job opportunities was increasingly being considered; Christy warned that nurses would have to engage in litigation if they were to change nursing and attract women to the profession. Such cases on discrimination against women nurses would also, if successful, help men, who were also deprived of certain benefits. For example, Patricia Forsythe (1971), an army nurse captain, reported that her husband was not entitled to medical benefits, but wives of male officers were. Sexist treatment of military nurses affected men as well; thus, the women's movement would, as in this situation, help both men and women. Christy's contribution to this conference was clearly the most feminist, marking a shift from her earlier published work.

Although not as overtly feminist as Christy, Rosamond Gabrielson took on the issue of nurses' subordination to physicians. She asked the nurses at the conference to imagine that a Dr. Smith, who is not known to the nursing staff, calls and tells the nurse to check the drugs to see if there is Astroten. Never having heard of this medication, the nurse finds the drug, returns to the phone, and is told by Dr. Smith to give the medication and he will sign the order on his arrival in 15 or 20 minutes. Gabrielson then reported that this scenario was part of research that found 21 of 22 nurses would follow "Dr. Smith's" orders, administering a medication they had never heard of, ordered by a physician they did not know and had never met. The drug did *not* exist, but the label showed the supposed maximum dosage; the women obeyed anyway. When presented with the same situation on paper, most nurses said they would not follow the order. Gabrielson believed that the very highly autocratic nursing tradition could be summarized in the phrase, " 'Born in the church, bred in the Army' " (Christy et al., 1972, p. 73).

Can we assume, from the feminist viewpoint, that the female nurse is less liberated? Are not nurses, asked Gabrielson, demanding that the traditional doctor-nurse relationship become liberated and collaborative? She asked nurses to remember that when physicians took power in hospitals, women had "neither voting rights, nor, if married, the right to own property in [their] own name" (p. 73). Today, the traditional relationships are no longer workable, not only because of women's liberation, but because of patients. To be liberated, free to practice without traditional constraints, the nursing service system must change so that nurses can actually nurse. Gabrielson said the hospital administrator, the physician, and the director of nursing are often blamed, but nurses themselves must take responsibility if they are to be unified and respond to forces external to nursing. For nurses to become truly liberated, they must take risks; there may be no tranquility, said Gabrielson, but the time is *now*.

Would nursing take the challenge and claim greater power and autonomy for itself? At the same conference, physician Leonard I. Stein asked, "Why do nurses continue to play the doctor-nurse game; a game which keeps them subservient and which inhibits the nursing profession from attaining autonomist status?" (p. 78). Stein reasoned that the game continues because of the system of rewards and punishments in which the nurse's feelings of self-worth and self-esteem come from physicians. As a woman looks to a man, a nurse looks to a physician to tell her how good she is. Stein encouraged nurses to stop this game, to look to their own profession and their colleagues for evidence of their own competence.

Focusing on individual, dyadic analysis, Stein did not provide a systemic analysis of nursing's subordination; nor did he discuss critical elements of reference group behavior, of a subordinated group that must look to a superordinate group for economic rewards. He did not clarify that physicians and hospital and agency administrators form the superordinate group, nor that nurses are trapped in a sexist system that they did not originate. Indeed, Stein expressly rejected self-pity and self-righteous anger: "I will not focus on those explanations falling into the category of 'How those bastards are holding you down'" (p. 75). Rather, he focused on how nurses themselves contribute to their oppression, inhibiting the achievement of an "autonomist" profession.

After stereotyping feminists as angry, then denying the validity of women's pity for each other and their anger at men or women who support discriminatory practices, Stein turned to nurses as the cause of their own oppression. He admitted that the penalties for not playing the game are severe; the physician is tolerated as a bastard and the nurse fades into the woodwork, or if she does challenge, she is a bitch, a castrator; she is unloved or is fired. Obviously, the penalty for the woman is far more severe than for the man.

Stein saw education as the culprit in the origins of the game, but failed to see medical and nursing training as part of a broader sex stratification system. He also admitted that physicians are not going to change the game since they do not feel oppressed, nor are they. Stein dumped the need for change in nurses' laps. Even though recognizing stereotypic male dominance and female passivity, he recommended that nursing education must change. Although he concluded that both professions must change their attitudes, there is little overt acknowledgment that, like race, sex discrimination is caused by those who gain economically through such bias. One wonders how a Black audience would have responded to a speech that accurately described the transactional analysis of a racist game, but told them that they, not their White oppressors, must change the game. Obviously, there is a moral imperative for change by those who have sustained and gained from prejudice. To tell nurses that physicians will not change their sexist behaviors is equal to telling Blacks that Whites will not change their racist behaviors.

Another panelist, sociologist and feminist Charlotte Wolf, focused on the inferior status of women as it has been institutionalized in nursing, in which the domestic role of women is simply extended to nursing practice. Wolf told of an intern who commented to her that surgical nurses were dispensable and could be replaced by male interns. There is, he admitted, room for a bright nurse, but "'how many nurses do you ever find that can innovate or can do anything on their own?'" (p. 80). To him, they could not do good jobs because they were not committed to careers; they were mothers and wives first. Wolf claimed he was a "nice young man," although his youthful arrogance and ignorance typified physician dominance, which to her represented a routine expression of a perspective rooted in the broader culture, having grave consequences for women's status, identities, roles, and occupations.

According to Wolf, nursing, one of the most necessary and important fields, is also "one of the most highly exploited, least rewarded and most inadequately appreciated professions" (p. 80). Gender and occupational status are unmistakably linked; the inferior status has been institutionalized in the whole of society. Wolf noted that nurses were originally brought to hospitals to perform usual family chores, an extension of the domestic role. This is a short view of the history of women healers, but even if one looks only at the past 100 to 150 years, it is probably not true that there was very little conflict between occupational and traditional roles or that nursing was simpler. It *is* true that the atmosphere of freedom initiated by feminism did influence women in nursing to attempt improvement. Wolf quoted Isabelle Stuart, who stated in 1934 that subordination to physicians must be replaced by equal partnership. That this had not been achieved was obvious in Stein's analysis.

Women's presumed conformity to social norms in the 1940s and 1950s was counteracted, said Wolf, by an expansion of nurses' roles and responsibilities, but not status or income. Caught between two conflicting authorities, most nurses work in hospitals characterized as multiple subordination systems, stuck between the heavy authoritarianism of hospital bureaucrats and free-wheeling doctors. With the latter, patriarchal relationships of unequals transfer to professions, but there are severe consequences of subservience, since nurses, focused on tasks demanded by physicians or hospitals rather than on patients, quickly become depersonalized. Nurses experience blocked mobility, few upward career paths, and few distinctions in rank, salary, or job specifications, regardless of amounts of education or experience. Indeed, Wolf stated:

> Nurses who are faced with the role of the lady of the lamp or with the imagery of bedside nursing find it very difficult, I think, to adjust to the highly technical atmosphere of the hospital. They're torn with two roles: those of healer on the one hand perhaps, or the mother surrogate role on the other hand. And so they feel quite confused in terms of what they ought to do in the hospital and the actual demands of the work load. . . .
> It is here where one's sense of identity comes in; what role is appropriate and what role is not? (p. 83)

Wolf concluded that traditional feminine virtues of obedience, passivity, and dependency and limited career commitments in nursing were disappearing. Constructing new identities called for courage to innovate and care, to redefine terms and perspectives, and to become involved in decision making. All this must be done without losing one's compassion for the patient. How could this be accomplished? Some, stated Wolf, think that men in nursing would lead women to the "promised land," one nurse even said, "they will never put up with the miserable hours and rotten wages . . . they will lift us up with them" (p. 84). But Wolf warned that when men entered the teaching and library science professions, internal segregation resulted, with the men taking power. She cautioned women to win the battle for themselves.

The women's liberation movement removes nurses from isolation and focuses on emancipation from old identities and subservience; through female solidarity, nurses can look inside and get the courage to change, then look outside to create institutional change. A continuation of smiles and lady-like tea-drinking, said Wolf, has never achieved freedom. If nurses remain individually isolated and powerless, "the whinning, [sic] the complaints, the clinging, the frustration, the hangups, and the deviousness" (pp. 84–85) will continue. Wolf urged nurses to break their isolation, join liberation groups, create strong local hospital groups, and coalesce as a professional organization with women's liberation groups. Only through unity, mutual aid, and loyalty to one another can women change: "No one else will do this for us, we must do it for ourselves" (p. 85).

Calling for feminist leadership among nurses, Joan I. Roberts and Thetis M. Group (1973) asked: "Why is it more nurses have not taken an active and consistent stand on the status of women in our society?" (p. 303). The authors agreed that "Nursing must take responsibility for needed changes in its own professional organizations. It is evident that strong leadership is needed— leadership from women who know what they are, not simply as nurses, but as women. The ultimate recommendation, of course, is that we *all* know who we are as women" (p. 321). To clear up the role confusion, there must be feminist analysis of gender roles. The authors claim that the major nursing associations have not been, as have other women's organizations, in the forefront of feminist change and thought. Indeed, the absence of large numbers of nurses in the women's movement left them still powerless to substantially reform health care. This is particularly ironic because the long-term history of women healers suggests they were relatively independent, actively participating in *both* cure and care; thus these "medical nurses" have only in the past century been sharply gender-stereotyped, differentiated, and separated with nurses increasingly ancillary to medicine (the Latin "ancilla" is related to maidservant).

Research conducted by Roberts' student, Donald Bille (1972), found the traditional attitudes of some nursing faculty to be incongruent with fundamental change. Instead of following Wolf's call for unity among women, half of the nursing faculty surveyed by Bille thought sex discrimination could be overcome by working with men in existing groups, and a third felt women working alone could change the problems of nurses as women. In contrast, only 19% of the nursing students believed working with preexisting organizations would lead to changing women's status substantially; they preferred feminist groups and the overthrow of discriminatory systems. Although faculty generally indicated approval of the women's movement, one-half of them, whether they identified themselves as traditional or liberated women, agreed with the statement that feminists exhibited sexual frustrations, aggressiveness, and castrating or neurotic behaviors because of discrimination experienced by them. In contrast, almost two-thirds of the students said feminists were well adjusted, with justifiable grievances, or were very healthy, but fighting a sick system. About half the faculty thought that the women's movement would improve their lives for the better; the other half thought it would be for the worse. In contrast, more than three-fourths of the students saw feminism affecting their lives positively.

Roberts and Group also referred to Cleland's work (1971), focusing on the lack of comprehension of the sexist system by nursing leaders, whose absence of real power sustains the discrimination they do not acknowledge. The authors also noted Stein's work (1967), stressing his view that physicians tend to develop a sense of omnipotence; for example, as private airplane pilots physicians have the highest accident rate because they take inappropriate risks, flying as if immune from harm. Fearing mistakes, a physician develops an all-knowing attitude, but he still needs the nurse's information; she, however, comes to believe that any recommendation she makes would insult him and leave her open to ridicule. Roberts and Group claimed that Stein still had a male bias because evidently he did not recognize that nurses constantly face life-and-death situations in which mistakes could have fatal consequences. Nurses also are legally responsible for correct administration of drugs, even if incorrectly prescribed by physicians. Why then do nurses not develop an equally high sense of omnipotence? Presumably, the gender-stratification system fosters their subservience, not their omniscience. With more research, the behaviors of female physicians could help sort out the analytic problems, but, warned Roberts and Group, women physicians, who have paid a high price to enter the male medical world, may also expect subordination from nurses, anticipating recommendations couched as nonrecommendations to an "infallible" superior.

How did this state of affairs originate? Roberts and Group turned to the historical account, *Witches, Midwives, and Nurses*, by Barbara Ehrenreich and Deirdre English (1972), who claimed the sexist battle was fought long before the development of modern scientific knowledge. They noted that in the medieval period, according to psychiatrist Thomas Szasz, the witch hunts were an early instance of physicians repudiating the rights of women healers. From the 14th to the 17th centuries, the witch-craze swept from Germany to England; 85% of those thousands or even millions tortured or killed are estimated by some researchers to be women and girls. Physicians, barring women from formal education, were the only ones "qualified" to judge women as witches. By the latter 18th century, the attack was so successful that midwives were in danger of extinction. However, Ehrenreich and English contended that women continued to give most of the medical and nursing treatments and, in the United States, were likely to give herbs and set dietary rules while men used more "heroic measures"—massive bleeding, large doses of laxatives, and drugs such as opium. By the 19th century, the popular health movement coincided with the earlier feminist movement. Women attended "irregular colleges," which were also later eliminated. With the advent of the germ theory of disease "scientific" medicine finally achieved some basis for the exclusion of uneducated women and was eventually successful in excluding even midwives, portrayed as ignorant, dirty, and incompetent women—the image of the independent female healer that we have inherited in this century.

Ehrenreich and English clearly perceived medicine not as a male prerogative, but as a masculist theft from women who had previously served as both physicians and nurses. The authors were not easy on early nurses, who were perceived as "mothers," instinctively doing servile work for small wages, giving complete obedience to physicians as noncompetitors. It is clear that they did not see early nurses as fighting successfully for an independent occupation for women outside of the home; for reestablishing the legitimacy of women healers led by women leaders; for developing public health and many other health reforms.

Although some nursing historians reject this early analysis by Ehrenreich and English, the transmission of this longer view of nursing history to nurses is important because it provides an alternative to the stereotyped nurse submissive to authority, the culmination of increasing male medical dominance. Roberts and Group insisted that nurses must change this situation by working with and through other women in the feminist movement and, if necessary, by leaving hospitals. Until they are freed from medical bureaucracies, nurses cannot be free of the control, authority, and power of physicians. Instead, Roberts and Group supported women nurses moving to community-based nursing to continue in the best historical tradition of women healers. This move should be accomplished by nurses joining with women from other health disciplines, thus providing a better knowledge base and, at the same time, associating with colleagues who would not tolerate "the subtleties and vagaries of the nurse-doctor game" (Roberts & Group, 1973, p. 320). Furthermore, interdisciplinary activities would make it easier for nurses to connect with other women professionals who support raising women's status. Breaking the isolation of the single woman alone in an all-male academic department, for example, can be seen as comparable to breaking the isolation of a whole department of women, who, as in nursing, may have been isolated and unable to compare their salaries and treatment to determine the extent of discriminatory practices against them. Finally, Roberts and Group suggested changes in professional organizations through assertive leadership by women who confront and demand changes in the existing power structures.

"THE UNPAID CONSCIENCE OF THE NATION"

Increasingly in the early 1970s women's and nurses' histories were reexamined, reinterpreted, and interrelated by nurses as well as non-nurses. The strength of these reconsiderations became stronger over time. Nurses such as Karen T. Lamb (1973) acknowledged that nursing confronted tremendous social change and could not take its rightful place among the professions until the status of women in the whole society improved. She joined others in her thesis that nursing and the women's rights movement were inextricably bound together. Lamb clearly stated that several alternatives for changes in women's individual development were feasible, but *not* within the current nursing curricula. To her, ignoring women's talents was a deplorable waste of human resources. In professional fields, opening to women after decades of struggle, and in women's professions, women were in the lowest-ranked and poorest paid positions, rarely in administration or management. In higher education, women PhDs were also in the lowest ranks, with women presidents "as rare as whooping cranes" (p. 329). In medicine, women, in 1973, represented only 7.8% of all physicians, most often in pediatrics, and least likely in surgery, despite women's stereotyped higher manual dexterity in small detail work. Similarly, in law, 3.5% of attorneys were women; there were no women senators at that time, and only fourteen (3%) female representatives in Congress. Only 150 out of 10,000 (1.5%) civil service appointments above GS level 14 were female. There was still a $4,000 difference between annual salaries of full-time working men and women.

Lamb concluded: "Wherever one looks the picture is equally bleak. In every area women are under-represented and underpaid" (p. 331).

In nursing, the terms "woman" and "profession" seem mutually exclusive to many, and it is, claimed Lamb, difficult to consider nursing a profession since less than 12% of nurses held baccalaureate degrees and only 3% held master's or doctoral degrees. To many in society, nurses are not professionals because they are women. Lamb cited research that indicated that nurses' conflicts with physicians are related to social class differences; nurses invest one-third to one-half the time in education as does a physician, but receive only one-fifth of a typical physician's salary. Nurses are still tied to their 19th-century stereotype: a tender, sympathetic, soft-hearted female is not the natural leader of the team. For women who deviate, terms such as aggressive and uppity should send them scurrying home, but if these fail, Lamb stated, more serious attacks are directed toward "our femininity, sexuality, morality, and finally our hormones" (p. 334).

Lamb interconnected gender and class perspectives, drawing from Raymond Birdwhistell's (1949) discussion of his anthropological study at a 1948 nursing convention which, she said, is still useful. In this study, the lower-income group perceived nursing as a noble profession. The nurse who had bettered herself was thought to be surrounded by interesting people and in a position to make a good marriage after her chaperoned training—a good technical expert, although she was also seen by the men as someone with whom the doctors had a lot of fun. Middle-class subjects saw the nurses as semi- or skilled women, working before marriage or widowed or divorced, or career women (unable to get a husband or neglecting him). Women saw nurses as husband hunters, employing unfair tactics; men saw them as easy marks, but respected their knowledge in a crisis. Those married to nurses saw their own wives as "different" from other nurses. Upper-class subjects had no ambivalence; the nurse was a skilled menial, located between a hairdresser and social worker, whose work was unpleasant. She was nice to men, cruel to women in childbirth, but no threat to women, because, though their husbands might have affairs with nurses, they would not marry them.

If social change begins at the top and diffuses outward and downward, Lamb stated that men in power would have to change things, but given the evidence, this would require a long wait. Another alternative is for nurses to invite men into nursing and promote them rapidly over well-qualified women to power positions in which the men will not stand for discrimination. The third option is for nurses to change things for themselves, to stop being "constantly buffeted and tumbled about" (p. 336). Given their subordinated status, can women really change things? This means getting nurses out of isolation in their institutions, stated Lamb, and, agreeing with Roberts and Group, she urged nurses to connect with women in allied disciplines to achieve a sense of sisterhood and collegiality, and to stop living in the "home of the enemy" (p. 337). Research suggests that Blacks' migration from the

South to the North raised their consciousness and cultural identity. Similarly, nurses who live in the shadow of physicians and male-dominated institutions must leave the oppressor's house to achieve a separate, more autonomous identity.

The assumptions underlying any strategy of change need to be articulated and Lamb's was to bring nurses as women and practitioners into the mainstream of society—not through radically restructuring society, or through revolution, but through reform that involved both more rights and responsibilities. Although the worldwide emancipation of women is the most radical revolution conceivable, Lamb limited her vision to individual and community reform, but at least went beyond the usual advice to individual nurses to change society by simply changing themselves.

Nursing must look more carefully at the quality of all women entering educational programs. Lamb wondered if the majority of students have any idea at all of becoming career women. Do students and practitioners suffer from the female malady, compensated volunteerism, being paid a small amount for a little work in order to be of some use to society? In 1965, noted Lamb, there were between 38 and 45 million volunteers in the United States, the majority women, who, if paid, would receive $14 billion annually. Women were the "unpaid conscience of the nation," and nurses were "a special instance of this phenomenon" (pp. 340–341). Do women themselves reinforce low self-worth by accepting no pay or very little for their labor, skills, and services, which are then further devalued?

Lamb advised nurses to engage in counseling or consciousness-raising to change destructive female brain-washing, stopping the attitude that career interruptions for women are normal. Instead, husbands must assume their share of work in families in which women are not expected to carry the full burden of the home. New students should be advised of alternative lifestyles; marriage and children need not interfere with professional goals; high school counselors must be retrained to stop sending uncommitted girls into nursing as a stop-gap before marriage. Surprisingly, Lamb made no demands for child care services at hospitals or different non-male-defined career patterns that would require significant institutional changes in policy.

Turning to the community dimension, Lamb urged nursing to prepare more than the one-to-one bedside practitioner: to develop a more comprehensive health-care system with women in key decision-making positions; to develop administrative and political internships; and to prepare women to be appointed to boards, commissions, and citizens' advisory groups. In short, she advocated clinical practice on the community and state levels.

On the governmental and societal levels, Lamb urged nurses to write and introduce legislation and run for elected office. To do this, either the number of legislative positions must be doubled or women must fight to unseat 50% of the incumbents: "A goodly number of male decision makers are going to have to step down. And it is unrealistic to believe they will retire gracefully.

We will have to fight to achieve the balance" (p. 346). In contrast to other writers, Lamb suggested that nurses begin in their own profession to give support to women equally qualified, rather than to men, until women have access to *all* top-level decision-making positions.

Lamb stressed the new powerful legal options under the Civil Rights Act of 1964, but claimed many women do not realize they have "worked their entire lives in employment situations that are in direct violation of their own legal rights" (p. 347). With thousands of discriminatory laws in a society that sees women as economic dependents and legal incompetents, is it any wonder that nurses are not empowered to manage the finances of their own departments? Protective labor laws have never applied to nurses, who have slipped through fair labor standards whenever expedient. This, stated Lamb, is "no cause for self-congratulation" (p. 348).

Nurses are familiar with more than equal responsibilities, but not with equal rights or authority for their decisions. Still many, despite supposed conservatism, "are proud that nursing has traditionally been close to the most critical issues and humanitarian objectives . . . certainly we see and care for the end products of an over-populated and environmentally contaminated world. Certainly we have been close to poverty and misery" (p. 350). Nurses have also been close to the major demands of the women's movement, such as safe child care, pay equity, and access to all levels of higher education. But if nurses do not expect to succeed, to lay to rest anatomy as destiny, then stereotyping will continue. Lamb concluded: "We have only to look around us at the achievements of women. We are learning that sisterhood is indeed powerful—for ourselves and for other women" (p. 351).

MOVING TOWARD THE FIFTH WORLD

To achieve feminist goals, the importance of resocialization for nurses is critical. Alice G. Sargent (1973) asserted that both nurses' and physicians' attitudes have been corroded by stereotypes. She conceived of an emerging "fourth world" in which women will question the assumptions of the division of labor, where women "will not continue to support the male-dominated political system, and will welcome women political candidates" (p. 17). Sargent gave credit to the Black movement, and recommended that women learn from the experiences with racism, thus avoiding a repetition of the same mistakes. Indeed, she hoped for interconnections between the Black and women's movements, but admitted that this did not seem likely because each movement seems destined to move through stages from dependency to counterdependency to independence. To Sargent, women are in the counterdependency stage, characterized by "rhetoric, anger, indignation, blame, and separation" (p. 16); meeting together without men present, women were relinquishing self-hatred, finding out who they are, and feeling good about themselves without living through and for others. Women were refusing to identify with men, just as Black people had rejected Whites as their models.

Perhaps when women recognize that their individual problems are actually social problems, then human choices can be made, leading to the third phase, independence. However, separation is necessary to reestablish in the culture the values of intimacy and connectedness as human values. Forcing people into sharply differentiated roles has been costly, claimed Sargent, and psychology has not reduced these but reinforced them. Going beyond Freud, Sargent denied even Erik Erikson's idea that women are defined by an empty anatomical inner space, the uterus; this theoretical position simply justifies pushing all child-rearing responsibilities onto women. She insisted this view does not provide women with open space for exploration and actualization.

In Sargent's Fourth World, division of labor will not be gender-defined and women political candidates will be welcome. In this world, nurses and other women will "avoid or desert doctors who do not consider the health of women in prescribing inadequately tested contraceptives, who convey incorrect sex information, who recommend unnecessary radical surgery, or provide poor information about abortion" (p. 17). Sargent expressed the hope of feminist women in the 1970s to change everything that separates women from each other: refusing the compassion trap that denies women a central focus for their lives; being wary of a sexual revolution that forces women to attend not only to one man's but many men's needs; redefining wives' and secretaries' positions as no longer auxiliary and nurses' roles as professional and as advocates for patients. Conversely, Sargent claimed that men are not fully aware of what their system has cost them: loss of sense of self, of purpose other than to achieve.

Sargent presented social science research findings on gender socialization, showing "the depth to which our attitudes have been corroded by stereotyped behavior" (p. 21), making change seem arduous. Indeed, as women in support groups change, men may become more aggressive, pushing women back to their "rightful" places. This can be seen in the increasing violence toward women in the media, of violence in hard core pornography, in the increased incidence of rape and child molestation. Alternatively, men may withdraw until women "get it out of their system." But some, stated Sargent, may recognize inequities and change their own attitudes and behaviors, moving to meet *human* needs for receiving and giving warmth, in a value system that goes beyond "their birthright of power and privilege" (p. 25). Someday, Sargent believed, much later, "we will welcome the human Fifth World" (p. 25). In retrospect, following the conservative 1980s a realization of her vision seems more remote and the backlash to feminism more apparent.

In a more pragmatic article, Virginia Cleland (1974) asserted that changes in the legal system make it possible for women to assert their demands for complete social equality; however, "women will be unable to make use of these legal means unless they free themselves psychologically and are able to insist that their employers comply with the existing laws" (p. 563). Cleland urged nurses and women to "agitate, educate, legislate and negotiate." In contrast to others, Cleland was very clear there have always been interdependent streams of feminist thought and action. Although it can be argued that there are more than two, at least Cleland did not make the mistake of trivializing previous feminists by seeing them as concerned only with suffrage.

One feminist stream focuses on social and psychological issues and educates the public; the other centers on legislation, administrative actions, and filing complaints to achieve legal enforcement. It is clear that women must first recognize and understand the problem before significant action can be taken. Self-education, a consciousness of oppression, arises from multiple sources. While it is debatable that curtailment of employment opportunities and rewards is the dominant cause, it is certainly the basis of Cleland's feminist consciousness.

Realizing that the personal is political, Cleland openly presented her own experiences, stating that as a graduate student in psychology, she recognized that female students were denied research assistantships and that married women students were given no help at all, not even an occasional teaching assistantship. Cleland had a federal nursing fellowship, but for others she "knew the situation existed and accepted the unfairness of it" (p. 564). This is a clear characteristic of discrimination: "Unless there is pathologic denial, the victim acknowledges the state but accepts it as inevitable" (p. 564). Thus, people make prejudiced decisions for the subordinated "openly and without shame" (p. 564). Discrimination is simply part of the system, seemingly a natural state, which women, even though they dislike the sexist prejudices, view as inevitable. Large numbers of women simply deny that a sexist system exists. To Cleland, feminists have broken through denial by reeducating women via books, articles, lectures, workshops, the press, and consciousness-raising groups.

With awareness, women can agitate, as Bernice Sandler did, for example, when she used the new executive order forbidding discrimination and filed charges against 300 colleges and universities in 1970. Quite accurately, Cleland observed the development of two interrelated organizations of women: one external to the system, usually the more radical, which applies political pressure; the other established by the institution, acting on particular issues but obviously under greater constraints to conform. Although Cleland did not make the radical/conservative distinction, she very clearly understood that agitators always risk their careers. The better the agitator, the more likely she is to incur personal loss, but simultaneously create societal change.

According to Cleland, the process of education is the most important function of the women's movement. The body of knowledge feminists were developing in the 1970s proved sexist biases existed. For example, she found practically no valid research about women managers or the effects of shift work on women and their families for the simple reason that women were excluded from the research. Cleland was probably unduly optimistic about the effects of the new knowledge on men's attitudes and behaviors toward women, but certainly right about the changes in women's.

Following her own advice, Cleland educated nurses on new legislation: the Civil Rights Act of 1964, Executive Order 11246, the Equal Employment Opportunity Act of 1972, the Equal Pay Act of 1963, the Higher Education Act of 1972, and the Comprehensive Health Manpower Act and Nurse Training Amendment Act of 1971. In February 1973 the ANA filed a complaint on pension benefits for nurse faculty, claiming the Teachers Insurance and Annuity Association (TIAA) paid lesser retirement benefits for women. Unisex benefits were finally established several years later. An equally positive conclusion for the ERA has not been reached, but Cleland's optimism in 1974 was shared by most feminists since the ERA had been approved by Congress and ratified by 32 states, with only six more needed to enact the 27th Amendment to the Constitution. With the collapse of opposition from organized labor, Cleland expected the amendment to pass in 1974, providing a "theoretical rationale for the interpretation of existing law and the development of new laws . . . [having] enormous moral and symbolic impact" (p. 568). But women did not accurately forecast the tremendous backlash that would occur in the late 1970s and become institutionalized during the conservative 1980s.

Cleland called on nurses to negotiate through collective bargaining, admitting that unions have historically excluded women from their contracts but claiming that this was no longer legal. Nurses had also been completely excluded under the Taft–Hartly National Labor Relations Act, which eliminated unionization of private nonprofit health institutions. This effectively eliminated from unionization millions of nurses and most other health-care employees who were also women. As Cleland expected, the act was amended and the ANA was able to enact their new programs for collective bargaining. As an example of action, Cleland pointed to the faculty bargaining unit of the American Association of University Professors at Wayne State University that assisted nursing faculty by establishing nondiscriminatory processes, such as child-rearing leaves of absence with fringe benefits, sabbatical leaves of absence, and leaves of absence with pay for pregnancy. Nevertheless, Cleland accurately concluded that the employment structure was essentially unchanged, with most women working at low levels, thus sustaining the wrongs of centuries—wrongs that cannot be undone by a single generation of activist women. Even if sex discrimination were eliminated, nurses would still have to use their new opportunities in the large task of developing a profession.

Will nurses agitate, educate, legislate, and negotiate? Gender role socialization involves a self-deprivation syndrome and subordination of one's own interests. Nurses must know who they are as women in order to create professional changes. Canadian nurse Dorothy S. Starr (1974) introduced the "poor baby" syndrome, claiming it made most nurses "ill-suited to the debate and demands of a push for women's rights and ill-equipped to organize on behalf of women's interests" (p. 21). To her, nurses depend on the maternal stance for their self-respect and self-image; consequently, they become hooked on self-deprivation and subordinate their interests to family, community, physicians, and nurses above them in the nursing hierarchy. "It is," said Starr, "not surprising that nurses are not noticeably active in the feminist movement" (p. 21). Nurses reason that they are in a woman's profession where there is no question of women's rights and no competition with men. But, said Starr, "If nurses lift their sights from the kitchen sink, the neatly made bed, and the problem-oriented patient records" (p. 21), the need for feminism is obvious. It is no longer appropriate to give priority to men's careers or to support their education at the expense of women's own development.

At the time of Starr's article, sexist legal restraints were crumbling in Canadian laws under the impact of the *Francis Report*, which made 167 recommendations for change that women were urging men to implement. Starr, however, stressed the self-imposed restraints: children's books that socialize girls for passivity and dependence; the double standard for sexuality, with flirtation mitigating against honest friendships and maximum professional contributions. Covert behavior and sly manipulation supported the status quo, failing to challenge subordination. Starr viewed all housewives, nurses, and secretaries as victims of a "fatal availability," an unselfishness that leads to nonpermanent achievements in jobs where tasks can be replaced easily by another worker. This behavior does not enhance power and, said Starr, nurses still do not have overt power. Indeed, nurses have supported men and physicians as "master and enemy, loved and despised, whom women cajole and trick, cosset and cheat but, when the crunch comes, to whom they defer" (p. 22).

Starr recommended five remedies for the poor baby syndrome. First, women must become aware, raise their consciousness, and refuse to laugh off humor that portrays women as sex objects. Second, women need to make personal choices to never belittle women or engage in sexist socialization of their children. Still another remedy is to develop confidence in other women, supporting their endeavors in the professions and in public life. Another remedy is to include men as nurses, not so they can hold the top nursing jobs, but to help break doctor-nurse stereotypes.

Starr believed that the women's movement not only freed nurses from subordination, but also helped them embrace the value system of a woman's culture. She concluded that the rewards for nurses' participation in the feminist movement would be a "more nearly autonomous profession with more open power . . . the liberation of women will result in freeing feminine qualities—the real feminine qualities, such as compassion, tenderness, empathy—in persons of both sexes. The feminist movement's message to the nurse is: Don't poor baby another person and don't be a poor baby yourself" (p. 23).

No problem could be resolved nor could public support for and recognition of the nursing profession be expected if the issue of "femininity" remained unclear. It is interesting to note that the stereotypes inherent within the concept itself, leading many feminists to refuse to use the term, were still accepted for debate by Judith Salmon Shockley (1974). To her, it is clear that changes in the concept of the feminine had affected nursing practice by dividing nurses themselves into opposing camps. "Some adhere to the traditional nursing role which correlates with the old ideas of femininity, including nonparticipation in decision-making and subservience to authority figures. They may thwart the efforts of their professional counterparts to gain acceptance as professionals in their own right" (p. 36).

With many other writers, Shockley turned to history to establish the perspectives needed for contemporary women in nursing. In the mid-1800s, noted Shockley, women were seen as "frilly, decorative, mindless and speechless, equated with uterus" (p. 36), while men were associated with intellect. Women who did not conform were seen as man-hating spinsters, who could not love. The reality was that women such as Mary Wollstonecraft, Margaret Sanger, and Lucy Stone were passionate in their relations, envisioning women as free human beings, demanding a voice in law-making, rights to property, and to higher education and the professions, and rejecting the requirement to submit to husbands in all things. Wars fought over civil rights taught the women who struggled for the rights of slaves that women must free themselves. Yet "the myth of feminist as a man-hater persisted" (p. 36).

Shockley relied on upper-class imagery; dichotomizing women in the 1920s as belonging to a group reared by mothers for gentility and a second group reared to believe that freedom of choice was the right of both sexes. But the images available, "fiery, man-hating, loveless career women, or gentle, soft wives and mothers, loved and protected by their husbands, and surrounded by adoring children" (p. 37), were so restricted that many chose the latter. Agreeing with previous writers, Shockley noted that the trend away from feminism was reinforced by Freud's theories, which made it harder to fight female "inferiority" because it was now proved by "scientific evidence." To avoid "abnormality," said Shockley, women stopped going to college; their numbers declined from 47% in 1920 to 35.2% in 1958, a time when marriage manuals emphasized passivity in sexual and social roles. The birth rate increased from 19.4/1,000 in 1940 to 26/1,000 in 1947 and these rates were sustained until 1960.

Shockley believed that there are two types of nurse in the profession: the first, a rigid traditionalist, somewhat similar in nature to the housewife of the early 1960s; the other, the fulfilled but frustrated individualist, similar to mid-19th-century feminists and liberated women of today. The existence of these opposing factions of nurses causes those who risk frustration and failure in order to gain concomitant success and self-growth to be thwarted by traditionalist nurses, who choose lack of involvement in decision making, but are still subsequently frustrated with the status of nursing and the quality of patient care.

Shockley claimed that Margaret Mead's research stressing women's unlimited human potential was negated by the aftermath of World War II; again women were forced into traditional roles, reinforced by sexist advertising on new labor-saving devices that fostered wifeliness and anti-intellectualism. Thus, at the close of the 1950s, fourteen million girls were engaged to be married by 17 years of age and 60% of college-age women dropped out for marriage reasons, with a birthrate close to that in India. For nursing, the result was severe personnel shortages.

Shockley, like other nurses, pointed to Friedan's book (1963) as critical in proving the happy housewife images to be mythical. Still, women were bombarded with traditional images now modified to make women better adjusted, but actually expressing the "housewife syndrome"—suicidal tendencies, depression, and somatic complaints. With the reemergence of feminism, women have discovered that only one-third to one-fourth of their lives are centered on housewife and mother roles. Now, noted Shockley, emphasis is on "the woman who is aware of who she is, who she could be, who others think she is, and who is attempting to close the gap between her several images" (p. 39).

These historical trends have profound implications for nursing, claimed Shockley. Nurses are able to handle patients in the reproductive phase of mother and wife roles, but what of women who are experiencing identity crises at menopause? Or older women, devalued by society as they age? Or adolescent girls, faced with new alternatives as well as continuing peer pressures? What of the increased openness about sexuality at all levels? How can nurses, who may have difficulty with their own sexuality, deal effectively with their clients? Increasingly, different lifestyles and sexuality require nurses to deal with homophobic thinking.

How, asked Shockley, will the traditional nurse, compulsive, ritualistic, subservient to authority, whose primary purpose is to complete a task, who is often fatigued, irritable, wanting to return to the old comfortable nursing ways, deal with the new problems and patients? How will the new nurse, actively involved in decision making, subject to harassment and firing, committed to full professionalism, but constantly taking risks, yet still insisting on equality with physicians, survive to effect needed change? More important, how will these nurses survive if traditionalist nurses oppose them? Shockley was hopeful that, with the support of women's and human rights groups, nurses who are committed to women's liberation could strive to create nursing, not as others define it, but as they themselves define it.

The questions raised by Shockley and other nurse writers in the early 1970s clearly reflect a heightened awareness by nurses of their subordinate status and the need to align themselves with feminist issues. The themes of the early 1970s centered on role change and empowerment. Nurses, most pointedly Cleland, made the case that sex discrimination was *the* most important problem in nursing. The interconnections between sex discrimination and the subordination of nurses and nursing were established, first by Heide, then reestablished and analyzed from multiple perspectives. A feminist reconstitution of nursing history, providing a more appropriate iconography, was urged by Edelstein, Roberts and Group, and Clemons. Resocialization, both personal and professional, of gender and nursing roles was demanded by Starr, who rejected the self-deprivation and subordination of self-interest. Stereotyped, conflicting, and contradictory roles were all analyzed by Mullane, Wolf, Wilson, Sargent, and Starr. The search for new identity demanded by Wilson required raising nurses' consciousness of oppression and its effects on nurses. This was particularly needed, according to Roberts and Group, among nursing leaders. The gendered artificiality of roles decried by Mullane, the transfer of domestic roles to nursing so disliked by Wolf, and the dichotomization of identity denied by Wilson all connected to a rejection of sex-stereotyped physician-nurse role relations by Heide, Stein, and Sargent. Wolf, Stein, and others called for greater professional unity among women and Shockley's important analysis keyed in on the influence of gender definitions on the incapacity of nurses to unite for political action: traditional versus liberated groups holding different views of themselves as women and thus as nurses, leading to lack of unity in perceptions of nursing. According to Christy and Edelstein, these gendered splits could be exacerbated and severe nursing shortages would result if feminists denigrated nursing while exalting medicine in women's move for power.

The political importance of the sheer size of women's groups in the health delivery system was emphasized by several writers, Mullane, Roberts and Group, More, and Lindabury, who called for greater political analysis and action by nurses who will question and influence public policy in coordination with other women's groups. Specific involvement in politics and in legal and economic systems was urged by numerous writers. More and Lindabury, for example, stressed economic injustice; Cleland focused on legal remedies to discrimination in work; and Golick and Edelstein stressed the passage of the ERA. These civil rights and libertarian approaches were paralleled by calls for reorganization of social values through the incorporation of women's values, a dominant motif of Heide and echoed up by others. Clearly, feminism had impacted nursing in the first half of the 1970s, but an even stronger feminist consciousness would emerge among some nurses in the latter half of the decade.

Chapter 7

Poking Heads out of Their Apolitical Bonnets: Nurses Zero in on Gender, Power, and Leadership in the 1970s

It was difficult for women in nursing to become more independent when the public, even in the turbulent 1970s, had not appreciably changed their traditional perceptions of nurses. By the mid-1970s the effects of gender stereotypes on the image of nursing became a major theme in the research and writing on feminism and nursing. To some researchers, the definition of nursing remained traditional because the presentation of nurses in literature and the media continued to be stereotyped in traditionalist images. To create the image of a new nurse heroine required a reinvention of nursing history. Furthermore, while some nurses in the 1970s clearly were concerned about nursing's image and women's lack of power, others focused more directly on issues of power, control, and leadership in nursing as the impact of the women's movement raised feminist consciousness. To construct a powerful profession demanded political action, even directed against organized medicine and hospital associations. New nurses—risk-takers and role-breakers—were required.

CREATING A NEW KIND OF NURSE HEROINE

Although a few analyses of nursing images could be found in earlier decades, the issue of public identity became increasingly important in the 1970s. Lucretia and Elizabeth Richter (1974), for example, examined the images of nurses in novels, analyzing 25 volumes from the young people's section in three libraries. The Richters found fiction that was outdated or misleading. Created in the 1930s and 1940s, the best-known nurse characters, Sue Barton and Cherry Ames, both attended hospital training schools, not universities; both learned to stand in the presence of a doctor, to memorize procedures, and, though committed to nursing, to remain more interested in romance or mystery. Nurse characters in romance novels had marriage as their major goal. For example, Tracy Crandell, who wept with pride on receiving her RN pin, later concluded that her training was the best in the world to become the understanding wife of a young doctor. Another character, Nina Grant, a pediatric nurse, was misinformed on theoretical matters and kept oxygen in a premature infant's isolette at a concentration that, in real life, is dangerous. The Richters marvel that Grant could be graded as the top student in her class when she was so abysmally misinformed about the facts of nursing.

The Richters were pleased with the more serious books, which invariably were written by nurses themselves; however, most of them were outdated. One story of two Black girls integrating a nursing school portrayed faculty and staff as stern and unmarried, a continuation of sexist stereotypes. In fact, most of this story focused on off-duty events. In a 1965 book all the characters were dedicated, but, as in 1945, believed they must choose between career and marriage and openly disparaged university-educated nurses. Indeed, the Richters did not find a single story about a student in either a baccalaureate or associate degree program: "Typically, students in nursing fiction work long, hard hours, are often left alone at night as charge nurses on busy floors, and live in dread of cold, harsh supervisors whose edicts they dare not question" (p. 1281). An unusual exception, noted the Richters, was a 1960 book that showed a nurse as mother of four, working toward a BA degree, and a warm-hearted director of nurses whom students could approach comfortably.

The women librarians who were interviewed by the Richters recognized that there were few good stories about nursing, except some biographies, but, as in the biographies on Nightingale discussed in Chapter 1, life histories may be very biased and sexist. The Richters concluded that the books set expectations of nursing education and practice that do not exist. They called for a new fiction with new nurse heroines. Neither nurses nor the public need the images of Cherry Ames or dependent "young ladies." To the Richters, it was obvious that the profession of nursing had undergone tremendous change in the past few decades. However, young people, if they considered nursing as a profession, would continue to read inaccurate fictional accounts about nurses: "If we are to satisfy these demands, a new kind of nurse heroine must emerge: one who can think and act intelligently, independently and creatively in a modern setting. She must be a person whose education has prepared her to function effectively as a member of the health team, who may be called on to use complex technological equipment" (p. 1281).

This call for changes in stereotyped perceptions was paralleled by increased research on occupations and professions by feminist scholars during the 1970s. Nurses' essays on the sexist images of nurses gave way to more specific inquiry. In 1977, for example, Drabman, Robertson, Cordua, Jarvie, and Hammer studied media influences on children's perceptions of gender roles. They presented a videotape about a young boy's visit to the doctor in which a female physician and a male nurse were depicted. When children were posttested, they reversed what they had just seen, claiming the male was the physician, the female was the nurse. This result was also found with younger children in a replicated study (Cordua, McGraw, & Drabman, 1978). Again, in 1979 Cordua, McGraw, and Drabman studied 128 children's perceptions of gender-typed occupations by showing four videotapes depicting all possible combinations of female and male physicians and nurses to children of five to six years of age. The researchers found gender-stereotyped thinking so strong, even at these early ages, that the children simply relabeled portrayals that countered usual stereotypes to conform to the typical view of male physician and female nurse. The relabeling was especially marked for male nurses even more than for female physicians. Clearly, gender stereotyping took priority over reality, occurring in *both* girls and boys. Although the researchers expected a decrease of stereotypic relabeling with age, this did *not* occur. The actual number of visits to physicians during the year did not affect the children's gender stereotypes. Exposure to male nurses did seem to improve the accuracy of the perception of reality in the films. Interestingly, children whose mothers were employed outside the home were less stereotypic in their perceptions.

The distortions are quite clear. For example, 53% of the children relabeled a female physician and a male nurse as a male physician and female nurse. Another 25% said they had seen two doctors. When the children saw a male physician and male nurse, 50% said that both were doctors; only 31% identified the characters as doctor and nurse. When viewing the videotape of a female physician and female nurse, 91% correctly identified the occupations. With the fourth film, male physician/female nurse, all the children correctly designated the characters. These findings clearly show the power of gender stereotypes. The children were asked how they knew the occupations, and they responded that gender was the major variable they used to classify them. The researchers also tested whether the children had paid attention and found that they had. Presumably, gender role regularities were seen by the children as lawful relationships, since most children, when asked, said, " 'Girls can't be doctors' " (p. 592).

RECONSTRUCTING THE PAST:
A NEW MYTHOS OF NURSING

A new image of the nurse requires a new mythos. This could only be achieved, according to Jo Ann Ashley (1975), if nurses knew their history as women. In agreement with other authors and researchers, Ashley believed that traditionalism had been maintained, in part, by nurses themselves: "Historically, it is highly significant that professional women were among the conservatives, with nurses no exception. Professional women joined all the 'good causes,' causes good not for them but for the male-dominated institutions that repressed them" (p. 1465). Ashley drew a parallel between the status of women in nursing and of women in general in the early 1900s and the mid-1970s, concluding that there was very little difference across the 60- to 70-year time span:

> If nurses are to prevent failure in the future, they must carefully evaluate their position of inequality in the social order and design public, political action to bring about improvements. Only by understanding nursing's history can nurses break the oppressive chains of the past. The main lesson to learn from history is how not to repeat the errors of the past. Today, identification with the feminist cause and obtaining equality with men in the health field is a must. (p. 1467)

So lost was the real history of women that Ashley had to remind nurses that they and all women were not free; even though early feminists achieved the vote, they were not as persistent in other vital areas, and thus equal rights for women was still a critical political issue. Although this view is often presented, a closer reading of early feminism shows it to be far less one-sided, but, as Ashley stated, the past is instruction for the present; women are still relatively powerless because of their lack of persistence in changing the social order. Ashley noted the dichotomization of women made by socialist-feminist Shulamith Firestone (1971): radicals were concerned for the total growth of women as equal human beings; conservatives, the larger number, were not deeply concerned with all aspects of liberation, and, while gaining the vote, did not support other changes espoused by the activists. After the vote was attained most women supported the political and social order, failing to make basic changes in values and institutions. Although subsequent research provides a more positive reading, Ashley is probably right that many women prematurely subsumed feminist issues in a vague humanism.

Ashley further claimed that professional women who joined "good causes" (good for others, but not for destroying repressive institutions) were conservatives who devoted their attention to narrow political, social, and professional issues, not to the social order itself. Subsequent research both supports and denies this assertion. The variation among women was far wider, and because of differential gender socialization, the professional women were to be found on a continuum from radical to conservative. But true radicals, such as Lavinia Dock, were not able to substantially influence others on more serious issues, even, for example, the Equal Rights Amendment (ERA), which could have created the symbolic and legal bases for a complete reconsideration of societal norms. Nor on issues such as prostitution was she completely successful. It is probably true that a number of nursing leaders were conservative, rejecting feminist leaders. Although some historians have argued that the rank and file were not represented by their leaders, the reverse is equally likely: some major leaders understood feminist issues, but their followers did not. Ashley claimed that "nurses were among the most conservative of the conservatives. With rare exception, they were nonfeminists" (p. 1465). To her, these women overlooked their second-class status, and helped develop hospitals as businesses. This, in turn, led to a failure to liberate nursing education and practice, which were absorbed into hospital management and sustained the institution's growth at the expense of nurses. Although women were central to hospital reform in the 19th century, and, one might add, their numbers made hospitals even possible, Ashley contended they have had little influence in this century. Ironically, histories of hospitals neither credit nurses with reform nor accept the fact that nurses provided care at minimal cost. The reason for patients being in the hospital at all was to receive care by *women*, not by physicians. This fact is consistently overlooked by medical historians.

Ashley believed that most nursing leaders "did not seriously question male dominance in the health field, nor did they question the serious and long-range effects of women's subjugation to men" (p. 1466). Another interpretation is that some nurse leaders saw themselves as women liberating other women by creating a profession, by insisting on decent salaries and working conditions, and by improving the standards of education for women. To what extent early leaders in university education differed on feminism from most of those in hospital nursing is yet to be fully analyzed. That all women in institutions were subject to dismissal by men surely must have watered down the activism of some, particularly those who came to identify with physicians. About one issue Ashley is correct: Lavinia Dock saw that the development of nursing would ensure male dominance, pointing, in a 1903 speech, to the determined movement of

> our masculine brothers to seize and guide the helm of the new teaching. . . . [They] have lately openly asserted themselves in printed articles as the founders and leaders of . . . nursing education, which, so far as it has gone, we all know to have been worked out by the brains, bodies and souls of the women . . . who have often had to win their points in clinched opposition to the will of these same brothers, and solely by dint of their own personal prestige as women. (Dock, 1904, pp. 78-79)

Dock knew that women in nursing had engaged in very real battles to keep their autonomy. Thus, it is clear that they did enact feminism in founding modern nursing in the 19th century. But did their efforts have a feminist basis and, if so, did they continue these efforts in the 20th century? Ashley thought not.

Despite Dock's urgent demand that nurses use their latent and even unsuspected powers to overcome threats of male dominance and to view overbearing physicians and administrators who inflicted injustices and indignities on women as no friends or benefactors of women—still she concluded that organized nursing was not effective on public issues concerning women. To Ashley, Dock's warnings were justified, and, by the second decade of this century, nurses were more concerned with seeking approval from men, not their own liberation. Thus, male dominance and control over nursing and health care have been sustained by women who comply in male-defined structures. This, said Ashley, allowed physicians to make rapid progress, but severely restrained women in nursing, in turn negatively affecting all women because of the substantial numbers in this one profession, becoming second-class by identification with women's subordination.

Ashley contended that the apprenticeship system of nursing education and early nurse practice acts, which specified the supervision of nurses by physicians and, thus, the legal subjection of nurses, resulted in second-class professionalism and sustained the myth of medical supervision, which to her was not often the reality in many practice areas. Ashley quoted Dock as saying that nursing had not made itself a moral force, or a public conscience, taking no position on large public questions; it was not feared by those holding low standards and it allowed " 'all manner of new conditions and developments in nursing affairs to arise, flourish, succeed, or fail' " (p. 1466). To Ashley, early nurses, without public protest, allowed legalized paternalism, with their oppression solidly built into the legal and educational systems, leading to low status and severe economic discrimination.

Ashley noted that Shirley Titus had told nurses in 1952 that they were yet to awaken from a "long social slumber"; they were still working 48-hour weeks or longer, suffering from the control of nursing by medicine and hospitals, who served their own interests by perpetuating the myth that women exist to be mothers and should not compete economically with men. To Ashley, the status of women was deteriorating, not improving, and unless nurses could understand their history, they would never be free from the oppressions of the past. On an optimistic note, Ashley noted that the American Nurses Association (ANA) had brought suit in nine cases against discriminatory faculty pension plans; nurses had joined "in fair numbers" the National Organization for Women, from which NURSES NOW had formed several chapters. Ashley's early death robbed her profession of one of its most courageous, outspoken feminists and critics since Lavinia Dock. We will never hear her assessment of effectiveness of changes wrought by current nurses and feminists. The bright horizon of which she spoke in 1975 was dimmed throughout the conservative 1980s, and the weather ahead in the 1990s is not as fair as might be wished.

PAST AS PROLOGUE: A LINEAR PROGRESSION?

If women's history is buried so are the actions of many of its leaders, particularly those who directly confronted sex discrimination and those who expressed anger or open dismay about women's subordination. Subject to ridicule, women leaders are too often denied or at least reinterpreted so they will not create discomfort for women conformists, who understand that men are not pleased with praise for females who have rejected patriarchal control. Karen L. Brand and Laurie K. Glass (1975) also turned to Dock to provide the historical, feminist imagery so often lacking in traditional nursing histories and to substantiate feminism today. In her early writings, Dock claimed that a nurse who knows only of her own time and surroundings is not able "'to estimate and judge correctly the current events whose tendency is likely to affect her own career'" (p. 161). She insisted that nurses must know how nursing arose, what lines were followed, and under whose direction it had best developed in order for nursing to be "'in harmony with its historical mission'" (p. 161).

Following Dock's admonition, Brand and Glass found that the social issues of the late 19th century and early 1900s were pertinent and relevant in the 1970s. From their historical search, they found that religion, war, politics, and scientific advances all affected nursing, but particularly influential was "the status of women in society and the degree of freedom which women enjoyed . . . the development of nursing and the status of women were interdependent and often parallel; the advances of one affected the advances of the other" (pp. 161–162). In many ways their research did not go deeply enough; for example, they asserted that religious orders in the Middle Ages provided women the first opportunity to leave home and that nursing was primarily limited to compassionate care. This, of course, is inaccurate in both timing and content of historical nursing, reflecting an absence of thorough knowledge of early nursing and an overreliance on standard nursing histories which, with few exceptions, have not incorporated women's history to any substantial degree. Further, their assertion concerning the reduction of Catholic nursing orders in the 17th century does not acknowledge the sexist bases for the exclusion of women's control by physicians abetted by civil authorities at a time when scientific superiority could hardly be attributed to the majority of physicians. To conclude that nursing care was "disorganized, degenerate, and sporadically provided by women who lived by gambling, prostitution, thievery, and bribery" (p. 162) is not so much evidence of what happens to women's history in the absence of feminist analysis as it is evidence of the total distortion of women's actual healing roles in their own homes and communities. (See Roberts & Group, *Nursing, Physician Control, and Medical Monopoly* for a thorough discussion of this issue.)

It is true, however, that women's *authority* in health matters was probably destroyed from the 15th to the 17th centuries. If the explanations by

Ehrenreich and English (1972) are even partially correct, the destruction of religious orders or the reduction of their power, coupled with the Inquisition and witch trials, produced severe disarray among women healers, only brought into some semblance of order by Nightingale, Barton, and other women in the latter half of the 19th century. Certainly, this is partially the view of Nutting and Dock (1907), which will probably be upheld in modified form in subsequent research.

One of the problems that nurses have in using historical information is not only the dearth or absence of data, but the assumption that progress is linear, going forward in direct improvements over time. Assuming male historical progression, which is questionable, women's history has no such easy linearity. Therefore, to interconnect women's status with the state of nursing can be more like putting together a complex quilt than a one-to-one correlation. Although Brand and Glass, as other thinkers, seemed to accept the assumption of linear "progression," they were certainly right about the appallingly low status of women and nurses in the early 1800s; however, more feminist research on nurses in surviving nursing orders must be conducted and then integrated with "lay" history before a comprehensive picture can be drawn. For example, at least one study on secular nurses in England puts some pre-Nightingale nurses in a more positive light (see Roberts & Group, *Nursing, Physician Control, and Medical Monopoly*). To Brand and Glass, the demands of humanism intersected with those of women and these in turn affected nursing, although reforms such as those at Kaiserswerth still followed monastic ideals.

As Clemons (1971) had noted, Brand and Glass too referred to the 1843 antislavery convention in London, noting its effect on women abolitionists but concluding that "effective action [was] impossible without the support of men" (p. 163). It is, of course, helpful to have men's support, but early feminists carried the burden of change then as they do now. Brand and Glass credited Nightingale for removing nurses from religious orders and from secular "debased care," for espousing equal rights, insisting on reimbursement for service and on women's control through their own leaders. Brand and Glass interpreted Nightingale's philosophy as classless in the sense that women from all classes were admitted to the nursing school at St. Thomas' Hospital. Nursing schools grew as more hospitals were founded and students were forced to provide care in exchange for their education, working "as many as 105 hours per week—and little or no pay—about $3 a day or 20c an hour" (p. 165).

Brand and Glass credited nursing leaders for trying to control admissions, curriculum, practice, and registrations, fighting the idea that nurses were "overtrained" and supporting the 1926 Committee on the Grading of Nursing Schools. But they also noted that "Women did not even control the only profession they had" (p. 167)—this, despite the fact that feminists directly influenced the women who provided the funds to open the Johns Hopkins

Medical School, only with the stipulation that women receive equal consideration, although they were subsequently allowed admittance only in small quotas. Information on the relationship of women to the founding of the nursing school is not given.

Brand and Glass pointed to the influence of Florence Nightingale on Elizabeth Blackwell's decision to establish a hospital completely managed by women; however, they did not discuss the differences in strategy, tactics, and goals between the two women. They again turned to Lavinia Dock (1908a) and her article on suffrage; the making of a new sacred icon, replacing other early American leaders, is clearly apparent. Thus, by the mid-1970s Dock had emerged as the new image of political power, although Isabel Stewart and M. Adelaide Nutting are credited for joining Dock and other women in the suffrage parade where "The forces of women and nursing had met" (p. 169).

The effects of World War I were presented by Brand and Glass as a test of nursing, not in zeal or devotion, as Nutting said, " 'but for our judgment and good sense and knowledge of our own situation' " (p. 169). The question of whether women as nurses want to be involved in war was not raised by Brand and Glass. Nor were the consequences of strengthening the power of medical and hospital men debated. The authors give the usual explanations of nurses' difficulties during the Depression, the Second World War, and the conservative years of the late 1940s and 1950s. Brand and Glass commented on racism in relation to sexism, noting, as had the Bulloughs previously, that nurses in 1946 were the first professional group to integrate racially and in 1947 began to meet at international forums.

In Brand and Glass's article, nurses' actions to achieve university education and to control their own institutions and practice are described as feminist efforts. In contrast, Ashley regarded some of these actions as inward withdrawal from women's actual subordination. Brand and Glass saw early nursing as providing women with opportunities to express and educate themselves, but by the 1970s, women's status and freedom were "no longer influenced by nursing. . . . Women no longer regard nursing as a necessary vehicle of their independence" (p. 173).

Brand and Glass advised nurses to remain consciously aware of women's problems, to work with women seeking equality, to keep up with the development of women in other professions, and to keep feminists informed of nursing activities and advances. Since one of every 40 women voters was a nurse (in 1975), Brand and Glass thought it probable that nursing was still critical to women's progress, if they would recognize and act on their mass political power. But they also seemed to expect non-nurses to take the leadership in feminist issues, with nurses paralleling the feminist work of others. A parallel model is not an interconnecting one, leaving many definitional and interactional questions unresolved. Nevertheless, Brand and Glass concluded: "Women in the movement must be kept informed of nursing's activities and advancements, so that each may augment the other's progress. . . . Nursing, therefore, is challenged to keep abreast with other professions while working in the general interest of women" (pp. 173–174).

RAISING THE CONSCIOUSNESS OF NURSES' OPPRESSION

Presumably, close interrelations with women in other professions could enhance feminist analysis. How this would occur if women have no consciousness of oppression remains the problem. Rosalee Yeaworth (1976), as others before her, points to the most fundamental problem in nursing—the lack of consciousness of nurses' own oppression that arises from nursing as a woman's occupation—but "the majority of nurses, along with the larger society, do not perceive this as a problem at all" (p. 7). Speaking at the national meeting of the American Association of Industrial Nurses, Yeaworth claimed that efforts to solve a problem that is not recognized as a problem by the majority are frustrating, ineffective, even seen as somewhat "strange" or "humorous."

Yeaworth states that a woman still gains status and power by aligning with a man, pleasing him, and supporting his upward mobility. Women who work outside the home must add these responsibilities to homemaking and child-bearing tasks, since public laws and policies still recognized (at that time) only a breadwinner with dependent spouses; all other cases were considered abnormal or deviant. Continuous and overt statements of traditional expectations reminded married women workers of their "real" responsibilities; consequently, those who achieved higher levels were often denied the usual signs of recognition. As an example, Yeaworth says she was regularly introduced as Ms. or Mrs., not Doctor or Professor—terms of respect normally given to her male colleagues. Women themselves reduce women's status: "Phone operators and secretaries make a thing of converting 'Doctor' back to 'Ms.' when it's attached to a woman's name" (p. 8). These daily reminders of subordination exact a cumulative toll. Yeaworth's son had an appendectomy with no notification given to his parents; yet she could not sign as responsible for her own hospital bills when she had minor surgery. Her husband accompanied Yeaworth to a National League for Nursing conference, but only he could buy a full price ticket and get a reduction in fare for her ticket. To Yeaworth, affirmative action had affected hiring discrimination, but institutional life was still structured to minimize women's influence and opportunities for promotion.

What does all this have to do with nursing, where women supposedly do not compete with men? Yeaworth asserts: "Unfortunately, despite a few courageous and perceptive leaders, nursing has done more to preserve the status quo than to promote the status of women" (p. 8). This has occurred because the image of nursing maintains the stereotype of the "nurturant, feminine, self-sacrificing person who meets the needs of others" (p. 8). Second, it has fostered work arrangements that allow nurses to supplement their family income, but persons not dependent on their wages for family survival do not have to be as concerned about salary and fringe benefits; this weakens the bargaining power of committed nurses.

A third way nurses have maintained stereotypes is by not publicizing the many decisions they make or their independent actions. When nurses write prescriptions over the physician's signature, or decide under various p.r.n. orders when medications or treatments are necessary, or obtain patient histories, observe symptoms, or suggest diagnoses and treatments, their acts are kept quiet. This silence is sustained by the laws in many states that prevent nurses from practicing independently or providing care for noninstitutionalized persons and receiving third-party payment; thus, most nurses practice under male control. Fourth, nurses are embedded in the bureaucratic hierarchy; many directors of nursing do not exercise control over their own budgets or rise to top-level positions in either service or administration. Their own nursing schools are often subsumed under colleges of medicine or education. Fifth, nursing education patterns have restricted professionalization, recognition for advanced practice, and educational mobility: "Nurses themselves have provided some of the greatest resistance to moving nursing education into the mainstream of higher education" (p. 8). A sixth factor, Yeaworth claims, is the persistent belief in nursing that other disciplines have the experts and the most worthwhile knowledge: "In nursing, we have a bad habit of calling in physicians, psychologists and other male experts from other disciplines to be the main speakers and teachers at workshops and special educational programs . . . we have nurses who are just as qualified or more so to do that teaching and speaking" (p. 9).

What strategies can nurses use to change the stereotypes? Yeaworth advocated emulating the Black power movement, to stop viewing Whites as models, or, translated, to stop using men or physicians as models: "We need to decide on the qualities and capabilities that are considered feminine that need to be valued, preserved, built upon—qualities in which women can take pride" (p. 9). Yeaworth warned of a backlash from universities and organizations as they tightened regulations, credentials, and requirements that would solidify barriers to women. To deal with this backlash, she said, would take determination; she urged the profession to "give women better psychological and educational preparation to equip them to exert influence, to gain status and to do so without turning off our would-be supporters" (p. 9).

Nurses were not the only health-care professionals subject to discrimination. Margaret Harty (1976) presented an update on health professionals in general. She detailed areas of discrimination that affected not only nurses, but pharmacists, chiropractors, social workers, physical therapists, and workers in other occupations in the health-care industry. Presenting a brief synopsis of the 1975 Health Resources Administration report on minorities and women in the health field, Harty stated:

> Relatively few women are found in primary decision-making positions concerned with health-care services, education or planning. . . . Although more than half of the world's people are women and nearly half of the paid working population in the United States, China, and Russia are women, unequal standards and opportunities are the rule rather than the exception. This unreasonable, unjust, and illegal partisanship extends into every field of human endeavor, including the field of health services where, traditionally, the majority of personnel (nearly 70 percent) are women. (p. 174)

Noreen Reavill (1976) reinforced Harty's message: "Nurses, the majority of whom are women, are the largest single force in our health system. Yet nurses do not have control within the system; rather they are controlled by it!" (p. 60). She emphasized the need for nurses to understand politics, the system of practices, attitudes, and beliefs that enable one group to maintain control over another. Obviously, two distinct groups must exist before dominance can be exerted by one over the other, either by consent or force. Although Reavill recognized nurses' consent to medical dominance, one might ask how many nurses have left the profession because they refused to consent, and how many others who stay fight male authority, at least covertly. Reavill stressed that in order to sustain the distinctiveness between two groups, families and all other social institutions must teach that the difference between the two groups is unchangeable; the penalties for member nonconformity must be severe; stereotypes must be well known and must "explain" the difference; a functional rationale must be asserted; segregation for differential treatment must be created; dominance relations must be specified; and institutionalization of difference must be established to sustain prejudicial treatment.

Reavill illustrated how change in gender difference is "proved" to be impossible, such as in biblical admonitions that man is not of woman, nor created for her, but woman is of man and created for him. God-given natural law is obviously hard to contest, but so is pseudo-scientific generalizations from psychiatry, particularly in Freudian theory—anatomy is destiny. Hormonal differences are also used to establish the immutability of change. Those who violate the gendered difference, "the feminized male and masculinized female" (p. 56), and particularly the homosexual person, have been severely punished. But, claimed Reavill, so have working women with children, who often are made to feel guilty for working, even though children can no longer be considered a lifetime occupation and despite research that indicates that under most conditions, children exhibit minimal negative, and often positive, consequences from having working mothers.

Stereotypes sustain difference by portraying the feminine role as the exact opposite of the masculine role. Media images express and foster this unattainable and unhealthy distinction. The stereotypes then are used to justify completely different functions, such as in traditional families, which, in turn, establish differential development in gendered roles. By segregating the sexes, it is difficult, noted Reavill, to discover human similarities and eventually this produces different interests, motivations, goals, and values, which are all reinforced in children's books and textbooks in public schools. Boys learn early in life the importance of winning, particularly over girls, who learn to fail. The difference of gendered types in families establishes dominance structures, which are then institutionalized.

Reavill cited Ehrenreich and English (1972) and their portrayal of women healers, which presents a history of nursing that cuts through so-called natural differences and shows how women in health care were limited or excluded. Unfortunately, Nightingale and Dix are seen as examples of women who merely transplanted the "natural" motherly role in the home to the ideal lady in the hospital, where care and cure were subjected to gendered dichotomization. Reavill claimed: "Ideally, there should be no reason to write on the subject of nurses and their kinship to those women struggling for equality. Nurses as an oppressed group should have long ago identified themselves with the women's movement. There should be no question in anyone's mind that the two—women's rights and nurses's rights—are actually one and the same" (p. 60).

Because nurses have been taught over time that medical knowledge is too complex and beyond their capability, their subservience has been strengthened by ignorance. Reavill could not keep track of the number of times over the years that her questions were answered with the dismissal that nurses do not need to know certain information. Why, she asked, have nurses not been involved in establishing women's clinics where medical knowledge is shared? At least the expanded role for nurses was seeded in the broader women's movement. In agreement with Roberts and Group (1973), she called for strong leadership by women who know who they are. But all nurses must develop their own awareness, must commit themselves to the movement, particularly in health care. Moreover, pseudocompetition rooted in stereotyped "femininity" must give way to a unified body of nurses working as a team.

Reavill hoped that the invitation to the president of the National Organization for Women to speak at the 1975 ANA convention might indicate that nurses were beginning to listen to feminist ideas and make the linkages, since "there is no way to separate the nurses' organization from the feminist organization" (p. 62). Control of the male-defined system is not enough; "feminine" insights and convictions can help humanize health care, said Reavill, who cited Wilma Scott Heide's (1973) call for "fully human and humane health practitioners," hoping that the women's movement would free nurses to be just that.

In agreement with Yeaworth and Reavill, Fran A'Hern Smith (1977) also believed that nurses must *understand* their oppression before they could do anything about it. As an example of the limited consciousness of oppression among nurses, Smith stated:

> Recently a woman used denial in a conversation with me. She said she had never experienced sexism. A few minutes later, she related that the dean from a community college at which she and her husband were employed told her that the reason she didn't earn as much as her husband was that her income was supplementary to the bread winner. I pointed out that was sexist and she said, "No, it was a reality." (p. 19)

Obviously, Smith said, this woman needed to change her conception of reality before she could understand oppression and discriminatory behaviors directed toward her.

NEW WAYS OF THINKING:
RISK-TAKERS AND ROLE-BREAKERS

In 1976 Marlene Grissum and Carol Spengler published *Woman, Power and Health Care*, the first book specifically devoted to nursing and feminism in the decade. Primarily utilitarian in orientation, it was synopsized by Grissum in a *Nursing '76* article. Grissum claimed that nurses have been socialized into rigid, inflexible roles that have channeled their goal-directed activity toward pleasing their superiors. Nurses must discard this female "virtue," but to do so would not be simply "committing a blunder . . . [but] deliberately moving counter to our traditionally acceptable role" (p. 89). Nurses must engage in more risk-taking and role-breaking behaviors to dissolve the stereotyping that has held them in a tight grip since the last wave of feminism in the late 1800s and early 1900s. The great task is to break the mold of handmaiden, nurturer, and *"beloved imbecile."* To Grissum, roles as women and nurses are so intrinsically woven together that nurses need not even designate which is being discussed. To take risks in breaking nursing roles, nurses cannot be submissive or passive in their personal worlds, because one change requires the other. Grissum clarified the essential problem: the compassion, tenderness, and nurturance needed in good nursing are the very traits used by men *against* nurses.

Demands for change may make nurses feel guilty, fearing harm may be done to patients because the nurses' demands are ego-centered. Thus, nurses are "torn between our desire to assert ourselves and our desire to remain self-effacing" (p. 90). To resolve this conflict, nurses will accept moderate success and give only superficial commitment. Role-breakers must be responsible and autonomous, but they must expect hostility and rejection will follow from those people who fear their own responses will be inappropriate. To counter predictable hostility, Grissum recommended taking the offense and attacking first, because nurses cannot allow a sexist society to dictate to nursing; indeed, nurses need to identify nursing leaders who are not afraid to be different: "Role-breakers (hence, our leaders) will be found in every health care setting, doing all levels of nursing care. They'll be the nurses not well liked by administration, not respected by peers, feared and distrusted by physicians. But they'll be loved and respected by fellow role-breakers for their courage, intelligence, and future-oriented outlook" (p. 91).

Nurses do not have time to consider whether behavior is masculine or feminine. What is important is whether it is human, in the best sense. Using the roles of mother, housekeeper, and housemanager at home, nurses have extended these to very similar roles in institutional settings, but the public must learn that these are now insufficient. Calling for unity of over one million nurses, Grissum stressed the need for women who will talk, not just listen; question, not simply answer; contradict, not merely acquiesce; and demand, not just comply. Affirming positive self-images, Grissum claimed the societal pay-off is better health care from nurses, whose traditional roles have kept them from a broad base of scientific knowledge and from accepting full responsibility for the well-being of their patients. Grissum spoke scathingly of the "Aunt Janes" of nursing who are simply assistants to physicians, taking blood pressures or giving medications previously only allowed physicians by physicians. Such rigidities must give way, not to nurses as pseudophysicians, but to women who have the skills to do far more than the dichotomized professions have allowed in the past. Until more physicians and nurses are educated together, Grissum expected the role-breakers to have to assume responsibility for leaders in correcting the injustices of a system that has been used against women, both as providers and patients.

Now that women are not totally economically and legally dependent on men, they can refuse, for example, the incarceration in mental hospitals of role-breakers for rejecting the happy housewife role. To change the sexist system, nurses must control their profession through *direct* access to patients, and control their lives by giving up traditional patriarchal views of family, which in turn reinforce powerlessness in nursing. To Grissum, the women's movement may pull nurses "into the real world," showing them that a woman's professional commitment is as important as her husband's. Until then, nurses are going to have responsibilities without formal sanctions and authority, acting as symbols without being able to function autonomously.

What makes some people capable of perceiving themselves as different, of having the strength to prevail against pressures to conform? For example, Grissum wondered whether Margaret Sanger, who endured hostility and anger, was a rebel or a woman who held firm because of a strongly held conviction that women had the right to birth control. Was Mary Wollstonecraft just a strange woman or a person who had aspirations beyond the usual societal demands? Where there is incongruence between self-image and self-ideal, between self and societal demands, role-breakers are likely to emerge. From this perspective, Wollstonecraft is a perfect example of the women who refused sexist limitations; independent at nineteen, traveling alone, teaching herself several languages, authoring articles, pamphlets, and books without a pen name, having a child out of wedlock, married but living in her own house—all these acts, rejected by society, made her, in a 1947 Freudian analysis, a severe case of penis envy, a compulsive neurotic. Considered crazy because she dared to be fully human, she, according to Grissum, is an example of a feminist role model. Margaret Sanger, herself a nurse, is another model; she was a woman who pressured society and refused to conform—ridiculed, arrested, shunned by other nurses and women, who now have her to thank for their better lives.

But must nurses look only to the past? Grissum thought not, pointing to Rena Murtha, who established a nurse-ombudsman for the New York City prison system, and Ruth Murphy, an expert nurse practitioner for Elk County, Kansas, or other nurses currently training for the U.S. space program. Grissum claimed that thousands of nurses are struggling to create health care that is more than "a pill to cure all ills" (p. 97). Grissum referred to her own family practice, expressing her joy and power when women seek her help, one even saying that it was the first time she hadn't felt "degraded, embarrassed, ignored, or a nuisance" (p. 97). When a physician thanks Grissum for a referral or consults with her about a patient, the change in the doctor-nurse game is obvious. The penalties and rewards are high for role-breakers, but Grissum concluded:

In the not too distant future, those of us who are now role-breakers will be seen as maintainers of the *status quo*, and the risk-takers of that age will be urging us to break the chains that bind us to the past. But until that age is here, we must increase our growing numbers of risk-takers, so that we can overwhelm (with sheer numbers if nothing else) the nurses and other health professionals who cling to the unreal roles of the past. (p. 97)

Earlier in the decade, Hildegard E. Peplau, in her 1972 presidential address to the ANA, had asked if nursing might be "phased out" eventually. Did the men in government who control public funds believe that nursing was an outdated female occupation? "If so," said Peplau, "the problem is greatly compounded if the women in nursing act as if they are in agreement with that view. Silence gives consent" (Peplau, 1976, p. 589). Why, asked Peplau, do nurses fear power? The reality of their socialization experience must be confronted, and inequalities that have been meekly accepted in the past must be rectified. Peplau asserted: "More women than not are fugitives from leadership and power" (p. 590). Too few recognize that benevolent relationships, for example, between physicians and nurses have elements of power. Some nurses transfer their behaviors with patients to colleagues and thus weaken their efforts to improve collaboration. To Peplau, the failure to develop and use fully one's power and authority was irresponsible. What is required is the willingness to stand together to sustain and strengthen the profession. "Courage is contagious, and we must show it" (p. 591).

AGGRESSIVE, MANNISH, STUBBORN, AND UNATTRACTIVE?

Sparked by feminist activism, a conference on leadership in nursing was convened at Yale University in 1971; three papers and reactions to them were subsequently published in the *American Journal of Nursing* (*AJN*) (McBride, Diers, Slavinsky, Schlotfeldt, Christman, & Kibrick, 1972). McBride claimed that most nurses were neither interested in being leaders nor educated to be leaders. She recalled one graduate student who thought that to be a leader must surely mean being mannish, aggressive, stubborn, and unattractive. While spending quantities of time on nursing care plans, faculty, according to McBride, "scarcely mention how an institution's organizational plan may crush any efforts . . . to be innovative" (p. 1445). To many nurses, there is a "masculine" flavor to political strategy, risk-taking, and other words describing leadership, but a "feminine" sense to empathy and emotional support, terms associated with patient care. These values, said McBride, are not enough when challenges to nursing are being felt from many directions. McBride applied Simone de Beauvoir's thought to nursing education, claiming that nurses are subjected to mediocrity; "pedantic blinders" and "methodical eagerness" cause a "tension and weariness of spirit" (p. 1446). McBride traced many of nursing's problems to the gender-typed nature of nursing education. Women often choose nursing in a negative way—as one of only three choices for girls: nurse, teacher, or secretary. As students learn about caring, they assume that the principles of good one-to-one care can be transferred to other situations with equally positive results. Lack of political education is decried: "We are the most feminine of professions, created in the image of the attractive, seductive, nurturing earth mother. Yet all of us have intense love-hate feelings about sex-directed education that encourages plodding rather than invention" (p. 1447).

Another speaker, Donna Diers, stated flatly: "Nurses lack a sense of themselves as leaders, potential or actual" (p. 1447). To many nurses, the term "leadership" is so myth-ridden that it is fearsome or inaccessible: Diers claimed that nurses even seem to undermine the work and influence of their own leaders. Why does this happen? Blaming shaky self-esteem and self-concepts, education that trains out independence and abstraction, and an unorganized and ambivalent profession, Diers hoped the women's liberation movement was raising the consciousness of nurses: "Perhaps a nurses' liberation movement would help raise our consciousness about ourselves as nurses" (p. 1448). Ann Slavinsky found it difficult to even name nurse leaders; indeed, most psychiatric nurses turned to men in psychiatry for models. "If we cannot understand that what we do as nurses is different from what others do, something has gone wrong" (p. 1448). To Slavinsky, the crisis in leadership was reflected in a crisis in theory development.

Reacting to the panelists, Rosella Schlotfeldt, in a very conservative mode, stated: "The emphasis on feminism at this point in time is terribly unfortunate, especially when we are attempting to attract more men in nursing" (p. 1449). But she was optimistic because feminism might open opportunities for both women and men, and women could take from the women's movement "that which is advantageous to all nurses" (p. 1449). On the other hand, Luther Christman believed that the usual leaders in nursing, those in the middle-range group, ages 25 to 55, had left the profession and were not there to lead anymore: "And that is going to last unless the feminist movement does find a way to create the means for two-career families to exist so nurses can continue to nurse" (p. 1450). In a misunderstanding of historical feminism, Christman believed that a "residual" of the early women's movement had led nurses away from competency in patient care to management. That Christman did not have a grasp of early feminism is clear, but Schlotfeldt's apparent need to advocate for male nurses is puzzling since proponents of the women's movement had always objected to single-sex occupations, and thus, were supportive of male nurses, as long as they did not disproportionately occupy the higher level administrative positions in nursing.

Ann Kibrick questioned the equation of educational credentials and leadership, and the validity of studies of personality characteristics of nurses, believing them dated when applied to current baccalaureate nurses, and insisted that clinicians, not leaders, were needed. In a restatement of stereotypes, Kibrick considered many nursing leaders to be somewhat mannish, aggressive, and stubborn. With no understanding of the societal critique of "feminine" as containing the roots of stereotypic thought, Kibrick claimed that "feminine" women could be leaders. What was really extraordinary about this symposium, conducted at a major university, is the lack of knowledge of women's history, psychology, and sociology. Without this background, a socially coherent understanding of power eluded a number of the participants.

NURSING HISTORY AS A CHRONOLOGY
OF GENDERED POWER STRUGGLES

In contrast, just one year later, Jo Ann Ashley (1973) published a social and historical systemic analysis of nurses' failure to recognize or use their power. According to Ashley, nurses felt powerless; thus, they focused on the negative, some even saying, as Peplau had wondered, that nurses would become "obsolete, replaced by something else, or cease to exist" (p. 637). Bemoaning one's lack of power was not likely to produce the "courage to act constructively at this significant time in our history" (p. 637). But Ashley believed that nurses have *always had power*, which derived from society's recognition of nursing as an essential service.

Ashley claimed that health-care systems are the result of years of change in ideas and actions originating in a basic system of values. Nursing's history could be described as a power struggle: "To obtain a proper education though opposed by more powerful groups . . . to throw off the burden of oppression imposed by those groups . . . to practice without numerous and professionally extraneous restraints and restrictions . . . to convince others of the value of nursing" (p. 638). Why had so few nurses examined the use of nursing power to maintain a system that oppressed them? Through cooperation and collaboration, nurses learn to support, not change the system. To Ashley, nursing power as a productive force was the *single most important factor* maintaining the health-care system. Without the pooled efforts of women, institutions would shut down, but nurses have "permitted themselves to be used as simply a labor force . . . to be controlled and utilized to keep the system and its various parts functioning" (p. 638).

In contrast to earlier writers, Ashley clearly recognized that nurses were in positions of potential leadership and power but were not recognized as logical participants in policy decisions. Power is relative: medicine is powerful, but was not previously, and is powerful now only because of the control and use of others—notably nursing—to strengthen itself. Ashley traced the historical aspects of nurses' power, accurately assessing the critical importance of women in lowering mortality rates, making hospitals acceptable for care, and establishing public health reforms. These nursing activities were essentially carved out *without* physicians' supervision. Nursing has lived with the myth that it is and always has been the dependent group. In reality, said Ashley, history shows that "physicians very early recognized their own increasing dependency upon nurses. This, and not the reverse, was true" (p. 639).

Talk of "allies" has led to a false sense of colleagueship, the nurse-doctor game, a peculiar form of communication that pretends that physicians make all the decisions while nurses make few or none. When women formed nursing organizations, physicians argued that nursing could never be a profession and would remain a form of supportive labor. To sustain this myth, the distinct contributions of nurses have been attributed to medical skill. To Ashley, the force of these traditions still weighed down nurses, limiting them as physicians' advocates, failing to effectively change health services to the public.

Nursing and the public seem unable to separate nursing care from medical treatment. The values on which the system is based are economic, reflecting a class ideology sustaining medical predominance, leaving nurses "so hidden and locked in organizations of various types that nursing's visibility is lost to the public" (p. 640). Ashley viewed hospitals as large industrial concerns with a nurse proletariat in which the traditional supervisory nursing roles are a holdover from earlier times when untrained apprentices, rather than fully qualified professionals, formed the staff. She stated: "I am convinced that the perpetuation of traditional supervisory roles in nursing contributes to the abuse of nursing power" (p. 640). Too often, nursing leaders identify with the medical and hospital administrators, thus crushing the development of power and leadership among nurses, whose pervasive feelings of inequality and inadequacy contribute to the formation of conflicting groups. Instead of forming a power base among nurses, many leaders make decisions in isolation and without consensus of followers, who then come to believe they have little or no power. Paradoxically, medicine has never really underestimated the power of nursing, but has effectively harnessed nurses' power to advance their own causes. According to Ashley, the myth of "medical supervision" will continue the attribution of nursing care to "medical skill."

Ashley's uncompromising socialist, feminist analysis affirms the power of nurses as women workers, marking a distinctive shift in nursing intellectual thought, a theoretical base that deals directly with power. Still, there was continued denigration of women leaders. Indeed, the social class analysis almost required the distinction between workers and administrators. But where do women *as a group* stand in relation to social class? This remained a problem in the analysis. Furthermore, where do feminist nursing leaders stand when their "followers" will not follow? Role-breakers need support, but traditionally defined women workers may be unlikely to give it to strong feminist women in administrative or supervisory positions. To the women who accept stereotyped roles, any woman moving toward power is a threat, not only to the subordinated nurse's role, but to the very definition of womanhood.

DISUNITY AND A DISMAL LACK OF INTERNAL LEADERSHIP

The widely variegated positions on nursing education in the 1970s reflected very different ideas of what a woman's occupation or profession should be. Marguerite J. Schaefer (1973) reflected on the diversity as evident in a national study funded by the ANA, whose board of directors voted to initiate research on nursing and education, resulting in an *Abstract for Action*, published in 1970. Schaefer specifically dealt with the political implications of the research, concluding that the profession could be characterized as politically and economically weak. Relying on traditional political science, Schaefer viewed politics as the act of an entire community creating actions by shaping many disparate social elements into joint action. "How," asked Schaefer, "can nursing create action when it can rarely even speak to an issue with a unified voice and continues to operate on a consensus-seeking base?" (p. 887).

To achieve consensus on the location of educational programs in collegiate institutions, a compromise allowed federal funding to be distributed *equally* to diploma, associate degree, and baccalaureate programs, thus reducing by 50% the funds for university-based students and maintaining the status quo, rather than supporting the National Commission's recommendation. To Schaefer, this lack of unity in political action is typical since nursing usually reacts to outside stimuli rather than creating actions. As a prime example, Schaefer pointed to the American Medical Association's 1969 invitation to nurses to assume expanded roles as physicians' assistants, which was rebuffed by nurses. Where, asked Schaefer, was nursing's initiative in developing nurses' expanded roles in the 1960s? Why did nurses again allow themselves to react to rather than create a new idea?

If women's political behavior is reactive, what are the economic consequences? Schaefer believed that hospitals would continue to replace nurses with licensed practical nurses, and that nurse practitioners, working at advanced levels of competence, would probably receive little or no substantial change in their salaries. For example, a pediatric nurse practitioner, reported by physicians as an economic asset netting them an additional $16,800 per year, received a salary of $7,620 in 1969. Formed of underpaid women, nursing organizations are "traditionally poverty-stricken" with lack of support from women who do not understand that effective political action requires powerful national organizations. Furthermore, the economic situation of nursing schools was going from bad to worse. Accurately predicting federal cutbacks, Schaefer warned of the financial disaster facing many collegiate programs in nursing.

What is the result of political and economic weakness? A vicious cycle of powerlessness, a "hang-dog-sorry-for-ourselves" attitude, and a low status public image. Is this state of affairs visible to non-nurses? Schaefer referred to Martha E. Peterson, then president of Barnard College, and her speech to the American Council of Education: "'Through intransigence, unperceptiveness, or preoccupation with other issues, the nursing community seems unable to recognize and take action in correcting the deficiencies in the nation's health care system . . . [reflecting] a dismal lack of internal leadership'" (p. 889).

In fairness, Schaefer admitted that women had not been culturally oriented toward leadership. Although this feminist point is made, it is not sustained in a systemic analysis. Schaefer instead called for individual moral courage from nurses to assume responsibility to the public rather than wasting time, talents, and resources on battles over turf, programs, and status. To Schaefer the question was: Do you confront your problems or conform to what others are deciding for you?

THE CONFRONTATION-NEGOTIATION ERA
AND NURSE LEADERS

Madeleine Leininger (1974) pointed to a leadership crisis in nursing, as women tried to cope with a "new order of phenomena . . . [caused by] technological advances, changes in social structures, shifts in moral-ethical values, and differences in the psycho-political strategies of management" (p. 29). According to Leininger, passive and nonaggressive nurse leaders working in most large and complex institutions have a low survival rate and impede rather than enhance nurses' position. They fail to see needed changes and continue to function in traditional and nonpolitical ways, conforming to old institutional values. Nurse leaders must grapple with the complexity of women's and minority rights; interprofessional competition; professional rights and autonomy; financing nursing programs; subcultural nursing values; and political pressures in relation to space, staffing, and resources.

Leininger distinguished between the confrontation-negotiation era and the previous establishment-maintenance era. The current situation required a position of strength, but some female leaders were reluctant to use the confrontation-negotiation approach because their perceptions of female leadership behaviors were too traditional. Leininger recognized that it *is* hard for women leaders to exert the required leadership in male-dominated and controlled institutions in which cliques, social linkages, and personal alliances are used to sustain masculist power. But women must learn to compete for money, space, status, and human resources; therefore, they must also overcome resistance that can be gender-based. Breaking male-dominated power cliques, women leaders cannot depend on "feminine charm," an unreliable way to deal with the competition for scarce resources. To initiate action, to confront openly, and to negotiate professional matters create stresses for traditional leaders because these processes require risk-taking, courage, and fearlessness, all incompatible with prior "lady-like" training to avoid fighting, or even the appearance of boldness or aggression.

Leininger claimed that the exaggeration of American egalitarianism had, by the 1970s, produced a negative cultural attitude toward authority in general. Thus, "any strong, aggressive nursing leader is likely to be distrusted and challenged, particularly in patriarchal situations" (p. 30). In addition, the cultural image of women's role continued to affect leadership in nursing: "Some nurses expect a core of active nurse leaders to uncover and deal with the sex discrimination problems as they ride in on the benefits of these efforts" (p. 31). As Leininger stressed, equal rights, pay, and privileges required all nurses to be committed to *continuous* affirmative action; unfortunately, many were too passive and not committed to changing the situation. Why was this so? Leininger blamed women's subordination and servitude toward males, which are reaffirmed in "assistant to" positions, excluding women from major decisions and planning. The cultural image causes "too many female nurses

[to] 'sell' themselves cheaply . . . willingly accepting *whatever* they are offered, challenging neither rank, position or salary" (p. 31). Males were placed in leadership positions without women being able to compete or even know how the appointments occurred. For those in administration, salary inequities were widespread; for example, nursing deans' salaries were considerably lower than those of other deans in academic institutions. But even worse, "nearly 50 percent of these deans had *not* taken affirmative action to change their salary" (p. 31).

All these issues were exacerbated by the size and complexity of organizational structures. According to Leininger: "To modify these complex systems is a sizable task that can never be done alone; it requires considerable knowledge, political power and support" (p. 31). With rapid institutional growth comes complexity shock or competitive shock. Nurses must understand power strategies, coalitions, caucuses, shifts, cliques, and games. Nurses' overreliance on interpersonal and persuasive techniques excludes many other organizational strategies.

An added problem was the ill-defined nursing role that some leaders actively worked on and others avoided. In the nursing subculture, lack of role clarity has traditionally fostered dependency, submission to authority, and humanistic and expressive care-giving activities. In contrast, medical subculture values independence, dominance, control of others, and scientific breakthroughs. Added to these problems are those of interdisciplinary interconnections, which in nursing are exaggerated because of the diverse interests and varying levels of educational preparation and experience.

According to Leininger, competent leaders were no longer staying in their positions until they retired or died. This trend would be exaggerated because dynamic leaders could be expected to cause ripples without which no change can occur. Leininger called for research on the role behaviors of female and male nurses. Nurses needed to know what happens in patriarchal versus matriarchal social systems. Mid- and top-level nursing administrative programs were needed to deal with the complexities of nontraditional authority and power.

POLITICAL ACTION: UNPROFESSIONAL, UNWOMANLY, AND UNNECESSARY?

To what extent did other nurses writing in the 1970s agree with Leininger? Marjorie Stanton (1974) claimed that nursing has been conspicuously absent as a political force, if defined as exerting influence: "Many nurses consider political action to be unprofessional, unwomanly, and unnecessary" (p. 579). These perceptions reflected a lack of understanding and sophistication about decision making and naivete about political action. A potential national health insurance system was at that time a real political possibility, yet, as Stanton noted, nursing seemed to have little or no input into how a new system would be shaped.

Since its founding in 1911, the ANA supported some social welfare legislation and worked for economic security for nurses. Over the past 80 years, organized nurses have engaged in numerous actions, often in conflict with the American Medical Association, which, for example, opposed Social Security and Medicare. Stanton claimed: "Nursing is the only humanizing health profession left. They [nurses] see people as total human beings, not as parts of the body or mind, or as disease entities" (p. 581). Yet nursing still seemed unable to exert enough power or influence to change the system to meet the needs of all citizens.

Agreeing with feminist Shirley Chisholm, Stanton insisted that politics is inherent in everyone's life. She called for a distinction between political and legislative action. She agreed with Ashley, stating that nursing has power, but it is unchecked, unleashed, and unharnessed, diluted by other professional groups, by legislators, and even by groups of nurses who compete with each other for status and recognition. Fragmented, nurses can be used effectively by the opposition. Stanton called for leaders to mobilize the massive numbers of women in nursing. She specifically supported the newly formed Nurses for Political Action, created as the political wing of the ANA: "No longer can we afford to wait to react to what is already a fact. We must take the lead—we must take the risk" (pp. 584–585). To do less, denied humanitarian care to the public and nursing its rightful place in history.

BARRIERS TO NURSING POWER: FEMALE SOCIALIZATION, LOW SELF-ESTEEM, AND MEDICAL OPPOSITION

In a more optimistic note, Shirley A. Smoyak (1974) argued that by the 1970s many nurses had a newly found sense of their own competencies and worth that fostered feelings of efficacy and power. In fact, nurses had been actively pushing for joint practice commissions of medicine and nursing in each state: "I can't think of a single instance, on the state level, when the *physicians* pushed for a joint practice committee. No doubt that's because physicians are comfortable with the status quo, while nurses are not" (p. 10).

Some nurses and physicians were trying to become more collegial, but the continuing difficulty and strain between the two professions could be traced to inequality. Though Smoyak believed that many nurses were becoming aware of their potentials and possibilities, major barriers to independent roles were still caused by the female socialization of nurses and the low self-esteem that followed. Furthermore, Smoyak stated, "Increased role responsibilities of nurses are an economic threat to physicians. . . . The most threatened physicians are usually the least competent—those who have not expanded themselves, and feel the nurses breathing hot upon their necks. The least threatened are the energetic, bright, active, expanding physicians who do not see change as so threatening" (p. 13).

Smoyak espoused the feminist version of nursing history: medicine did not precede but emerged from nursing. Now women must demand equality in status, power, prestige, and access to information. Smoyak credited the women's movement for boosting nurses' self-esteem and their assertiveness in claiming more independent work roles. By providing new versions of competence, "feminists have succeeded in getting women—and men—to consider how differently the two groups have been socialized to undertake their human roles" (p. 11). Time and effort were needed to socialize nurses to create new alternatives and actions, but nurses of all ages were using meetings and other encounters to begin their resocialization; indeed, said Smoyak, the "sharpness of insight and self-expression of nurses today are impressive" (p. 12).

Still, nurses often improperly extended the patient role to co-workers; for example, surgeons with violent tempers were still being pacified. To not lose the battle before it began, Smoyak insisted that nurses must differentiate patients from workers in relating to each: "A large part of the work ahead is to convince nurses and physicians still locked in master-slave, king-handmaiden or authority-subordinate relations that there is a better, more productive way to work" (p. 13). With pointed satirical humor, Smoyak offered "A Nurse's Psalm," a few lines of which said:

Colleagueship is my guide: I shall not want.
This maketh me to demand equal pay for equal work.
To visualize a new day of equal exchanges; it comfort my soul.
Yea—though I walk through the valley of the shadow of medical male domination, I will bear no long-lasting grudges—
Retribution for past grievances is not my aim—
Only acknowledgement as a colleague in health care delivery. (p. 13)

THE RIGHT TO DO:
GOING BEYOND A SUBBRANCH OF MEDICINE

By the mid-1970s the idea that nurses had rights was gaining momentum. Claire Fagin (1975) credited her mentor, Hildegard Peplau, with introducing the idea that nurses had the *right* to follow their beliefs in patient treatment. To Fagin, "Nurses have the established right *not* to do; now it is time to grasp the right *to* do" (p. 82). Traditionally, nurses have delineated rights and then presented papers filled with statements about responsibilities, but Fagin reversed this process by differentiating between the *meaning* of rights and responsibilities: "The word 'right' is defined as a just claim to anything to which one is entitled such as power or privilege. A 'right' is that which one may properly demand or claim as just, moral, or legal" (p. 82). Society appears to grant rights for a service that is given directly, rather than a service delivered through an intermediary. Without this direct relationship, it is difficult for people to become aware of what a group has to offer. "The public is for the most part unaware of what nursing has to offer in the improvement of health care. The public sees nursing as a sub-branch of medicine, ordered and controlled by physicians. If they have received good nursing care in a hospital, for example, they frequently believe that this is the result of physician's orders or some other control outside the realm of nursing practice and decision-making" (p. 84).

This image is further enhanced by nurses, who, for the most part, play the role demanded of all women by being submissive, dependent, indirect, manipulative, perhaps even frightened. Fagin stated: "Failure to act on behalf of our rights increases our guilt and low self-esteem and compounds our problems by discouraging the development of enabling behaviors to achieve rights. In seeking security, rather than satisfaction, we are, more often than not, unaware of our lack of achievements" (p. 85). Rather than focusing on "acceptable" responsibilities, Fagin encouraged nurses to use their rights to act politically, becoming involved in a wide range of activities calculated to affect law-making groups, acting to improve the professional interests of nurses and, through these actions, enhance their responsibilities to the people they serve.

Fagin's espousal of feminism was unambiguous; she supported and used the Statement on Rights produced by the National Organization for Women (NOW) in which equality is a birthright of human beings, who must have the opportunity to develop to their fullest potential through complete freedom of choice in their lifestyles and goals. Nurses' rights do not differ from human rights or women's rights. In the NOW Statement on Rights, the word "nurse" could be easily substituted for "woman"; thus, nurses would gain most by acting now and speaking out on behalf of their own equality, freedom, and dignity. More specifically, nurses have the right to self-expression of their abilities and backgrounds; to recognition of their contributions and professional economic rewards; to a work environment minimizing stress and health risks; to control professional practice, to set nursing standards, to participate in policy making affecting nursing; and to social and political action in behalf of nursing and health care.

A LONG WAY TO GO: WOMEN AND THE UPPER ECHELONS OF HEALTH-CARE LEADERSHIP

Though the women's movement had opened opportunities for women in many fields previously closed to them, how much change had occurred in opportunities for women in traditional health-care administration? Alan Appelbaum (1975) had predicted that women in medical schools would increase from 18% to 30% by 1985. He was correct: in 1985, total enrollment in medical schools was 32.5% female and 30.1% of those graduating were women (*On Campus With Women*, 1986). Despite the impact of the women's movement, Appelbaum warned that women still had a long way to go to achieve top positions in health-care management, particularly in the male-dominated hospital field. Appelbaum recognized that historically hospitals were matriarchal: 70% of the Catholic hospitals, which included 25% of all nongovernmental hospitals, had women administrators. However, in 1973 the Dixon Commission found that only 23% of students in health administration and only 15% of both graduate and undergraduate faculties were female. Of the 47 graduate programs in health administration, half were developed in the first half of the 1970s. At the same time that federal funds for graduate programs in nursing were cut, new programs in health administration were opening. In 1965 only 34 women were in health administration programs, but by 1971, 119 of 933 students were female. They were enrolled in 31 of the 36 programs available at that time, compared to being enrolled in only 9 of 18 programs in 1965. There was, however, no expectation that the number of women at the top would rise in proportion to their increased numbers; thus, more women would go into government, planning, or education. Women, whether nurses or not, were still rejected for the more powerful positions.

Marcy Sheinwold investigated the initial employment experience of the 1973 and 1974 female graduates of 30 programs in health and hospital administration, finding that women were less likely than men to secure hospital positions; more likely to be unemployed; less likely to hold line positions; more likely to be in peripheral jobs; and more likely to be older and single. For those employed, the administrative ranks were one to two levels below chief officers. Although middle-management salaries were roughly equivalent, nurse administrators were substantially underpaid and found upward mobility outside of nursing difficulty (Appelbaum, 1975).

Limited upward movement was closely related to a lack of role models at the top in hospital administration, which was still a "man's world" where little equality existed for women. Florence Gaynor, president of the National Association of Health Services Executives, recalled that for some time she was the only female member. Ruth Rothstein, director of Chicago's Mount Sinai Hospital, did not believe there was an organized women's movement in hospital administration. Without organization, she did not expect any breakthroughs since "'hospitals are open to women only in a token way'" (cited in Appelbaum, 1975, p. 55).

Administrator H. Robert Cathcart noted that there were a large number of women already working in hospitals so there must be some numbers of qualified women, but hospital executives interact primarily with other male executives and often see a woman leader as "acting like a man" or "acting just like a woman." One of the few nursing administrators interviewed stated that she was annoyed with women who demand high-level positions but have not demonstrated competence in administration; she admonished them not to rely on the women's movement. This stereotyped prejudicial thinking, stressing individual action, was contrary to the fact that any subordinated group must act *cooperatively* to achieve social change. Other male administrators admitted that women were likely to be in middle management, but not at the top levels. One male executive believed women were not as likely to be top executives because the pool of women was smaller than that of men! He overlooked nurses completely, implying that the needed training programs for upward mobility would not be available for nurses, even those at supervisory levels.

A study by Edward J. Spillane (1973) revealed that not only is top-level management a man's world but that the " 'same is true to a lesser but still an overwhelming degree in the assistant administrator or upper management level. Sex per se is a significant background factor in an individual's chance of achieving an occupational level above the department head in the hospital industry. . . . It must be pointed out that, at the present time, the opportunities for female hospital executives to reach the top of the hospital organizational structure are indeed very limited' " (cited in Appelbaum, 1975, p. 59).

Women outside nursing were discovering what nurses had experienced for decades: a system of gender segregation allows women leaders only lower-level administrative opportunities; does not recognize the qualifications of nurses for general hospital administration; and, to the contrary, has historically usurped whatever hospital leadership nurses originally had. Evidently, hospital administrators had to be reminded that they could draw hospital administrators from the ranks of nurses already in the system.

COMMITMENT TO COURAGE AND THE QUALITY OF FEARLESSNESS: A DISCUSSION AMONG NURSE LEADERS

What were women saying who did have power in nursing? In 1975 the *AJN* invited some nursing leaders to talk candidly about nursing's potential for leadership and for changing the health-care system. According to Jo Eleanor Elliot, former ANA president and then president of the *AJN*, the *same* issues and needs of 25 years before were still unresolved: more research as a base for practice, university-based education, and the redistribution of nursing skills and services for better care for more people. Ingeborg Mauksch, chairperson of the ANA Congress on Nursing Practice, replied that these issues emerged in the 1950s as symptoms of problems that nurses were unable to pinpoint, but by the 1970s they could now isolate two basic issues: "One, of course, relates to the role and to the nature of the woman who is a nurse. This has changed. The self-concept of persons who are women has been an underlying problem in many nursing issues" (p. 1848). To this, Mauksch added the shift from reaction to action, from doing what was ordered to practicing according to the needs of patients. Rosamond Gabrielson, president of the ANA, agreed, noting the shift from issues on salaries and fringe benefits to practice and authority. For example, in Youngstown, Ohio, nurses were striking to incorporate their professional code in their contracts. Agnes Flaherty, chairperson of the ANA Commission on Nursing Services, agreed, noting the demand for third-party payments.

Virginia Cleland, chairperson of the ANA Commission on Nursing Research, returned to the feminist issues, claiming that the recent emphasis on shared decision making and governance was due to changes in the role and nature of the woman who is a nurse. But, she noted, "Nursing service administrators have not clearly understood this. They consider efforts in this direction to be an infringement on management's rights, rather than the legitimate professional sharing of governance" (p. 1849). Cleland also saw a change in male nurses, who were more aggressive than those 20 years earlier and were often placed in positions to effect change. To this, Pam Cipriano, president of the National Student Nurses Association, replied that 27% of the delegates to the 1975 NSNA Convention were males—a big proportion: "We find that women are reluctant to run against them and that usually a male will be elected over a female opponent. That shows how far we still have to go as liberated women" (p. 1849). Clifford Jordan, president of the Pennsylvania Nurses Association, responded that the male-female issue was related to a lack of unity and accountability.

The participants wondered why nurses turned away from the profession for answers rather than to it. What would it take to organize nurses collectively to advance their purposes? Why did nurses seek hospital legal counsel rather than their own counsel on interpretations of the law and the National Labor Relations Act? To this Mauksch said, "We need to understand the lack of feelings of self worth which is still rampant among women, therefore, among nurses" (p. 1850). Only when a woman as a nurse has a sense of self-respect would she be able to respect her peers and create cohesion and unity. Cleland emphasized that this meant trusting the "sisterhood." This was particularly difficult given the distrust in the "system" of organizations that emerged in the 1960s. In addition, some nurses were now aligning themselves with specializations and looking to physicians as their employers rather than to nursing services. With decentralization, directors of nursing were nonexistent in some hospitals; there were no nurse leaders to turn to. Mauksch, however, defended nurses who sought professional identity within a clinical specialization, claiming, for example, that they were *medical* nurses. To them, the director of nursing does not represent professional *nursing* practice. Mauksch's own vision of a nursing organization was of a *practice* department, similar to other professional departments, and "divorced from . . . counting the towels and chasing the false teeth that went down the laundry chute" (p. 1851). The kind of department leader needed was a manager who was not loaded down with management problems unrelated to the delivery of care. Mauksch rejected the "interchangeability" of nurses; for example, when the ward clerk is sick, nurses often take on the clerk's functions. Mauksch said she would compromise if "On day one, you, as the director of nursing, tell the head nurse to go ahead and ask the staff nurses to take on the chores of the clerk . . . [but] on day two, you will call the medical chief and say, 'Please send an intern to mind the telephone because the ward clerk is sick'" (p. 1851). And on the third day, the director calls the dietary head and asks her to send a dietician because the ward clerk is sick. Why should it be the nurses who give up nursing care to fill the little cracks?

Would overemphasis on organizational development skills produce nurses without leadership skills? What would happen to those nurses who refused to count paper clips or shuffle papers? Jordan said, "I know of summary dismissals in places where directors of nursing have stood up and said this is what will happen in this department" (p. 1852). Nurses had to learn not only how to function in bureaucracies, but also understand health economics and labor relations. Cipriano agreed that most new graduates had not been introduced to administration. Jordan claimed that many do not understand organizational complexity. Kathleen Hoover, a member of ANA's Commission on Economic and General Welfare, warned that a clinical nurse acting on her own could find herself being ushered out the door; even directors were being fired when they should be assured of their job security. Instead of building a power base of women nurses, said Cleland, the director of nursing "looks at her power as though it's delegated from the hospital administrator, unfortunately" (p. 1853). But Jordan disagreed, stating that without organization among nurses, the fact is that a nurse's power *does* come from hospital administrators.

Jessie Scott, then assistant surgeon general, argued that nurses were not being prepared for leadership positions; Gabrielson replied that many people in these roles were stepping down. Scott noted that greater government intervention forced more demands on nursing leaders to think in terms of people's problems in varied populations and develop a nursing system, not simply a profession. Hazel Blakeney, chairperson of ANA's Commission on Nursing Education, returned to the issue of lack of leadership, and asserted that leadership skills can be taught. Another problem, however, was harder to attack and that was a lack of backbone. Mauksch agreed that numerous studies on nurses' characteristics in the late 1950s and early 1960s suggested that "nurses then were basically people who lacked backbone. But I have great faith that today it is different" (p. 1854). Elliot recommended that admission criteria should include assessment of the quality of fearlessness, which must be fostered, not systematically taken out of students.

Mauksch asked: "Who determines nursing leadership? Nurses still are not in the position of determining it . . . it is still determined by administrators in the hospitals, by administrators of community health organizations . . . and by academic administrators" (p. 1854). The only response to this was talk of leadership development through the ANA, career development, mentor and preceptor systems, and collaboration between education and service. Blakeney returned to the problem of low self-esteem and Elliott to the lack of decision-makers and risk-takers, but noted: "We are now having assertive training workshops conducted by nurses for nurses as well as women's awareness groups" (p. 1855). Stressing support systems, she related these to sisterhood: "We don't support each other in terms of decisions made and risks taken. We have not developed support systems for the director of nursing service or anyone else. I believe commitment is tied to courage" (p. 1855). Cleland agreed, claiming that nursing pays a big price for lack of commitment. Some married women who work do have commitment, but Mauksch believed that most nurses mirror societal perceptions that claim women lack commitment.

Cleland had a vision of all nurses moving into hospital and agency staff associations, developing criteria for quality control with mechanisms for shared governance with nursing administrators; creating nursing care committees, many under collective bargaining, but focused on shared policy making. Scott demanded a focus on nurses in communities, and Mauksch wanted to focus on the promotion of health, not simply on institutions for the acutely ill, which, she predicted, were likely to sharply decrease. After much debate, Elliot concluded that any major change in the health-care system would have to be made by nurses. She recommended "think tanks" where nurses could retreat to design a new health-care delivery system: "We've not made it worthwhile to keep people out of hospitals or raised enough hell about it to make a difference" (p. 1857). She insisted that nurses have to make home care acceptable and get rid of the cult of going to the hospital: "We've rewarded illness and we have rewarded physicians for putting people into hospitals" (p. 1857). She claimed that nurses cannot wait for a change in the overall system, but must design for themselves what can be done.

How could this be done if nurses could not get paid directly for their services? Cleland cautioned that this might incorporate the same problems in the existing system. Gabrielson agreed that fees for service certainly had not made medicine accountable and nursing would be foolish to follow the medical model. Cleland called for abolishing physicians' fees for services; only when nurse practitioners worked with salaried physicians was there a successful working relationship. Others, however, pointed out that nursing services were not perceived as producing revenue and often were not even known. Mauksch looked to the year 2000: She saw about half the labor force being female; tremendous changes in the nuclear family; the spread of day care centers; population stabilization; and an increase in the aged population. All these changes had not been anticipated by physicians: "Nurses are simply way ahead of physicians in looking at societal needs. . . . I am hoping that nursing can take the leadership and plan for health and illness care delivery" (p. 1859).

THE MACHIAVELLIAN MANIPULATION OF
POLITICALLY NAIVE NURSES

Could nurses create a better health-care system? Were they sufficiently political to do it? According to Beatrice and Philip Kalisch (1976), nurses were one of the most neglected groups in the voting population. Politically, most nurses were unorganized and few were in government; yet nursing was becoming more and more influenced by political decisions. Clearly, the separation of nursing and politics was no longer possible, but most nurses rejected the idea that politics influenced policies, deliberations, or activities. Surely nursing must be above favoritism, corruption, or specialized interest, committed only to the patient's interests. The Kalisches argued that this was illogical because decisions are not made in a patient-interest vacuum.

Politics is too often a dirty word to nurses. The Kalisches admitted that allocating resources can be a hard and cruel business, but so is health care in matters of life and death. Promotion of one's interest group and the use of resources to advance self-interests run counter to the political naivete of nurses, which is based on the traditional worship of authority; socialization to institutional mores; reliance on those above for decisions; and fear of questioning and controversy. The Kalisches did not connect these to the general characteristics of women's roles; they perceived a female workforce as a transitory population of workers concerned with families. Whether this interpretation can be sustained, given recent data, is questionable (see Group & Roberts, *Nurses as Caregivers at Work and at Home*). What is needed is further refinement and a more systematic analysis of gender segregation within the health-care field.

Lack of political education of nurses produces political neglect. The Kalisches noted that this was represented by President Ford's veto of the Nurse Training Bill in 1975, a reduction of $650 million over three years. In comparison to the $115 billion spent on health services, this rejection of comparatively small amounts of desperately needed funding in nursing, particularly at a time when nurses were trying to establish more sophisticated nursing educational patterns, represented a severe lack of governmental concern for nursing's interests. Misinformed outsiders, improperly suggesting an oversupply of nurses, effectively influenced politicians who would continue to make decisions damaging to nursing unless nurses themselves were involved in the political process. But how nurses could break the male control of political structures was unclear in the Kalisches' analysis.

Institutional politics too often require "selling out" nursing to advance a career. The nurse may identify with men in authority at the expense of other nurses. Turning to Machiavelli, whose name has become synonymous with amoral manipulation of power, the Kalisches suggested replacing "physician" or "hospital administrator" in sentences extracted from *The Prince*. For example, "A Prince (physician) should be concerned for the people he governs only to the extent that such concern strengthens his hold" (Kalisch & Kalisch, 1976, p. 31). The exercise is salutary, an abbreviated lesson in male-defined medical power over women. The Kalisches maintained that manipulation of nurses is evident in the selection of nursing leaders by non-nursing individuals or physician-dominated committees; the failure to include nurses in budget decisions; the expectation of absolute acceptance of directives from above; the excessive obedience and lack of constructive criticism by nurses. Tersely stated: "The price of silence is deadly high" (p. 32).

The Kalisches believed that challenges to the status quo were being met by raising women's political consciousness through the Nurses' Coalition for Action in Politics, the National Organization for Women, and the Women's Equity Action League. Many nurses, however, were so caught up in their day-to-day lives as nurses, women, and mothers, that the Kalisches despaired that their consciousness would change at all, or, if altered, would lead to any action. But perhaps as reality became discordant with social myths, power would not seem "masculine," but a simple requirement for personal and professional life. The Kalisches suggested that women come to a sophisticated understanding of traditional male politics and become adept at the men's game. Although this first step is mandatory, the question remains: What is a woman's version of politics? How can or will the political process be changed by women who may have very different values? Ironically, the impact of feminism was apparent but the full implications for values transformation were yet to be explored.

Jacqueline R. Hott (1976) also stressed the need for political awareness in the struggles inside the body politic of nursing. She, too, believed that nurses are politically naive and agreed with the Kalisches that "although nursing is being shaped more and more by political decisions, nurses generally have not had either the time, energy, available resources, confidence, assertiveness, self direction, or the will needed to move into active [political] roles" (p. 325). Hott believed that unity among members of the profession is a most elusive achievement because "Politically, the independent nurse is not quiet and submissive, but one who seeks power—power to help determine her own and others' action for improving patient care" (p. 337). Hott quoted Thelma Schorr, editor of the *American Journal of Nursing*: " 'There is no way we can educate anyone to the potentials of this profession unless we demonstrate in the work situation that we mean what we say in the political situation. . . . Nurses can't be Gloria Steinems at a meeting and Phyllis Schlafleys on a ward' " (p. 337). It is fatal for nurses to support the status quo, warned Hott; if they do the profession will fail to become a viable political force for patient care.

Diane F. Powell (1976) agreed with Hott, and examined the struggles *outside* nursing's body politic, warning that nursing for too long had behaved as a separate system. Echoing Lavinia Dock's plea of 60 years before, Powell called for nurses to become more active in political groups external to nursing.

According to Powell, nurses throughout the country had become more involved in legislative issues, meeting with varied success in their attempts to become members of federally mandated health-care policy-making boards. Now, Powell said, "The time has come for nurses to poke their apolitical heads out from under their caps and recognize that politics is the only route to take if nursing is to command the respect of other professions and the attention of legislators who represent 'we, the people,' including nurses" (p. 354).

UNDERRATED AND UNDERUTILIZED: SPLIT PERCEPTIONS OF NURSE ADMINISTRATORS

How would women be able to use political forces to redesign their roles as leaders? If nursing is a microcosm of women, how, indeed, were women in authority actually seen by men in authority in the system? In 1977 the results of a survey on the perceived relationship between hospital chief operating officers and directors of nursing was published in *Hospital Topics*. Five problem areas were reported. First, half of the respondents agreed that the director of nursing was at the first level of management and below the chief operations officer; however, "the other half either failed to agree or viewed the Director at one or even two levels below the first line" (p. 38). For her informal role, about half saw the director as first line management in institutional problem solving and in the informal communications network; but "the other half either failed to agree, or to realize, that the power held in that role was less than the first level" (p. 38). Obviously, there was considerable confusion about women leaders in nursing. The report concluded that the position of director of nursing was underrated and underutilized in half of all institutions.

The level of female-male agreement was high (87%–89%) on the director's right to make binding decisions on new patient care programs and on her authority to hire and fire. But on her authority in budget preparation, administration, and flexibility of budget spending, the agreement varied from 62% to 73%. Much lower agreement, from 32% to 49%, was found on whether a nursing director could determine starting salaries; act as a member of budget approval groups; substitute LPNs for RNs or allow LPNs to give medications; initiate new coronary care courses; or decide on the use of space. On union contract negotiations, only 16% agreement was found.

The actual and implied authority also differed, showing *less* authority as the director's role moved from clinical to fiscal officer to division administration: "This implies that the Director is viewed by the Chief Operating Officers more as a nurse than as a director in about half of our hospitals" (p. 38). In rating functions of the director, higher evaluations were given for patient care (69), quality nursing (56), and leadership (45) than were functions involving changes in nursing (17) and fiscal matters (12). The survey revealed relations between physicians and the director that signal a conflict situation. Two-thirds of nursing directors thought their positions should be equivalent to medical directors, but currently they were not; in fact, one in ten nursing directors reported their positions were inferior. Thus, status conflicts and conflicts of unfulfilled expectations often existed. Only 17% of the sets agreed that nursing-medical relations were excellent.

Finally, the survey showed "distinctly different perceptions of the role that the Director of Nursing should play in the institution" (p. 39). There was not even agreement on the time consumed in job functions. Despite a moderate to strong agreement on some functions of the director, "they failed to agree on the significant problems relating to nursing in their institutions. . . . They even appeared to speak different 'languages' when referring to nursing functions" (p. 39). Clearly, the director's role is ambiguous and her job is not clearly defined by the institution or fully understood by the chief operating officer. She performs many diverse functions and these produce role conflicts. From the survey it was clear that the director's role is complex, requiring a woman to "slip in and out from a multitude of subroles—from clinician to manager to educator to human relations expert to mediator" (p. 39).

From the research, recommendations for change suggested that the formal position of the director should be elevated to a top management position with commensurate power and authority recognized by the entire hospital staff. Further, chief operating officers and medical staff should learn and appreciate the multifaceted role of nurses and of the director. Directors should improve their fiscal administrative skills and actively participate in hospital management as first-line managers. The report placed key responsibility on the chief operating officer to solve the problems in relationships with the nursing leaders, but did not specify how the entire gender-stratified structure should be changed in order for perceptions of women leaders to be genuinely modified. Nor did it suggest how nursing leaders, as women, might want to reconceptualize the meaning of power itself.

DENYING NURSES THE EDUCATIONAL PREPARATION NECESSARY TO FUNCTION AS EQUALS

How power itself is conceptualized is a feminist issue, one that Claire M. Fagin (1978) discusses in perceiving knowledge as a professional and political force. Knowledge might provide personal power to an individual, but, claims Fagin, only *sharing* of knowledge brings political power. She looked toward the year 2000 and, as Mauksch had done, predicted dramatic changes in the population. Projected increases in the number of aged from 11% to 22% would require a significant shift from cure to care, particularly given increasing deinstitutionalization and an emphasis on health maintenance rather than medical intervention. Fagin predicted significant shifts in the traditional balance of power, which, accompanied by "the resurgence of public acknowledgement of women's rights can only facilitate nursing's efforts to assume its legitimate rights and responsibilities" (p. 11).

According to Fagin, history was on the side of nurses because their traditional emphasis has been on humanistic, holistic care of patient, family, and community. However, physicians were beginning to stress these issues and increasing their numbers; for example, there were 156 physicians for every 100,000 people in the United States in 1966; 194 per 100,000 in 1976; and a projected 222 for every 100,000 by 1985. Thus, warned Fagin, a glut of physicians might lead them to simply take over nurses' functions. To counter this, nurses must share their knowledge, become a public presence in the solution of problems, as Florence Nightingale, Lillian Wald, Mary Breckinridge, and Margaret Sanger had done in previous decades. Fagin believes that most nurses have shared their knowledge with each other, but have had little or no impact on the external world, leaving nurses outside of power brokerage. How, she asks, did nurses come to deny their own power? Certainly, nurses' collective efforts to insure direct patient access to nurses have been thwarted at various levels.

What if women cannot agree on their base of power? Where does this leave their leaders? Fagin examined what had happened since the passage of the New York State Nurse Practice Act in the early 1970s and the consequences of the changed definition of nursing practice. The crux of every challenge to nursing's autonomy or power has been the assertion that nursing can be learned on the job; thus, nurses need not be educationally qualified to do much of any significance. By delaying action on passing the 1985 resolution, Fagin believes nurses were showing agreement with these assertions. Thus, she urged speedy passage of the 1985 proposal, which was to establish the baccalaureate degree as the minimum requirement for professional nursing practice. As we know, this still has not been realized.

Fagin insists that nurses could not claim equality with other practitioners without the educational preparation required to function as equals. Nor could students be admonished to assert their rights and be accountable in the exercise of responsibilities and then "subject them to an educational system from which they emerge feeling less educated, less informed, less articulate, and less self-directing than either their clients or other members of the health care team" (p. 14). In a classic feminist assertion, Fagin states that nurses must get rid of the comforting but paralytic notion that their "only option as a predominantly women's occupation is to serve as the noble, long suffering, sacrificial lamb of the health care system" (p. 14).

By refusing to agree on the basic level of knowledge required, nurses have vacillated for decades and were, even in the 1970s, still engaged in a fierce internal struggle over educational requirements. The public has been aware of nurses' indecisiveness, which, of course, produces a lack of public confidence in nurses' credibility and competence. The sorting out between types of nurses and their education has been "deferred time and time again because we simply did not trust ourselves and each other. Collectively we have been directed by fear—fear of being underestimated or undervalued; fear among some of being labeled elitist; among others of downgrading credentials or programs; fear of being unable to create something at least equally good if not better than the creations of the past; fear of being separate not equal" (p. 15). But how can society allow nurses direct access to clients if nursing does not declare its knowledge consistently and clearly? Fagin warned that nurses cannot blame others for restricted practice if they are unwilling to be accountable and that nurses must share the blame for whatever waste of talent has occurred. Political and professional power, she claimed, would be achieved through sharing knowledge and through a unified decision about the educational base required for the acquisition of that knowledge.

THE ANDROGYNOUS LEADER:
MODIFYING THE ENTIRE ORGANIZATIONAL CULTURE

Certainly, clarity and unity on nursing preparation and knowledge would affect women's power and authority. However, there are more basic differences in the gendered perceptions of what constitutes knowledge, power, authority, and leadership. Traditionally, administrators have been valued for their coolness, competitive power, toughness, resilience, and reliance on extrinsic rewards; thus, organizational norms have been synonymous with male norms. In contrast, women's values and the redefinition of power were central issues addressed by many feminists in the 1970s. Alice G. Sargent (1979) a management specialist, focused on the feminist concept of androgyny and suggested a values fusion in an androgynous leader.

Sargent divides cultural norms into organizational (male) and family (female) norms, based on male socialization to task-oriented styles and female socialization to expressive-oriented styles. This division, traceable to sociologist Talcott Parsons, cannot be supported as actually enacted in daily life. Nevertheless, Sargent uses it to trace the shift from the organization man of the 1960s to managers in the 1970s, who were expected to combine both human relations and problem-solving skills. Appraisal forms and on-the-job training formats now included, said Sargent, items pertaining to communication at all levels, openness, and mentoring or molding others' skills. To express feelings, to behave sensitively, these were now further supported by the radical shift in the workforce to include women and minorities in management.

Sargent was optimistic, but also realistic; she recognizes that tokenism and restriction of women from upper-level positions continues: "If women managers are not simply to be forced into the mold of male management styles and black managers to become carbon copies of white managers, then the entire organizational culture needs to be studied and modified" (p. 23). How, she asks, could female characteristics and behaviors be encompassed in management without getting rid of the best in male managerial style? Since women and minorities bring different values and behaviors, could new attitudes toward the place of work in life, the role of intimacy, the conceptions of time and success be included in organizational values?

According to Sargent, shifting expectations demanded androgynous managers who could combine the so-called masculine and feminine, or fatherly and motherly, or competitive and cooperative modes into one. Sargent perceived a new set of characteristics: independence and nurturance, dominance and yielding, assertiveness and concern for others, rationality and intuition. To her, the manager had to shift from achievement to affiliation motivation, which is more compatible with women's caring values. Clearly reflecting the influence of feminist theory, Sargent states: "In a number of areas it is as if women and men grew up in two different cultures" (p. 25) in which rewards are allocated for dissimilar values. Now, as women and men become integrated, at least three aspects of institutional life would be affected by androgynous management: self-expression and assertiveness, power relationships, and communication processes. In the transition, "women in their quest to be taken seriously go through the stage of becoming like the archetypical man before allowing themselves to recapture or reintegrate some of the tenderness and playfulness that they have abandoned" (p. 25). After initial awkwardness, women would move on to the next stage, being assertive without being oppressive or uncaring. In process, women would give up being excessively pleasant; preoccupied with the integration of people at the expense of substance; smiling too much; allowing themselves to be interrupted; letting their voices trail off when making a point; and laughing at the end of an important sentence. Women would have to repudiate passivity and denigration, abandoning a position of strength in conciliation, and giving up credit for their own work. Men, also awkward in their shifts, would need to be more collaborative and less competitive; become more aware that their own power needs may supersede the job to be done; and modify their tendency to exclude their needs for approval, closeness, liking, and spontaneity.

According to Sargent, power relations would be expressed best in situational leadership and participatory styles. Women, however, must learn confrontation in decision making in relation to power dynamics. Rather than giving away power and "making do," they must learn to demand adequate resources and appropriate training. In contrast, men slip "naturally into one-up, one-down interactions, . . . they also distance themselves" (p. 28); they need to be less in control, more reflective, refusing to fear self-disclosure by acts of aggression and victimization.

In mixed groups, women speak much less than men, who normally dominate the interaction. As the single man in a woman's group, he dominates; as a single women in a male group, she experiences isolation and feels unsupported. Sargent uses the transactional model of patient, adult, child, and the crossed interactions that can occur. For example, men use women managers as mothers; women engage women in negative girl-girl relations; and women managers defer, as little girls, to "father" managers. Sargent calls for adult problem solving, combined with parent nurturance and child spontaneity.

To support and create change, women must unite and organize to change institutional culture: one woman, alone, cannot take on the magnitude of change envisioned by feminists. As an example of nurses' power through unity, Madelon M. Amenta (1977) reported on NURSES NOW as a model of worksite organizing for specific change. Amenta acknowledged the gains made by feminists in the 1970s: degendering the help-wanted ads, more equitable pay for equal work, affirmative action settlements, and substantial increases of women students in law and medicine. However, she believed there was "only minimal effort at improving the working conditions of the greatest number of women employed outside the house—teachers, nurses, nurses' aids, clerical workers, factory operatives, domestics, salespeople, waitresses and cashiers who neither can, nor wish to advance" (p. 343).

How many of the issues espoused by feminists affected *all* women, regardless of the level of their work? Amenta recognized that interrupted work life, child care, maternity leaves, insurance plans, control of working conditions, and increased power and status were early supported by women activists. NOW promoted worksite organizing, and feminist caucuses composed of members from the same occupations were to help women in all female-dominated occupations. NURSES NOW, the first occupational task force, was founded in April 1973 by five Pittsburgh nurses who were acutely aware of the parallels between feminist and nursing issues. The nurses' task force subsequently expanded to 35 chapters; their goal was to enhance "nursing's professional status in the male-controlled health care system by revising the traditional image of the nurse as the 'handmaiden' to the physician and surrogate of agency or hospital administration" (p. 344). Amenta noted a large variety of activities designed to change social and professional roles, rejecting the perception that nurses were apathetic to women's plight. In fact, by 1975 NURSES NOW had already opposed suspension of nurse licensure in test hospitals in a pilot study on institutional licensure. Over time, however, the organization did not bring together large numbers of nurses and feminist leadership in nursing remained diffused.

While feminist activism among nurses in the 1970s never became widespread, well-organized, or unified, it is clear from their writings that nurses' consciousness had been raised significantly by the women's movement. The themes of role change and empowerment, so evident in the early 1970s, continued throughout the decade. The feminist reconstitution of nursing history was continued by Ashley and Brand and Glass. From content analysis of fiction, the traditionalist image of women as nurses in the public imagination was detailed and decried by the Richters, who called for new nurse heroines. Research conducted by Drabman and his associates and Cordua and his colleagues illustrated the strength of imagery in children's gender stereotyping of nurses and physicians.

Resocialization of gender and nursing roles was again emphasized by Grissum, who stressed the emergence of role-breakers and risk-takers. Stereotyped, conflicting, and contradictory roles were decried by Sargent and Grissum who, along with Yeaworth, rejected gender-stereotyped physician-nurse role relations. This was particularly necessary among nursing leaders according to Harty and Appelbaum, who called for more women in top administrative positions. Indeed, the issue of empowering nurse leaders was a consistent theme of McBride and her colleagues, Leininger, the Kalisches, and others. Stanton, Amenta, and others called for greater professional unity of women and important analyses by Schaefer, Ashley, and Fagin keyed in on the influence of gender definitions on the incapacity of nurses to unite for political action.

The political importance of the sheer size of women's groups in the health-delivery system was emphasized by several writers, Ashley, Harty, and Reavill, who, along with Fagin, Hott, and Powell, called for greater political analysis and action by nurses who will question and influence public policy in coordination with other women's groups. Specific involvement in politics and in legal and economic systems was called for by numerous writers, and the reorganization of social values through the incorporation of women's values, a dominant motif of Heide, was picked up by Reavill and others. Clearly, feminism had impacted nursing in the 1970s, but the depth and breadth of change would be severely challenged in the conservative backlash of the 1980s to civil rights and liberated women.

Chapter 8

"Ride the White Horse Yourself!" Women's Culture, Feminism, and Nursing in the 1980s

Many themes of previous years persisted in the 1980s, but some of these by now reflected more forceful analyses of the oppressive systems that affected nurses. The political conservatism of the Reagan era led many feminist scholars to warn of a backlash to women and their fight for equal rights. Some nurses were aware of the social and political mood swings and warned of the misogyny inherent in the patriarchal system. Others wondered exactly how much progress women and nurses had made toward economic equity and professional independence. Perhaps the most thorough and revealing analysis made of nursing's status in the 1980s was of the profession's image and the public's perception of nurses' roles. Analyses such as this led some nurses to question feminism's impact on nursing. Had nursing rejected feminism? How had feminism influenced nursing? Were nurses becoming more assertive in their demands for equity? Were they more politically active? And, most important, how could nursing change its public image to reflect more accurately what nurses do, especially if freed from excessive medical and institutional control?.

ARE WE BLIND TO THE SUFFERING AND DESTRUCTION OF OUR OWN KIND?

Typical of the more forthright, direct, and unambiguous feminist thought emerging from nurses in the 1980s was that of Jo Ann Ashley (1980), who claimed that misogyny, the hatred of women, is structurally historical, but now the problem was to see how it affected the current politics of care: "Remaining deaf, dumb and blind to the suffering and destruction of our own kind is agreeing to the political dominance of those who wish to continue destroying the strengths of women" (p. 4).

Agreeing with feminists Mary Daly and Rosemary Ruether, Ashley claimed that men's hatred and fear of the expansion of women's potential beyond the male-defined limits of serving males finds greatest support in religious traditions and institutions. Legitimizing women as property, who are made for dependency and service, religion has defined women as the source of evil. Woman as inferior is, according to feminist church historians, overwhelmingly evident in Christian tradition and thought, which historically dehumanized the female sex. To Ashley, woman as servant was philosophically believed to be the "natural state" because of innate female inferiority, requiring constant restraint of girls and women by men. Indeed, philosophers believed that women had "no sense of justice" because they showed more sympathy for the unfortunate and treated them with more kindness and interest. This was proof that they were less honorable and conscientious than men!

Both Ashley and Daly (1980) claimed that patriarchy is the prevailing religion of the planet. Structured misogyny is sustained in systems of beliefs and psychological theories that affirm, as Freud did, that females are mutilated defectives since they lack penises. Freud's views of women's development claimed first, a withdrawal into neuroses, burying feelings of deprivation; second, a refusal to accept "castration," creating the "masculinity complex" and emulation of men; and third, an acceptance of biological inferiority, producing a baby to compensate for the lack of a penis.

It is the centuries-old tradition, rephrased by thinkers in the current era, which underpins and exaggerates the problems in nursing. Ashley stressed that in nursing curricula most nurses were still taught to accept, absorb, and believe Freudian theories. Even humanist theorists, such as Maslow, reaffirmed the old patriarchy, believing women to be profoundly and deeply unhappy without a man, while men must overlook the "basic nature of evil in women in order to 'love' them" (Ashley, 1980, p. 11). These contradictions appear in images of nurses as witches, bitches, whores, or saintly angels of mercy. Ashley called on nurses to take apart the subtle misogyny in curricula and to engage in research designed to analyze and correct masculist ideas in theories and bodies of knowledge.

For nurses, coming to grips with the politics of care requires a feminist consciousness, found, for example, in the analysis of more than a century of medical advice to women, in which men's creation of sickness in women is repeatedly evident (Ehrenreich & English, 1978). Ashley claimed that nurses have swallowed the misogynous beliefs about themselves and other women, still striving for the illusion of power by attaching themselves to men, acting as their assistants. In fact, she said, the longstanding close relationship of nursing to medicine, psychiatry, and gynecology has destroyed the potential power of women in nursing.

How often, asked Ashley, has the professional model negated the value of nursing? Instead, the priority should be to nurture women, which negates the male model. How often has nursing been at the crossroads and chosen to continue its subservience, rather than shedding its petty and childish fears of feminism, instead of embracing the powerful insights from it? By accepting token generosity from medical father figures, nurses lose the validity and power of their own experiences. Rather, nurses should refuse to be divided and conquered, reject hostility and the devaluation of the work of other women. To Ashley, it was truly shameful that nurses do not care for other nurses sufficiently, or create a community of shared caring. She concluded: "Women nurses are *women* first. If we consistently remember this, accepting our heritage and strengths as women, our politics of care can begin" (p. 21).

Carrying the burden of caring and the virtue of selflessness, nurses like all women are caught in a compassion trap. Margaret Sandelowski (1981) warns that the burden of caring shouldered by the nurse extends beyond ministering to the patient to protecting the God-like position of the physician. Calling nurses the "unsung heroines" of health care, she claims that nurses live in an "occupational ghetto," unaware of a bond of oppression among them: "Nurses have paid and are still paying an exorbitant price for not recognizing and not acting against the sexist ideology that keeps them down. . . . Women in nursing have allowed themselves to be exploited in every way imaginable because, like being a woman, to be a nurse means to be exploitable" (p. 158).

Sandelowski's critique seems correct when one analyzes the actions of some nursing organizations, for example, in regard to their nonsupport for the Equal Rights Amendment (ERA) and its principles. As in the earlier part of the century, women in the 1980s were still trying to obtain passage of the ERA, which remains today an unrealized goal. To put pressure on nonratifying states, feminist leaders used the loss of economic gain as a threat to force ratification. A substantial number of national organizations agreed to not hold their national meetings in any state that had not passed the ERA, but in 1981 the National League for Nursing (NLN) met in Nevada and, in 1983, Missouri, both nonratifying states. Penny A. McCarthy (1981), editor of *Nursing Outlook*, says that the NLN, in a "fitting flash of unwitting inspiration" (p. 347), chose the "man's town" for its latest biennial convention. Setting, she claims, is symbolically significant and communicates something important about the inner life of the individual and group. As a setting, Las Vegas "says some things quite dismaying about the inner life of the League" (p. 347). She further claims that the NLN had lost significant revenues from nonrenewal of the State Board Exam contract, representing about one-third of their usual annual income; thus, because it reflected men's money, the choice of Las Vegas was, as sarcastically stated, "perfect."

To this editorial, the president of the NLN, Elsa Brown, responded in a deeply distressed letter (*Nursing Outlook*, September 1981) in which she charged McCarthy with providing misstatements, innuendos, falsehoods, and a complete disregard of previously published facts. Brown claimed that the 1977 convention delegates voted against changing scheduled meeting sites, including Nevada and Missouri, because of severe economic consequences.

Furthermore, she pointed to published balance sheets of the NLN, showing that McCarthy's assertions about the league's financial losses were false. A retraction and apology from McCarthy were demanded, but an editorial note stated that a correction of inaccuracies had been printed in the previous issue of *Nursing Outlook* (August 1981). Even so, several letters from readers (*Nursing Outlook*, September 1981) followed Brown's critique.

New York nurse Susan Talbott pointed out that only one year (in 1981) remained of the seven-year period during which states could ratify the ERA. She had written the NLN every year to urge holding conventions in ERA-ratified states and to work for ratification: "I know other League members who feel as I do, and many have written to express their views. Still nothing happens, and many of us believe the NLN leadership is out of touch" (p. 492).

Connie Vance's letter said McCarthy's editorial struck at the "very heart of our profession's problems and those that we experience as women" (p. 492). To Vance, it described "the despair and outrage many of us feel over the lack of responsiveness of some of our organizations and their leaders" (p. 492). She claimed that the profession showed a persistent lack of courage and vision to deal with issues directly affecting nurses' lives and an inability to make changes to help nurses and their clients. Vance had dropped her membership because of the anachronisms of the NLN.

E. Gayle Strelnick, a nurse from the University of Wisconsin at Milwaukee, wrote of a resolution to join the National Organization for Women (NOW) boycott of nonratifying states that was passed overwhelmingly by her nursing faculty; the resolution was also sent to the American Nurses Association, who immediately responded, saying the executive committee had voted to join the boycott and change their convention site. Strelnick continued: "I also sent the resolution to the League. I never received a response" (p. 494). To her, the league's problems were not surprising: "It is out of step with nursing" (p. 494). If the ERA was not ratified (and we now know it was not), Strelnick said, in words reminiscent of Lavinia Dock, that nurses with their lack of political interest will have played their part in keeping women second-class citizens: "I have seen few nursing journals address this issue, yet it seems that nurses should have been in the forefront" (p. 494), since they could not be frightened of the one, major argument against the ERA, that of drafting women into the armed forces. Obviously, nurses would not be as concerned since they have been in every war healing and caring for soldiers. Strelnick urged more editorials and articles to force nurses to understand that they would be the losers with the defeat of the ERA; this would turn back the clock for all women. Strelnick was prophetic; nurses and all women have lost because the ERA was not enacted.

In Jean Kijek's letter, she exclaimed: "The very idea that the NLN, an organization representing a profession of women, would continue to hold its convention in non-ERA states is beyond me" (p. 494). She noted in contrast that even the American Congress of Rehabilitation Medicine had moved its convention to California! To her, the NLN's choice of convention site was symptomatic of other NLN organizational problems and she questioned how representative it was of its own members.

Helen Margaret Archer, former president of the National Student Nurses' Association, wrote to say that McCarthy's editorial "captured and clearly elaborated on the concerns of many young nurses. Professional organizations that fail to address the reality of the crises in nursing today, yet claim to be representative of the profession, do us a great injustice" (p. 494). Previously a member of NLN, Archer terminated her membership because of the organization's insensitivity to current social issues and its seeming unwillingness to respond to concerns of the membership. In contrast, Marjorie M. Luc was disappointed with McCarthy's "divisive" editorial, saying her perception of the Las Vegas convention, as a participant, was different and stressed the need for a united front in nursing.

The wide disparity among nurses on professional issues can certainly be traced to their differing perceptions of themselves, not simply as nurses, but as women. While it is true that most women's organizations are lacking in substantial funds, compared to men's, the central symbolic and legal import of the ERA to women and nurses should have been an event of unusual significance. By holding conventions in unratifying states, the NLN broke ranks with women in general and with the majority of major professional associations, making nurses question, as McCarthy said, the theoretical bases about women and nursing in the inner life of the organization.

THE BREADTH OF DISCRIMINATION:
UNEQUAL REWARDS AND OPPORTUNITIES

The heightened consciousness of nurses led some to critically examine how well women/nurses were faring as the 1980s began. Shirley A. Smoyak (1982), for example, recognized that it was the women's movement in the 1960s that uncovered the social, professional, and economic disparity between men and women. Why, she asked, is the work that women do in their homes not recognized as contributing to the Gross National Product? "The parallel to why nurses' work has not been billed separately in hospitals (i.e., why nurses' work is a part of the bed fee) is so striking that it needs no further explication" (p. 9). Economists see households as noneconomic units, presumably because they are regulated by altruism and affection. The parallel to the arguments for paying nurses such low salaries is obvious. Relying on Claire Fagin's (1981) analysis, Smoyak pointed out that not only the public, but nurses themselves are unaware that salary expenses for nurses as a percentage of hospital expenses had *declined* since 1968.

It is not only economic, but social, religious, and other systems that are affected by the worldwide phenomenon of sex discrimination: "everywhere there are social and legal arrangements tilted in such a way as to produce unequal rewards and opportunities for men and women" (p. 10). Seventeen years after the passage of the 1964 Civil Rights Act, nurses in Denver had a starting salary of $1,064 a month; the men who trimmed the trees around the hospital earned $1,164 a month. It was clear that redistribution of existing sources from men to women was needed, and this meant that nurses must see themselves as competitive with other health-care providers, particularly focused on substitutability of services, as proposed by Fagin. "Clients and third-party payers must be shown that hiring a nurse is a far better idea than hiring a physician to do specifically defined things—such as delivering babies or providing primary care for a wide variety of clients" (p. 10).

While it might be true that the opening of other career options would draw away bright, young women from nursing, Smoyak believed the resulting shortage of nurses would lead to a positive long-term effect as salaries rose to compete for a diminishing pool of women. As comparable pay was achieved, self-esteem would grow. Smoyak warned that the work of consciousness-raising is endless, and that nurses were getting tired of fighting for equity and professional autonomy. Yet, after eight years on the National Joint Practice Commission, she reported, "we did persuade them [physicians] that collegiality was a better game than domination" (p. 11).

Centrally important was Smoyak's concern for the multiple ideologies and theories produced in the explosion of literature generated by the women's movement. Smoyak recommended the usefulness of G. G. Yates' (1975) typology of feminist, women's liberationist, and androgynous ideologies to understand how change is differentially described, how the enemy is typified, and what techniques are used with what results. Concerned with Reaganism and conservatism, Smoyak contrasted these with research that indicated a "steady relaxation of traditional definitions of work, marriage, parenthood, and self . . . a personal liberalization that runs counter to the apparent growth of political conservatism" (pp. 12–13). Smoyak and others feared that the conservative social and political mood of the 1980s was leading to an erosion of humanism and caring values—values inherent in women's culture. Smoyak said, "Women *are* different from men. How can we hold on to those positive, humanist attributes in the coming years?" (p. 13). Nurses' (women's) humanitarian qualities needed to be protected against erosion and included in the socialization process of new nurses.

PREVIEWING THE FUTURE:
CHANGES IN VALUES AND SOCIAL STRUCTURES

Preserving positive, humanist attributes was also the concern of Madeleine Leininger (1981), who assessed the issues women would face in the new decade and delineated key areas for accomplishing future goals. To her, clarity was needed about objectives in the 1990s and beyond, particularly in occupational roles. If women assumed more of the political and economic roles of men, what would they seek next? What changes in social structure and organizations would be needed to sustain change? Leininger believed that women must face the critical problem of the devaluation and denigration of women's roles. To do this, women's behaviors in top administrative positions needed to reflect the "humanistic values and contributions of women such as sharing and caring for others in need . . . we need to put into perspective the past male values of conquest, dominance, and aggression in our society with the essential female caring values of support, humanness, protection" (pp. 206–207).

Speaking as a futurist, Leininger predicted several trends. First, with increasing cross-continent transportation and communication, intercultural contacts among women might lead to cultural shock, but eventually expansion of knowledge would lead to a transcultural worldview of women. Second, women from minority and third world cultures would challenge Western women, leading to increased confusion. Again cross-cultural knowledge, particularly transcultural nursing knowledge would be needed to reduce tensions and build common strategies.

Leininger forecasted a major increase of women in key leadership positions, particularly in public offices. At the same time, male administrators in academic, state, and federal positions would remain threatened by competent women leaders, who, unable to rely on affirmative action, would turn to women's support groups, which, however, would still be marked by internal covert, destructive problems. In apparent agreement with Campbell (1981), Leininger predicted another trend: a major increase in inter- and intragender problems, related to increased terrorism, violence, killing, and law suits. "Humanism and feminism will need to go hand in hand to prevent social violence" (p. 211). At the same time, Leininger predicted that "a new era in social structural theory and research will gradually evolve due to women's experiences and insights" (p. 211). These will be necessary to deal with another major trend, an increase in the abuse and neglect of women, the elderly, and children.

Leininger further predicted increased attention to the means to get qualified women into leadership positions through processes other than tokenism or the widow's mandate. These women would be necessary to deal with the increasing problems of youth and the aged that she saw emerging. Nursing must take steps, said Leininger, to deal with these worldwide trends.

To do this, women will be best guided by new theories and ideologies that may emerge in the years ahead. However, as the year 2000 nears, there seems to be no consensus on explanatory systems that would connect nursing and women's issues in a coherent theoretical manner.

Yet some women did take up the challenge of creating experimental structures to express a new version of organization and action. On June 27, 1983, a group of nurses met or, in their terminology, "gathered" in San Francisco, where they created Cassandra: Radical Feminist Nurses Network to end the oppression of women in all aspects of nursing and health care through commitment to woman-centered analyses. They hoped to create local and regional networks of nurturance for radical-feminist nurses and recommended creating environments for communication, support, and safety for nurses of all races, classes, creeds, abilities, and sexual preferences. They espoused sharing and passing on leadership, analytic, and communication skills to other women; urged strong public actions on nursing and health-care issues; emphasized preserving and publishing significant works of nurses and feminists on women's health; supported feminist nursing research and the development of feminist educational materials.

A report of the "Gathering" by Peggy Chinn and Charlene Wheeler (1983) contrasted the words from women's poetry with those from men, whose stereotypes disclosed "patriarchal lies and myths." On masculist definitions of the ideal nurse, Chinn and Wheeler said, "we have heard these voices all too well, internalized them and even spoken them to each other" (p. 4). Rejecting these voices, the nurses turned to the words of foremothers, to wise women, as a means of "uniting with our history . . . [and] getting off our knees!" (p. 4). Clearly, this meeting of nurses was *distinctly* different from the usual national meetings.

How did these efforts to create a different mode of organization and interaction affect the nurses so accustomed to male bureaucratic structures? One woman felt a special closeness to the women in the circle, realizing she was not alone. Another wrote: "The most profound and lasting phenomenon for me was the process by which the meeting evolved. The consensual process has always seemed, in theory, to be simple and clearly desirable. I now consider it even more desirable, but certainly not simple" (p. 9). Still another wrote: "I've been involved in many nursing and non-nursing organizations. Never before have I been so touched by each person. Each person had input. No one dominated or controlled the agenda. It was amazing" (p. 9). Another said that "some women felt the group was much too radical for them, others felt that we were not radical enough! . . . We emerged, not necessarily of one mind, but with clarification, a core of purposes and beliefs" (p. 10). Clearly, not all women were happy with the experiment, which may, over time, fail. But the important point is that nurses were attempting new structures.

CHANGING SEXIST TERMINOLOGY:
MIDWIFERY "MAN"POWER? SHE IS A MAN?

Some nurses were aware that new theories and processes could not be easily expressed in the traditional, patriarchal language. Christine Webb (1983) affirmed this view from a British perspective. To her, language was not "mere words" but conveyed particular ideas or judgments and reflected stereotypes. The terms used reflect judgments: nurses as "girls" connotes immaturity and irresponsibility—complex stereotypes, not merely words.

Nursing, a woman's profession, still has *man* as the central concern in the standard terminology of traditional textbooks. Webb pointed to nursing periodicals that discuss "midwifery manpower" with no realization of the irony. "Man" is presumably used generically in a neutral way, but this does not logically follow: "Man is a mammal. Mammals breastfeed their young. Therefore man breastfeeds her young" (p. 65). Webb claimed that parallel words do not exist (e.g., eligible bachelor/eligible spinster). Webb builds her case on the work of feminist Dale Spender (1980), who described a "downhill slide" of words when applied to women; for example, tramp, a man who travels, becomes derogatory for a woman, for whom tramp means prostitute or one with loose morals. Webb asserted that sexist language places limitations on both women and men, creating inaccurate distinctions between people and denigrating women. She concluded: "We who have been taught to care must care enough to be brave in asserting our feminism" (p. 66). Nurses' image as women extends to the structure of language itself; thus the problem is profound.

Ashley (1980), too, believed that language and ideas are alive, shaping lives and serving political ends. Nurses need to create new words and ideas that will reenergize women's psychic and mental health. "The power and political use of words," said Ashley, "cannot be overemphasized" (p. 14). The historical opposition to women's education is proof of the power of languages. In agreement with Webb and Ashley, Suzanne Smith Blancett (1989), editor-in-chief of the *Journal of Nursing Administration*, presented a hypothetical paragraph that included terms such as manpower, man-hours, to "man" a clinic, chairman, male nurse, layman's language. Reading the paragraph, some, said Blancett, might wonder what the point was, but others might bristle. What was surprising is that *any* nurse by the end of the 1980s could fail to get the point!

At the seventh annual meeting of the International Association of Nursing Editors, Blancett led two well-attended sessions on sexism in writing. Nursing editors were concerned with the amount of sexist language in nursing literature, but agreed that it was the result of ignorance or indifference. The challenge was to educate nurses to recognize and avoid biased writing. Since language is powerful, what message is transmitted by a nursing philosophy that states "Man has 10 basic needs?" To this, Blancett retorted, "If man has 10 basic needs, how many does woman have?" (p. 5).

To become sensitive to stereotyping in language, the speaker or writer must find nonsexist ways to verbalize or write and may then be required to explain or defend why traditional usage is inaccurate or inappropriate. It is equally important to be aware of the male minority in nursing, not referring to nurses as "she" unless, as in this volume, there is a reason to consider the effect of the female gender on nursing.

To Blancett, the clearest example of sexist language is using "man" as a generic term. This evolved "from a time when women were chattel, a dependent, subspecies. . . . Today, using man to generically refer to females is inexcusable sexism" (p. 5). Creative solutions, said Blancett, exist to replace this and other sexist terms. Man becomes person, individual, human being, or people. Man-made may be fabricated or machine-made. Chairman can be leader, presider, moderator, head, or chairperson. As Blancett noted, chairman has been used since 1654 and chairwoman since at least 1694. If nurses accept the premise that communicating with a total group cannot be successful if a substantial part of it is offended, they will try hard to avoid stereotyped speaking and writing. In comparison to Webb's earlier emphasis on changing the structure of language itself, Blancett was more concerned with the appropriate application of language. In both cases, the imagery evoked is important.

FRUSTRATED BATTLEAX OR IDEALIZED WOMAN? NURSES IN FICTIONAL IMAGERY

Concern about the public image of nurses received much more attention from nurse scholars in the 1980s. Stereotypes of nurses as passive, obedient females, or sexually promiscuous women, or even sadistic caregivers persisted in literature, film, and television. Linda Hughes (1980) presented a historical perspective on how poorly the public has understood nursing. As early as 1928 the *American Journal of Nursing* (*AJN*) requested readers to define the major professional aim for the coming year. Hughes noted: "Public cooperation and understanding of the nursing profession was identified by many of the respondents as the major aim toward which the nursing profession should address itself. As one nurse commented, 'the task of obtaining community understanding and, through it, community cooperation is indeed a challenge for, as nurses and as a profession, we are still poorly understood'" (p. 57). Despite the passage of 52 years, said Hughes, the nursing profession was *still* poorly understood, noting that public opinion was a powerful factor in how consumers utilized nursing care. The mass media had created a mythical image of the ideal nurse, based on the stereotyped conception of women. The image of the "ideal" nurse, projected through popular magazines and other media forms, was really a figment of public imagination, creating an unrealistic expectation of a practicing nurse. Thus, young women might still be encouraged to enter nursing as a road to marriage or a way to become physicians' helpmates. Hughes stated: "If the nursing profession believes that it has a valuable service to offer in the area of health care, this must be communicated to the public through the mass media. . . . By openly communicating with the public, nurses can dispel the myths that have long surrounded the nursing profession and begin to project an image that accurately and positively reflects what nursing is" (p. 70).

In an analysis of work and gender in the post-World War II hospital, Barbara Melosh (1983) provided historical depth to the study of fictional imagery. She claimed that nurses' increasing skill and competence put them in conflict with the postwar ideology of domesticity, later called the "feminine mystique." This is apparent in the literature after 1940, which portrayed nurses as "failed women, sometimes pathetic, sometimes dangerous in their distance from proper female activities and aspirations" (p. 165).

Melosh studied prescriptive literature, professional manuals, sociological studies, and didactic fiction, all of which focused on nurses at work and at home and provided a look at nurses as women. Didactic novels with "exemplary" nurses, fiction with nurses as characters, and the nurse in the romantic genre—these together represent a large literature. Melosh excluded men's portrayal of nurses in so-called lesbian stories and in full-blown pornography.

The 100 novels and short stories analyzed by Melosh represent a form of cultural history. Of course, the unanswered question is: Whose culture and whose history? Men's or women's? Melosh traced the patriotic call to "femininity in foxholes" to encourage nurses to enter the military, which was later replaced by the demand that they leave the labor force and return to domestic labor. Although Melosh believed this last call went unheeded by most women, there is evidence that some did leave their work in the public sector. For nurses, this was especially contradictory; while told to return home to their wifely/womanly duties, they were also urged to work as nurses by both hospitals and nursing schools.

Melosh found that the most negative portrayals of nursing "suggested that the authority of the nurse's position was anomalous and unnatural . . . a new and threatening posture of dominance" (p. 168). She claimed that the sentimental fictional images reversed the "proper" dominance of men over women. Men's dependence as patients on women as nurses stressed male vulnerability. Ironically, even though they anticipate all the men's needs, nurses found themselves perceived as man-haters. The literature showed that, "In a world turned upside down, men lose their power to women, and women with unnatural power abuse it" (p. 169). In the literature researched by Melosh, nurses alternately ordered men about and then ignored them; seduced male patients or abandoned them for lesbianism or celibacy. To the writers of these fictional accounts, nurses simply "unbalance the proper relationships" (p. 169).

Melosh found that prewar fiction showed nurses as marginal women doing marginal work, on the edges of social life. But postwar fiction showed competent nurses as questionable women. Once idealized, women now did work that perverted or unsexed them. The conflicting demands of work and womanhood are depicted in stereotyped images of head nurses or supervisors who are seen as unmarried, frustrated battleaxes, whose "competence, altruism, and devotion to duty are all potentially suspect, evidences of incomplete women" (p. 171). The message, said Melosh, is that Old Ironpuss may have a heart of gold, but she should not be emulated.

Melosh found that sociological critiques were equally damning, while genre and didactic fiction showed increased pressure on working women to choose between professional commitment and "femininity." In the romantic version, nurses wanted pretty clothes, ribbons, laces, and cologne. On the other hand, nurses committed to their work had to be set straight by male suitors and advisors, who berated or simply dropped those girls who cancelled dates for hospital emergencies. Melosh concluded that although nursing, the perfect preparation for wife and motherhood, was acceptable as women's work, women learned that marriage and motherhood came first since love and work are "mutually exclusive." Some nurses actually attained both career and marriage, but usually with young doctors. The manuals warned nurses to balance female feeling with male thinking, a "precarious juggling act in managing 'male' work and 'female' personality" (p. 174). Melosh noted: "Without the defense of an articulate feminist ideology or the support of an active women's movement, nurses often met this attack with rhetorical efforts to accommodate their work to the demands of the feminine mystique" (p. 175).

WE'RE NOT ANGELS, WE'RE WORKERS: BRITISH STEREOTYPED IMAGES OF NURSES

Nurses' distress with distorted images crossed cultural boundaries and Britisher Jane Salvage (1983) connected the stereotypes of ministering angel, nymphomaniac, or more recently, militant nurse to economic conditions. One nurse, at an emergency pay conference, said: "'We're not angels, we're workers . . . and here's one angel who's going to take his halo to 10 Downing Street and strangle Mrs. Thatcher with it'" (p. 13). The exasperation and frustration of being overworked and underpaid are directly connected to the trivial and demeaning ways in which nurses and their work are portrayed in the media. In agreement with Melosh, Salvage claimed that heroines in doctor-nurse romances are "identikit angels, docile, compliant, tender, dedicated . . . devoted handmaidens (making tea and scuttling a respectful 10 paces in the rear pushing the notes trolley) whose virtue is usually rewarded by marriage to one of those brusque, lantern-jawed, green-eyed masterful monsters" (p. 13).

With the emergence of feminism, Salvage claimed that the nurse as angel had a corollary, the "naughty nurse," who appeared in comedy films, Soho pornography shops, and as sex objects in every local newspaper; photos of nurses in low-cut swim suits were accompanied by headlines proclaiming them " 'Just what the doctor ordered' " (p. 13). Another stereotype in British imagery that accords with Melosh's analysis of American portrayals is the battleax-dragon matron. In fact, the blurring of cross-cultural imagery is represented by both researchers, who look at the sinister shift in Big Nurse portrayed in *One Flew Over the Cuckoo's Nest*, which shows a woman nurse as "obsessive, ruthless, and power-hungry" (p. 13), justifying the male patient's misogyny. Further, nurses fall within the male-defined framework of women's imagery, which creates a travesty of what nurses really do. In this structure, said Salvage, any male who identifies with women or their work automatically fits into the derogatory female imagery; thus, the male nurse stereotype, limp-wristed and feminine, arises from the same oppressive system.

Salvage warned that nurses cannot dismiss these myths as simply inaccurate, ludicrous, or trivial. Even if nurses fail to recognize themselves, seeing haloes as ridiculous after a grueling night shift, nurses ignore imagery only at their own peril; they can be drawn into the trap of enacting roles as expected by the image-makers. How much do nurses come to share common illusions that nurses are female, poor, born rather than made, existing to carry out physicians' orders, and having little to do with education, research, or politics? Salvage believed that nurses are basically flattered by these myths, particularly if they emphasize dedication and self-sacrifice.

Salvage claimed that a new image, the militant nurse, has emerged. The image arose during recent pay disputes in which nurses are photographed on picket lines, waving placards. According to Salvage, press photographers snap these shots because "they are incongruous, because political activity is seen as incompatible with femininity, compassion or dedication" (p. 15). In this sense, the new imagery is equally selective, and still distresses some nurses, who see it as unprofessional. Trade unions also create stereotypes in their recruitment materials, one being particularly fond of militant Black nurses who are used as a left-wing cliche. But at least, said Salvage, the new images are overt: "More dangerous are the myths which are so familiar we drink in their political message unawares" (p. 15). In agreement with some researchers on Nightingale, Salvage noted that the Nightingale statue, emblems, and even jigsaws puzzles depict an angelic woman, which denies her pragmatism and political shrewdness. Salvage warned that one single new icon could not represent the variegated work of thousands of nurses, but how nurses are to change the traditional images of nurses, as well as the new militant one, remains unclear.

SEX OBJECT OR MAN-HATER?
AMERICAN MEDIA IMAGES OF NURSES

Probably the most thorough research and best recommendations for change of imagery have emerged from Beatrice and Philip Kalisch. With funds from the United States Public Health Service Division of Nursing and other sources, these researchers established the Image of the Nurse in the Mass Media Research Project, out of which a number of research publications have emerged. (Two of these on Nightingale were considered in Chapter 1.) With Mary L. McHugh, the Kalisches published an article in 1982 specifically on nurses as sex objects. This work, in conjunction with other research reports, represents the best work on gender stereotypes as they affect nurses.

Conducting content analysis of 191 motion pictures featuring 211 nurses as significant characters, the researchers attempted to identify how the depiction of nurses as sex objects changed over time from 1930 to 1980. In a patriarchal society, control of the media is within men's hands; thus, in the motion picture industry, males can and have presented women as they see them and want them seen. The researchers found that in 73% of the nurse roles the women were characterized as sex objects. Worse than this finding is the fact that the frequency and intensity of stereotyped nurses as sex objects *rose significantly* during the 1960s and 1970s. Only in films emphasizing professional nursing in the story or character development was sexist stereotyping uncommon. The researchers concluded: "the image of the nurse as a professional care giver was incompatible with that of the nurse as sex object . . . the motion picture industry has opted primarily to present the latter image" (p. 147). They were particularly concerned about the extremely negative sexual stereotype during the previous two decades and urged the profession to act to counter the continuing unfavorable portrayal of nurses.

No other media offers sexuality as explicitly nor intertwines this so overtly with the images of nurses as does the film industry. This in turn manipulates audience needs and beliefs and affects public opinion. Referring to feminist research, the Kalisches and McHugh found increasingly degrading depictions of women in general in other studies reviewing movies over time. Clearly, African and Native American groups have protested the racist stereotypes of members of their groups. Similarly, women, particularly nurses, must stop the film industry from negative stereotyping, which can contribute to a shortage of talent for the profession. The researchers claimed that women teachers have not been the subject of negative stereotyping, but a fuller feminist analysis would probably find that these women, too, are sometimes portrayed as low in the gender-stratification system of occupations.

Although the Kalisches and McHugh chose to exclude all pornographic films but one, it is inaccurate to assume that these films have limited appeal and distribution. The most recent government report on pornography verifies that it is a multimillion-dollar industry; extensive distribution outlets exist for pornography; it is very likely to be "hard" pornography, involving violence against women, and is now more likely to involve children than in the 1960s. If nurses portrayed in pornography had been included, the already devastating findings from the Kalisches' and McHugh's research would be much worse.

Using the Sex Object Index, the Kalisches and McHugh studied types of dramatization and audience, aspects of the character's position and behavior in nursing, nursing activities, professional power and leadership, and qualities of the nurses' personal characters in terms of constructs, such as nurturance, value for work, home, family, and control, and traits such as intelligence, submissiveness, vulnerability, ambition, and femininity. (It is unclear how the last stereotyped construct was conceived.)

As noted, only one in four nurses portrayed in the films analyzed were presented *without* an emphasis on woman as sex object. Few films from the 1930s, 1940s, or 1950s portrayed nurses predominantly as sex objects, and when romance was present, rarely was overt sex shown. From the 1960s on, however, overt depiction of nurses as sex objects rose sharply. Thus, it can be concluded that sexism is an increasingly dominant aspect of American culture. Given this research finding, "You've come a long way, baby," the theme of recent advertising, should be reversed. Nurses may have gone a long way *backward* in the public imagination, especially since the 1960s and 1970s, when blatant sexual activity was increasingly depicted at the expense of portrayals of nursing professionalism. The nurse-as-sex-object theme was even more apparent in films produced for male audiences. That sexuality is connected with actual or implied violence can be inferred from the higher likelihood that nurses were sex objects in movies that focused on fright, horror, or criminal themes.

The Kalisches and McHugh found that films that emphasized the professional work of nurses usually showed them in smaller roles. Indeed, the larger the role, the greater the emphasis on sexual attractiveness and behavior. If older, nurses were further stereotyped as nonsexual. Younger, predominantly blonde nurses, were shown as married during some part of their lives or were likely to give up nursing for marriage. The researchers were not surprised, since nurses were presented as having a strong value for home life and a low value for work, fitting the traditional female stereotype —submissive, nurturant, vulnerable, feminine, not very intelligent, and lacking in ambition. With nurses in higher positions, ratings on the Sex Object Index declined, and the women were shown as having leadership qualities, valuing control, and directing others or managing organizational units. Evidently, power and sex appeal are antithetical, at least for females. The authors noted that only six characters (2.8%) combined the qualities of leadership and sexual attractiveness during the 50-year period studied.

The researchers found a most disturbing phenomenon in the 1970s—a continuation of nurses as sexual playmates, but the emergence of sadistic nurse characters, not as sex objects, but "cruel and abrasive . . . who held

positions of power that permitted free reign to their abominable behavior"
(p. 152). It should not be surprising that these negative images emerged at the
same time the women's liberation movement gained strength. Men in control
of the media often show women with power as sexless man-haters; for
example, in films such as *One Flew Over the Cuckoo's Nest* and, most recently,
Misery. The moral is obvious and so is the effect on the younger generation,
who may turn away from or even against their feminist mothers and
grandmothers, as some did previously in the latter 1920s. Now, as then, with
no proud history, these women are left with no theoretical or conceptual
gendered framework in which to position their individual lives.

In nursing, the lack of generational consistency and congruence between
gender and professional roles leads to loss of power over time and lack of
cohesion among nurses in their own organizations. To find images of strength,
young women nurses would have to go back to a 1946 film on Elizabeth
Kenney, to two 1950s productions on Nightingale, or one in 1953 on a nurse
fighting to bring health care to African villages. The Kalisches and McHugh
point to only one antiwar film in 1971 that portrayed a nurse who, unlike the
physicians, "never lost sight of her patient's humanity" (p. 152). From these
findings, it is clear that nurses must attack sex discrimination (although this
term is not used by the Kalisches and McHugh) in a way analogous to African
Americans and other minorities who have attacked demeaning and
stereotyped images of their groups. The researchers recommended media
awareness groups that would monitor, react, and foster more positive images
of nurses. Although not stated, these groups *were* formed in NOW in the early
1970s and did influence to some degree a few television programs. This
strategy requires nurses, as women, to have a developed consciousness of sex
discrimination. A second strategy demands action, letters, and protests in large
numbers and positive feedback for accurate portrayals. These tactics require
nurses who value political action, who understand and use power effectively.

The Kalisches and McHugh point to a successful example of political action
used by nursing students who picketed a university campus that was showing
the R-rated film, *The Student Nurses*. The film depicts young women who are
told they cater to more than their patients and are further told they will be a
great addition to the decor! A poll conducted by the School of Nursing found
that 94% of the university students objected to the film; both students and
faculty wrote letters to the campus newspaper, placed an ad, and protested in
front of the theater. The researchers urge using nursing consultants to the
media, giving awards for those who produce positive and accurate images of
nurses, and finally, that nurses, such as Mary Roberts Rinehart, who had
previously written novels on nurses, write their own novels, plays, and media
productions.

On the basis of their research, the Kalisches and McHugh believe that
nursing shortages and scarcity of health resources for nursing will continue as
long as the media are allowed to denigrate women nurses. Although the term

is not used in the article, sexist presentations of women in general will have to stop, but this requires an understanding that sex discrimination is built into the structure of *all* patriarchal institutions, into the culture itself.

NURSING AS METAPHOR

What is the more fundamental connection between images of women and nurses? Claire Fagin and Donna Diers (1983) considered the image of nursing itself as a metaphor. They were curious about the reactions of others who, when told in social situations of their professional identity, responded with "I think I need another drink" (p. 116), or "I never met a nurse socially before" (p. 116), or related their latest experiences of hospitalization, surgery, or child birth. The authors conclude that "nursing evokes disturbing and discomforting images that many . . . find difficult to handle in a social situation" (p. 116), and this cannot be simply explained by labeling an attitude a stereotype. Fagin and Diers look for underlying metaphors, beginning with nursing as a metaphor for mothering—nurturing, caring, and comforting are maternal behaviors seen as "essentially mundane." But the thought of a nurse standing over a prone patient may evoke regressed feelings, since adults in social settings do not like to be reminded of "the child who remains inside all of us" (p. 116).

Fagin and Diers also see nursing as a metaphor for class struggle. As the underdogs in the health-delivery system, women struggle for equality, to be heard, approved, and recognized, but they work in settings where physicians, the upper and controlling class, dominate and do so by stereotyping nurses as satisfied with their jobs, not members of a prestigious profession. On the other hand, nursing is a metaphor for equality, since little social distance separates the nurse from the patient or a nurse from other nurses, since few distinctions are made, for example, by levels of education. Fagin and Diers point out that nurses, as members of the working class, may comfort sick patients, but "it may be awkward to encounter one's nurse at a black-tie reception, where working class people do not belong" (p. 116).

Nursing is also a metaphor for conscience since nurses see the neglect, the cures, and the reasons for both, as well as knowing that physicians' attempts to conquer death often fail. Nurses are, thus, a reminder of fallibility: "The anxiety, not to mention the guilt, engendered by what nurses may know can be considerable" (p. 116). Fagin and Diers believe that nursing is also a metaphor for intimacy, because nurses are involved in the most private aspects of life, doing for others in a public setting what is usually done in private at home, and hearing secrets expressed from vulnerability. People do not want to remember vulnerability and loss of control, but nurses are clearly identified with those personal experiences. This connects with yet another metaphor, nursing as sexual; nurses see and touch strangers' bodies, and are often seen as willing sexual partners who, unlike prostitutes, are "safe," in clean white uniforms, with professional demeanor.

Fagin and Diers claim that nurses live and work in a psychological milieu that is the sum of these images. Little wonder, they say, that nurses are badgered about their choice of career. "Why would anyone with a brain enter nursing?" Nurses respond to questions like this with talk about roles, variety, mobility, and changes in the profession, but they need to address the metaphors, the *real* reasons for such questions. Why shrink from the word "intimacy," instead of affirming equality, conscience, and motherhood, separated from the usual stereotyped meanings? Fagin and Diers urge nurses to be "wistfully amused" by evoked reactions, rather than defensive since nurses must be advocates even for those who stereotype them.

"LOOK! ISN'T SHE TYPICAL?"

Clearly, changing the image of nurses involves changing the pictures of women at a very deep cultural level. So widespread are the negative perceptions of women in nursing that even get-well cards foster sexist derogation, ostensibly under the guise of humor. Jacqueline Rose Hott (1984), in her informal research on this matter, related a personal experience of entering a male patient's room and seeing him gazing at a get-well card that depicted a flaming redhead with hair flowing over her shoulders, cleavage showing between voluptuous breasts, white dress tight and soiled, and droopy white stockings hanging over dirty clogs. Carrying a tray covered with cigarette butts and a beer can with a straw in it, the "nurse's" face showed disdain, almost a snarl; her namepin said "Flo," and a white starched cap was tipped on her head. Hott looked at the middle-aged patient, who held up his card, smiled, and said, "Look! Isn't she typical?" (p. 46). Hott gulped and said, "Tell me about it" (p. 46), sitting down to talk with him about nurses' images.

What is humorous when the butt of sexist jokes is women? Hott questioned her own sense of humor. Was she overly concerned? But after collecting cards for three years, there was nothing funny about the insidious, subtly hostile message about the woman nurse (and she found it always was a female) as seductive sex object, sadistic, or stupid. When the nurse was sweet or caring, she was drawn as a "cute animal, usually a kitten, puppy, bird, chicken, teddy bear, mouse, bunny, pig, or elephant" (p. 46). On a less friendly note, one card depicted a nurse as a gorilla in a hospital zoo. More usually, patients, "sick as dogs," are cured by pussy cat nurses.

Hott found that the human caricature of a nurse pictures her in white, tight, short uniform with cap on messy hair, carrying an enema bag, bed pan, thermometer, stethoscope, or threatening hypodermic syringe with a very long needle. In contrast, physicians are seen as money-hungry and incompetent, always a male, the ultimate authority figure, the punitive father. Patients are depicted as young to middle-aged males, helpless and weak. Hott noted that she saw no cards showing Black or other minority characters.

Hott found that patients receiving these cards are usually hospitalized for acute medical/surgical problems; psychiatric patients seldom receive these cards, perhaps because, as Hott speculated, people do not know what to say, or fear the card's meaning will be distorted, or do not expect the patients to get well! Children receive cards with gender-typed animals on them. Critically ill people are usually spared sexist humor, receiving quiet landscapes with no hospital personnel or equipment shown. Hott satirically notes that these seem to say, "You're not long for this world. No more jokes about doctors and nurses for you. You're going down the tube" (p. 47). Only at the point of death does the gendered parody of women nurses stop.

Greeting cards, initially sentimental, were originally postcards, and did not become popular until after the First World War. Currently, 85% of cards are bought by women, but most of the artists who create them are men. The caricatures, grotesque or ludicrous, exaggerate human characteristics for satirical purposes that ridicule, aggressively and derisively, the incongruencies and discontinuities of life. Humor can be an expression of fury, according to psychoanalytic theory, at the meaninglessness of life, a defense against pain, expressing emotions in a socially acceptable way, circumventing overly rigid taboos. Although Hott stays within this interpretation, it is very difficult to assume such cards are expressing gender taboos, since depictions of women in all kinds of advertising, publishing, and other media presentations are also often demeaning and sexist. Thus, in get-well cards, the nurse as woman is used in a specialized way to tell men there is nothing to fear from their vulnerability. Women are ridiculed to put them in their place as care-givers, who might have temporary power over hospitalized men; they are not to be seen as any lasting threat.

Hott's initial response to her analysis of greeting cards was to boycott the card companies, write letters, or set up a contest for the best presentation of a woman nurse as intelligent, empathic, sincere, and the like. Although she took no action, she did begin to ask patients how they thought of nurses, talking about the stereotypes. She hopes that the "sick card industry eventually gets well" (p. 48), but this is unlikely if nurses do not act politically on Hott's findings and other media distortions.

In fact, some nurses did quite the opposite, encouraging further sexist stereotyping by posing for the November 1983 *Women in White* issue of *Playboy*. Joyce E. Dains (1984) states:

The nurses who appeared in *Playboy* chose to do so. I defend their right as individuals to do so, but I condemn their misuse of the privilege of professional representation as an abhorrent misrepresentation of nursing. To display oneself publicly as an individual is a personal moral choice. To display oneself publicly as a nurse is a violation of professional ethics.

Such a violation profoundly affects nursing because an act that demeans one of us demeans us all. (p. 20A)

Both women and men in the profession are insulted, but short of creating a more professional climate, Dains states there is little that can be done about this particular issue of *Playboy*. A second, related issue, however, *is* subject to active pressure. The sexist advertising in medical supply and hospital apparel catalogues can be changed by mobilizing nurses to protest and boycott. Two recent examples of exploitation are described by Dains: "In one case a product was displayed on a naked female manikin; in the second case women were portrayed in subservient roles, positioned in provocative poses, and presented in inappropriately frivolous settings" (p. 20A). To Dains, these and many other ads exploit women and insinuate sex to sell products: "As a woman, and as a professional, I am enraged. We *should* be enraged" (p. 20A). Indeed, rage is needed to create constructive action to support a collective vision of the nursing profession. Dains is not sanguine about the speed of change, understanding that sexist cultural values are so pervasive that it will take time to create a society in which women are respected and nursing is seen as a legitimate and powerful profession. She calls for letters and large-scale protests from several hundred nurses, admitting that this means time and energy and risk, but claims the battle is worth fighting. The alternative is to wait for feminist groups or other professional nursing organizations to do the work for us. Dains says nurses can choose to act for themselves and shape their own destiny or sit back and claim the battle does not really affect them. To her: "this battle is one that we cannot afford to lose, because at its heart is the very crux of the issue: if we are professionals, then we should expect and demand to be represented as such. To do anything less is an act of betrayal—of nursing and of ourselves" (p. 20A).

FANTASIES, MYTHS, AND STEREOTYPES: MORE SEXIST IMAGES OF NURSES

Janet Muff (1982; 1984) is very clear on the power implications of imagery; the key issue is the image nurses as women hold of themselves. She bases her thinking on four ideas: that image problems of nurses come from image problems of women; that origins of nursing stereotypes are far more extensive than mere media phenomena; that changing nurses' images of themselves will alter how they behave; that change is predicated on nurses' attention to personal and professional socialization and to sexism in health-care systems.

Muff (1982) categorizes nurse stereotypes into six areas: first, as *angels of mercy*, of selfless devotion, affirming compassion but negating nurses' own interests; second, as *handmaidens* to physicians, involving traditional "feminine" deference and submission to masculist authority, to the exclusion of autonomy; third, as *women in white*, emphasizing uniforms and caps, or purity and cleanliness in a simplistic, limiting, and impractical way; fourth, as *battle-axes*, confusing assertion with castration and organization with domination; fifth, as *sex symbols*, perverting scientific into carnal knowledge, degrading professionalism, exploiting humanness and sexuality; and sixth, as *torturers*, expressing calculated sadism, mocking nurses, as agents of pain, who derive pleasure from hurtful and embarrassing treatments.

Regardless of the stereotypes, nurse equals woman, whose "natural" femininity, not intelligence, allows her to care, for little financial reward, but not cure, for considerably more money. Muff warns, however, that Mother Nature can be loving and also violent, so myths of women healers partake of the dichotomy of madonna and whore, exemplified in the broader mythology of women. A curious mixture of reality and fantasy, images are deeply woven into the fabric of institutions, even expressed in female socialization by some mothers to daughters and by some nurses to their students, by rewarding obedience and dependence and discouraging assertiveness, teaching them to say "yes" when they mean "no," to sacrifice themselves, to keep the peace, to play the doctor-nurse game. These sustain a gender-segregated system with discriminatory salaries.

In a gender-segregated labor market, to keep the subordinated in their places, it is important that what women do remains vague; indeed, most non-nurses, according to Muff (1984), do not comprehend the breadth of nursing practice. And nurses, twice socialized to subordination, are plagued by problems of identity and low self-esteem, causing them to turn on each other in bitter fights or to battle others over disciplinary boundaries, attempting to resolve them with "the often arbitrary and isolating use of 'nursing' theory" (p. 44) that has insufficient substance.

Muff further warns against the false belief that "paternalistic systems will recognize and reward dutiful daughterhood" (p. 44), which only produces naive or self-destructive, powerless dependence. To Muff, public images will change only when nurses change their own imagery by understanding their gender and nursing socialization, seeing the parallels in nursing history with the status and problems of women, and widening their vision. They need to be proactive, not reactive, by accepting nurses' power and using it. To sum up, Muff claims: "It is no longer enough to expect that if we do a 'good' job, we will be adequately cared for. Our lady-in-waiting days are over. Prince Charming may never come, and in any case, real self-esteem comes from learning to ride the white horse yourself!" (p. 44).

Accomplishing these changes will not be easy. When women and nurses are completely excluded from any public presentations, one must question which is worse: being completely ignored in the media or being presented as sex objects without the intelligence or assertiveness to do anything but support a few men. Eleanor Turnbull (1986) studied nurses' responses to their *complete* absence in a 1984 NBC television series of twenty, ten-minute health sequences of four weekly topics on health assessment, disease prevention, detection, and nutrition. Physicians, psychologists, dieticians, pharmacists, safety council representatives—all were represented, but "nurses were neither involved as presenters nor pictured in the series. The word 'nurse' was used only once" (p. 5). Thus were 1,600,000 nurses, mostly women and the largest group of health workers, blithely ignored.

Connecting to earlier research conducted by the Kalisches (1980; 1981; 1982a; 1982b; 1983c; 1983d) and by Gerbner, Gross, Morgan, and Signorielli (1981), Turnbull asked 300 student nurses, nurse educators, and service nurses what they thought of the absence of nurses from the NBC program. The majority of respondents (75%) reacted unfavorably to their exclusion— "disappointed," a "gross injustice," and "astounding," given that nurses play a major role in health care and spend more time with patients than any other health-care provider. Neutral responses were more resigned—"not really surprised," the "public does not understand nursing," or the media does not see nurses as important to disease prevention.

The nurses recommended that television programs present more specific knowledge of nurses' roles, functions, responsibilities, and scope of practice, such as medical-surgical nursing, hospice care, research activities, mental health, and industrial nursing. Furthermore, they wanted the truth told about their service in hospitals, the fact that nurses make 90% of the day-to-day contacts affecting patient well-being and the promotion of health and wellness. In lesser numbers, nurses wanted their intellectual abilities and complex responsibilities presented to the public. For example, nurses are usually the primary person on the scene during life-and-death crises, making several decisions before the physician appears. Others wanted the media to show their professional organization, higher levels of education, problems with autonomy and ethics. The nurses wanted the public to understand the functions of visiting nurses, involvement with complex machinery, the reality of nurse-patient interactions, the need to upgrade all levels of nursing and to achieve autonomy. They wanted in-depth profiles shown of nurses giving support to persons who were told they have cancer, providing well-baby check-ups, and so forth—in short, real footage of what nurses *really* do.

GENDER STEREOTYPES IN PUBLIC PERCEPTIONS OF NURSES

Whether the information proposed by Turnbull's subjects would indeed change the public's attitudes toward nurses is not certain. Would the public, as Lisa H. Newton (1981) claimed, refuse to accept the new autonomous professional role of nurses because it is in opposition to the traditional public ideal of a nurse that focuses on nurturance and service? In fact, Newton argued that the public's view of women as nurturers, servers, and a subservient group could *not* be changed; therefore, nurses should remain in their traditional roles. Actually, numerous studies comparing nurse practitioners' competence to physicians' on the same functions found patient acceptance of nurses to be very high and results of health care to be as good and often better than for patients seeing physicians only (see Roberts & Group, *Gender and the Nurse-Physician Game*). As in studies of race discrimination, actual changes in behavior in new settings could result in a faster rate of reducing prejudicial attitudes of patients than simply providing new information aimed at altering their attitudes.

Many nurse scholars reacted negatively to Newton's thesis, leading some researchers to investigate the nature of stereotyping of occupational role information by evaluating perceptions of personality traits (Kaler, Levy, & Schall, 1989). Kaler and her colleagues asked 110 subjects drawn from the public, half female and half male, to rate the degree to which 12 personality characteristics typified individuals in 14 professions. On the 1 to 7 scale, the men and women rated gender types of occupational categories (e.g., enterprising [lawyer], conventional [secretary], artistic [actor]) and also rated low- and high-status occupations. Personality characteristics presented in polar opposites, such as leader/follower, feminine/masculine, cold/warm, were then judged in relation to the occupations. The researchers found a horizontal dimension of achievement versus helping orientation that was clearly gender-organized. Business executives and lawyers, for example, were seen as masculine, cold, competitive, self-concerned, and as leaders. Librarians, clergy, nurses, and homemakers, at the other end, were seen as feminine, generous, honest, and idealistic. It was obvious that nurses were evaluated in relation to "clearly defined and consensually endorsed norms governing the appropriate masculine and feminine images" (p. 87).

A second vertical dimension, representing the academic preparation of each occupation, was found, with physicians perceived as having the highest, and nurses having a middle level of education, but more than teachers and clergy. Nurses were seen as educationally equivalent to librarians or therapists. Of all professions, nurses ranked highest on concern for others, as cooperative and generous as clergy, as warm and as much followers as homemakers, and as feminine as librarians and secretaries. Furthermore, nurses were seen as occupying the midrange on intelligence, with physicians highest and athletes lowest.

Kaler and her colleagues concluded that their research supported Newton's concern that nurses' move for autonomy would eliminate the emphasis on human needs, best met by persons imbued with culturally stereotyped feminine tenderness, warmth, sympathy, and expressions of feeling. They noted that "the public image of nursing and medicine continues to be firmly sex-role stereotyped" (p. 88) and that nurses are still seen as less intelligent, independent, and achievement-oriented than physicians. In opposition to Newton, Kaler and her colleagues concluded: "the results underscore the need for nursing to assert the right to practice so that the stereotype of the nurse as being intelligent and autonomous can exist in the public's mind" (p. 89). This underscores the need to change attitudes through actions, rather than by information only.

CROSS-CULTURAL PERCEPTIONS OF NURSES

In other countries, too, concern and dismay about nursing's public image led to several research studies. In Britain, for example, Margo Mapanga (1985) asserted that the media influenced the spiritual, political, and intellectual development of audiences, but in an unequal and biased manner. European research showed that television upholds the traditional, while ignoring changing relationships between the sexes. As in previous decades, nurses are seen as angels, dragons, or sex symbols. Furthermore, women in media industries hold predominantly low-level positions in which little influence on programming is possible. Advertisements sell not just women as commodities, but women's relationships. British nursing recruitment advertisements present neat, tidy women with motherly, caring attitudes. Mapanga noted that nurses are rarely heard or seen in public debates on health issues, and feminist women, who attempt to change their subordinated status, are portrayed as hostile, aggressive men-haters.

A study on cross-cultural comparisons of nursing's image, conducted by Austin, Champion, and Tzeng (1985), analyzed conceptual ratings for "Nurse" and "Feminine" across 30 language/cultural groups, using data from 1,200 young males, previously collected from Osgood's 1975 *Atlas of Affective Meanings*. Three independent factors—evaluation (E; good/bad), potency (P; strong/weak), and activity (A; active/passive)—were used as affective meanings on judgments of diverse concepts in a variety of human societies, appearing fairly stable cross-culturally. The researchers used previously collected data on "Nurse" and "Feminine" and retrieved the mean scores on the E, P, and A factors. The scores on evaluation were positive for the concept "Nurse" in 29 of 30 cultures, excepting only Greece; thus, nurses are perceived generally positively worldwide. On the potency factor, reflecting strength and power, "Nurse" was rated negatively by 50% of the cultures. The least powerful ratings were from Germany, Finland, and the Netherlands; positive ratings from other countries were relatively small. In the activity domain, the majority of countries rated "Nurse" as very active, with six of them giving negative values—Greece, Japan, Brazil, Germany, Romania, and the United States, where an African American subgroup had also been studied.

The researchers concluded that "Nurse" is rated good and active, but not powerful. How, then, would the values of "Feminine" look in comparison? The evaluation domain for "Feminine" was positive, with only three countries giving small negative values: the United States (African American group), Iran, and Afghanistan. As with "Nurse," the term "Feminine" on the potency dimension was rated negatively in 22 of 30 cultures; thus feminine characteristics are seen as weak, not reflecting much power. The activity dimension indicated positive values, but not much beyond neutral, with only three cultures rating this dimension below neutral. The problem, of course, with the term "Feminine" is that it is so stereotyped as to be rejected by most feminists themselves. It is, therefore, not surprising that a stereotyped term produces a stereotyped response.

The good news is that women and nurses are perceived as good, and to a lesser extent active, but the bad news is that they are seen as weak in potency or power. Why, then, asked the researchers, are the negative public images, described, for example, by the Kalisches and others, so frequent? Presumably, the view of nurses as powerless and weak substantiate the handmaiden role image perpetuated by physicians, in which nurses "are not perceived to be able to function in a position of strength or independence . . . [perhaps] a consequence of the dominating role of males in society" (Austin et al., 1985, p. 237). Clearly, a dependent image does not contribute to independent or interdependent functioning. The researchers wondered if physical differences in strength could have spilled over into professional roles, giving a false conception that women are equally less effective professionally.

Are the linkages between "Nurse" and "Feminine" so close because nurses are usually female or because nursing is so related to the act of mothering? Can nurses change their image without changing the traditional woman's image? If nurses increase their power, would they be seen as more masculine, and would their other rankings drop? The most critical question is how nurses can maximize the traditional values of women while gaining more power. This, of course, is at the heart of debates in feminist theory and involves all women, but nurses exemplify this issue most clearly. How to be perceived as both good *and* strong, according to Austin et al., is the dilemma.

HOLDING ON TO OUR FEMALE VALUES: THE WOMEN'S MOVEMENT IS STILL NECESSARY

With the rising conservative backlash to women in the 1980s, there were fears that nurses' activism and support for feminist goals would weaken. In an interview with Canadian nursing administrator Alice J. Baumgart, Margaret Allen (1985) asked whether nurses had rejected feminism. Baumgart claimed that nursing had been somewhat tardy in feeling the impact of the women's movement. But although the media presentation of "bra burners" had made some nurses uncomfortable with feminism, the feminist movement had made a significant impact on nursing practice, education, and activities of the professional nursing organizations. The impact of feminist scholarship had provided nursing with a different lens to view the world: "We owe a tremendous debt of gratitude to the feminist movement for helping us analyze what power is all about. It is not a destructive force" (p. 20).

Allen asked Baumgart about the impact of feminism on nurse-physician conflicts, and she noted that "doctors and nurses were on a collision course long before the feminist movement began. . . . It all translates into 'women's proper place.' . . . Nurses' place equals women's place in these nurse-bashing exercises. . . . In the health-care system, doctors have been regarded as the only 'rightful knowers.' What the doctor-nurse game is really all about is that nurses know, but can't let the world know that they know" (p. 21). And what of the relation between education in nursing and feminism? Besides influencing trends in nursing practice, increasing professionalization, research, and autonomy, Baumgart claimed that feminism had contributed to a new understanding of women's health. Recognizing that textbook descriptions and treatments of health problems are often male-biased, Baumgart concluded that sex discrimination was still nursing's most pervasive problem.

Other nurse scholars examined the impact of feminism on nursing, acknowledging that feminism had helped nurses develop and use power and politics, but also noting the historically "uneasy alliance" between nursing and the women's movement (Vance, Talbott, McBride, & Mason, 1985). For example, Judy Chicago's acclaimed art project, "The Dinner Party," paid tribute to hundreds of women including Nightingale and Sanger, but neither of these woman was explicitly recognized as a nurse. Deploring a 1980 report that the National Organization for Women neglected to include nurses in their local conferences, the authors did not mention that a NOW nurses group was formed as early as 1975. During that same year, feminist Florence Howe urged women to focus on women's professions, emphasizing nursing. Although they may have exaggerated the exclusion of nursing, Vance et al. recognized that feminist scholarship and activism has helped nurses "understand and reject the heavy burdens of sexism . . . , destructive images, and devaluing of women's work" (p. 282).

How do women in nursing hold on to the best female values, while changing their roles? Vance and her colleagues quoted Carol Gilligan: " 'It is precisely this dilemma—the conflict between compassion and autonomy, between virtue and power—which the feminine voice struggles to resolve' " (p. 282). These tensions are experienced in nursing. Values are in transition as nursing struggles with a history of submission and male domination. Vance and her colleagues denounced sexist language, improper media depiction of nurses, disparities between government funds for medicine and nursing, stereotypes of the intellectual male and emotional female, inequities in salaries—all these issues were seen as infuriating and frustrating in the 1980s as they were in the decades before. But Vance and her associates looked to feminist solutions developed and refined in the 1970s. Equal pay for comparable worth seems one way to stop the trivialization of nurses as women. Still another way is to separate nurses' costs from general hospital accounts in order to assess the value of women's work in nursing. Still another is to attack the increasing inequity between nurse and physician salaries. In 1945 nurses' salaries were one-third of physician incomes, but in 1981 they had dropped to one-fifth! Nurses must turn to feminist solutions and organizations to rectify these inequities.

In agreement with Baumgart and others, Vance and her colleagues concluded that feminism has influenced the perceptions of women's health, causing nurses to redefine health-care priorities and to attend to women as patients. In fact, "Nurses have come to realize that they may be the health care providers best suited to meet consumer demands for self-determination" (p. 285). Although new nurse-managed centers have proved to be effective alternatives to traditional care, legislative rights to autonomous practice are critical to nurses' practice. To achieve this, the authors maintained that the women's movement was still necessary.

WHAT CAN NURSING CONTRIBUTE TO FEMINISM?

There has been a long-standing debate about the relationship between feminism and nursing. Although nursing evolved parallel to and was interconnected with the earlier women's movement in the mid-19th century, nurses have never organized against sexism in the health-care system. This has led some critics to conclude that nurses are unwilling to embrace feminism, because they have not wanted to give up the image of themselves as "ideal women" and of the physician as "ideal man." However, in a discussion of the role of feminist ideology in the quest for professionalization, Sandra Speedy (1987) could find only one author "who openly rejected feminism as a useful strategy for the development of nursing" (p. 25). Indeed, there were twice as many writers who believed feminism could and had contributed more to nursing than nursing had to feminism. For example, feminists have laid bare the realities of unequal opportunity; analyzed and supported unions' and/or professional organizations' actions for improved economic and job standards; questioned the values system underpinning health care; provided impetus to regain and reinterpret nursing and women's history; and created the possibility of health care emerging from a woman-defined value system, going beyond patriarchal institutions.

Two major goals in nursing, obtaining autonomy and receiving adequate reimbursement for services, required an alliance with feminism, which had already legitimized the development and use of power and politics to redefine nurses' roles and women's health care. As noted earlier, Wilma Scott Heide had urged a massive consciousness-raising effort among nurses to accomplish a values transformation that could lead to human liberation. But in Speedy's literature review she could find only three papers that called for nursing to put its "own house in order" without relying on feminist ideology. One author decried the energy expended fighting for women's rights (Seigel, 1984). However, Lamb's (1973) assertion that it was up to nurses to put nursing in order could hardly be placed in the antifeminist camp with Seigel. Nor could Wolf's (1972) article, which emphasized nurses' needs to create their own power by using the feminist strategies of group solidarity, mutual aid, loyalty, and sisterhood.

If there was consensus at least in the published literature on the positive effects of feminism on nursing, what of nursing's contribution to feminism? In 1986 a national conference on nursing and feminism was held at Yale University, attesting to the continued importance of the women's movement to nursing. Speedy reports that a number of the conference delegates felt that nurses had been slow in internalizing "the feminist's underlying message of self-determination and commitment" (p. 26). Other participants, such as Caroline Whitbeck, asserted that feminism "needed the input of nursing theory to ground it in the experiences of *all* women" (p. 27). Patricia Benner believed that theory always derived from practical knowledge and that nursing practice could contribute to feminism; observing and valuing the context of care marks the women's unique approach. Although Speedy claims that Benner recommended not feminist principles, but the rejection of masculist science and scientific method, this principle had been enunciated for many years by a number of feminist theorists.

Ann M. Voda said that nursing could offer feminism the power of care in the real world, but both nurses and feminists tend to be unaware of each other's scholarship. Nevertheless, she asserted that nursing research and feminist consciousness must be combined if nursing was to achieve its full potential. Donna Diers rejected the theory of oppression, asserting that nurses did not fight because they were oppressed, but because the divide-and-conquer strategy had been effectively used by other groups to divide the women. If feminists used nurses for self-serving ends, then nursing could be damaged. What these "ends" were remained unclear. However, Speedy concludes that nursing needed to confront the fear of feminism: "If the opportunity for an alliance between nursing and feminism is rejected, nursing may spend its future fighting the same battles it has for decades, and nothing could be more wasteful" (p. 27).

Peggy Chinn, nursing professor and feminist scholar, agreed with some of the presenters at the Yale conference, noting there are many theoretical parallels between the domains of nursing and feminism (Henderson, 1988). Both have been concerned about nurturing and the quality of life and are committed to a holistic view of human experience, holding a value of respect for the individual. Both feminists and nurses have public image problems that tend to discredit or trivialize the women involved. In the public imagery, nurses and housewives are both incorrectly seen as menials to physicians or husbands and are often dichotomized into good or bad images. Attacking the man-hater image used to discredit feminism, Chinn states this was like saying if you like apples, you must hate oranges! The fact that feminists such as Chinn value women, women's writings, their history, and what they do in the world, and focus on females rather than males is interpreted to mean feminists hate men.

When Chinn was asked if the next 15 years would be spent fighting for equality, she responded that many feminists now question if they want equality in the system as it presently exists. One might remember that Nightingale's initial refusal to focus on suffrage was that the more fundamental issue was that women's economic situation must change. To Chinn, as a radical or cultural feminist nurse, "It is critically important to understand that something is wrong in the system and simply trying to emulate it will not create the kinds of changes that need to happen" (p. 8). She urges nurses to achieve power in the larger political arena to obtain public support and funding, currently controlled by physicians. To equalize power imbalances, for example, does not mean that everyone enters a situation equally capable or achieves an equal level of attainment, but everyone has equal involvement and access to resources for development within a caring and nurturing environment.

Some critics say that nurses are not very caring to each other; that there is too much competition among them and too little support. Chinn, however, points to the Friendship Survey that appeared in the November 1987 *AJN*. Derived from a project by Chinn with Charlene Eldridge Wheeler, Adrienne Roy, and Elizabeth Mathier Wheeler, the survey asked nurses to share both their good and bad experiences with friendship and caring. Believing, as did feminist Janice Raymond (1986), that support and friendship between women make their work in the world possible, Chinn and her colleagues wanted to know how nurses felt about the support they received in order to learn about barriers to female friends so nurses could learn how to care for each other and give and accept support. Nurses' behavior can often be destructive and, states Chinn, when women are hurt they often react like victims and become confused with hurtful behavior. So far the research showed that most of the nurses received support and encouragement from other nurses, and "the more we focus on how to do this better, the more this will become our reality" (p. 9). From a cultural or radical feminist perspective, Chinn attempts to focus on creating the liking and loving needed to translate feminism to nursing. But other feminist nurses are less optimistic about nurses' capacity to change.

THE TIME FOR PASSIVITY IS OVER

If nurses see themselves as members of an oppressed group, would they be able to act effectively on the insights of feminism? Janet Muff (1988) is not so sure and reaffirms Cleland's early contention: "The problems facing nursing—lack of autonomy, role confusion, disunity, stress, job dissatisfaction, and high turnover—are related to the fact that nursing is a traditionally 'woman's job' in a traditionally 'man's world' " (p. 197). Even by the end of the 1980s, Muff claims that nurses' progress was slow; they continue to suffer dual socialization to traditional "feminine" identities and this, in turn, contributes to status and power inequalities. However, Muff says, "Nurses, themselves, are responsible" (p. 197).

Muff believes that it is not experiences that induce stress, but *perceptions* by nurses of their experiences, and these perceptions influence their responses, which in turn influence others' reactions. She claims that women, and nurses as women, although acknowledging the impact of history and culture, cannot afford to blame others for their problems any longer. While Muff says that she is not blaming the victim, it is unclear whether nurses even know their culture and history as women or as nurses. Certainly, their formal education has not normally included feminist histories of nursing or analyses of the profession, nor have external women's studies courses been required of nursing students. Furthermore, if the sexist structures of hospitals and agencies are not changed by legal means, then faculty will continue to teach what they have to in order to adapt to male control. Although Muff does not focus on the practical compromises demanded, she claims that most students are given a conflicting message: "learn to be an autonomous professional, but follow the rules unquestioningly. Nothing could be more crazy-making" (p. 200).

Muff warns that, as a "caricature of femininity," nursing is subjected to sexist beliefs that it is not an intellectual discipline, does not require higher education, can be taught through apprenticeship, requires no special skill, that any woman can do it and should because it is ideal preparation for marriage, and after having children, a woman can easily return to work. The goal of this mythology is to maintain the status quo, and unfortunately, says Muff, it works. She accuses nurses themselves of repudiating the need for advanced education, dropping out, and seeing nursing, as Linda Hughes (1982) states, as a "stopgap to marriage." Research findings, of course, vary on these and other reasons for turnover; it is clear that powerlessness of nurses, their inability to take care of patients as they wish and to provide the best nursing care possible, are major reasons why nurses leave the profession (see Roberts & Group, *Gender and the Nurse-Physician Game*). It is the sexist attitude that nursing is "natural," requiring little education, that establishes it as not worth much, needing minimal remuneration, and supports a gender-stratified marketplace. Ironically, states Muff, "the only reason a person need be hospitalized is to receive nursing care" (p. 209), since laboratory tests and even surgery can often be done on an outpatient basis. Yet nurses do not bill for their services, are included in the "room rate," and cannot prove the revenue they produce because of their failure to set budgets and have access to funds. As targets of sexist propaganda, nurses either accept or are confused by it, rarely rejecting it because the process is covert, not recognizing that they are being manipulated.

It is quite likely that increasing numbers of nurses do recognize sexism, but have no clear vision of how to change large bureaucracies to express women's values of caring and curing. The overwhelming control of all aspects of women's lives in large and interlocked institutional structures makes it difficult to know where to start. Instead of carrying out a systemic organizational analysis, Muff claims that the idea of "professionalism" is used to get women to wear uniforms, even though service workers usually wear them, to work double shifts, to engage in the doctor-nurse game, which, although resented, is continued because of fear of conflict over change. Altruism and selflessness, so deeply ingrained in women's socialization, make nurses particularly vulnerable to flattery as a means to divide and conquer: day nurses are told they are better than night nurses, critical care nurses are better than their medical-surgical counterparts. Some women believe such manipulative flattery, which is then used to obtain compliance to others' needs.

Divided, nurses cannot organize against sexist propaganda and their salaries will continue to defy the law of supply and demand. Shortages should result in larger salaries, but claims Muff, hospital administrators have agreed to standardize nursing salaries in their communities, using shortages to reduce nurses' hours and employ ancillary staff instead. Although Muff believes that nurses have not acted on their discontent, even when they see funds expended for costly hospital expansions, equipment, and "perks" for physicians, some nurses over several decades *have* fought for better salaries and working conditions, but usually have not been unified in their demands.

How, asks Muff, can nurses value others if they do not value themselves in a society that does not value women? Muff believes that the oppressed group behavior of nurses leads to self-hatred, but she does not seem to credit nurses with their constant struggle to improve their circumstances, or their survival despite their situations, or their care of the sick and dying, despite societal devaluation. Muff's charge against nurses has to be said, but so does the opposite. How much self-hatred is there in the accusations nurses hurl at each other in writing? Only out of self-affirmation can come power. Critical analyses that are devoid of loving, mutual regard based on an equally honest appraisal of strengths as well as weaknesses cannot suffice. While Muff places the ball in the women's court, one might ask why the perpetrators of sexism, the men who gain from female subservience, are not held to the same level of accountability required of women. Why must nurses be held almost solely responsible for change? At what point do the victimizers accept responsibility for their own biases, their own immoral or irresponsible behaviors? Still, Muff focuses on what *nurses* must do: first, recognize women's issues as their own, become aware of sex discrimination, create androgyny by valuing women's traits of compassion and caring while combining them with assertion, analytic ability, and independence, refuse to put down women or find humor in being demeaned, and identify sexism in women's health care; second, recognize their identity problems and define their boundaries; third, recognize dependence-independence issues in relation to paternalistic and maternalistic figures and accept the risks and trade-offs of assertiveness, using support groups, if necessary. Most important, Muff recommends that nurses recognize perceptual distortions that force them into modes of powerlessness and pessimism. She urges recognition of interpersonal difficulties, the development of business acumen, perceiving and acting on sexist propaganda and stereotypes, actively engaging in professional issues, and warns, "The time for passivity is over" (p. 218).

THEMES OF THE 1980S

Several themes from the 1980s were sustained from the 1970s and continue to influence nurses in the 1990s. Changing the public image of nurses requires gender reeducation, because female stereotypes continue to overwhelm nurses' reality. Mapanga and the Kalisches and McHugh extend Hughes' analysis to television and the film industry, finding stereotyped imagery that can only lead to low-level public perceptions. Indeed, the Kalisches' and McHugh's analysis attacks the nurse-as-sex-object in films, noting that sex stereotypes of nurses have increased, not decreased, over the past two decades. Muff extends the Kalisches' and McHugh's analysis by exploring the fantasies, myths, and stereotypes of the public's image of nurses, claiming that the origins of these stereotypes are far more extensive than mere media phenomena. Blancett critiques the pervasive use of sexist language in speaking and writing, while Webb deepens the analysis by examining the sexist structure of language itself. And Melosh finds sexist, demeaning imagery in fiction, but points to feminism as providing a framework for analysis that was previously missing. Salvage is in agreement with Melosh, while Hott deplores the sexist imagery of nurses in greeting and get-well cards, noting the hostile, subliminal messages that are fostered about nurses. Dains, too, attacks the sexist portrayal of nurses in critiquing *The Women in White* issue of *Playboy* in which nurses posed nude. These protests against the biased media representation of nurses escalated in the late 1980s. Turnbull, for example, reports on nurses' responses to their complete exclusion from the NBC television series on health issues. Recognizing the increasing importance of worldwide connectedness, Austin, Champion, and Tzeng focus on cross-cultural comparisons of images of nurses; their findings, not surprisingly, reveal that from a global perspective, nurses are perceived as "good" and "active," but certainly not powerful. From a more theoretical perspective, Kaler, Levy, and Schall question whether nursing's goal of increased power and autonomy will succeed, claiming that perceptions and images of nurses are processed by the public according to ingrained, gender-biased, stereotyped schemata, totally opposite to images of power and influence. Fagan and Diers indirectly support this claim by recognizing images of nurses as metaphors for mothering, class struggle, intimacy, and conscience.

A key aspect pertains to differing values inherent in the imagery and this finding continues a second ongoing trend extending from the 1970s, in the work, for example, of Smoyak, who calls for positive women's and humanitarian values; in Leininger's analysis that stresses humanist and feminist values, such as support, protection, and humaneness; and Vance's contrast between autonomy and compassion. Women's values are central to the development of Cassandra as a new nurses' structure, even involving an evolution of women's spirituality. Although a variation of the previous feminist NURSES NOW, this conscious attempt to create a woman's organizational process around the woman's metaphor, weaving, gives credence to Leininger's forecast that new organizational and social structures must emerge to facilitate women's changes.

In this regard, a heavier emphasis on social theory emerges in the 1980s. With Smoyak, the practical implications of feminist, women's liberationist, or androgynous theories are indicated, but are not analyzed. Speedy looks at feminism and the issue of professionalization, concluding that nursing will not be a true profession until it embraces feminist concepts and theories more completely. Leininger also calls for better explanatory bases, but brings in a new theme, the development of a transcultural worldview of women, a system of values heavily influenced by minority and third world women that requires a transcultural nursing knowledge. The international emphasis in the 1980s reflects the worldwide growth of feminism and the concomitant need for nursing to shift to a wider women's perspective, clearly recognized by Smoyak, Muff, and Vance, Talbott, McBride, and Mason, who all call for unity among women's groups as well as unity among nurses in order to strengthen the "uneasy alliance" between nursing and the women's movement. Parenthetically, one may remember Lavinia Dock's international concern for women of the war-torn countries affected by World War I. Similarly, Chinn urges unity among feminists and nurses, and focuses on the caring and support nurses need to give to each other and to all women.

The effects of feminism on nursing show through clearly in Smoyak's analysis of nursing leadership, the move to mentorship and mutual recognition, and in Leininger's prediction of more women in power positions— not through affirmative action, but through women's support groups. Muff contends that nurses continue to suffer from sexism and stereotyped socialization patterns, struggling with their identities, role confusions, and institutionalized powerlessness. That nurses who demand change continue to be seen as threats by men is attested to by Smoyak, Leininger, and Muff.

Role change continues as a theme in the 1980s, with Sandelowski, Salvage, Hott, and Dains rejecting the equation: woman equals exploitable. Nurses' selfless and caring values have led to protection of physicians and rejection of women's control of their own health. The rejection of traditional womanhood in nursing by feminists is also the refusal of powerlessness. The attack on physicians' power by nurses, extensively covered in two separate volumes by Roberts and Group (see Introduction), represents a major and continuing trend over the past two decades. Smoyak reflects on the collapse of the National Joint Practice Commission, but remains hopeful that women can work with equality with physicians. However, she calls for the redistribution of existing resources, a trend supported by Baumgart, who claims that men as the only rightful "knowers" can no longer continue to dominate. To her, feminism has helped nurses in professional development, in research, and in autonomy.

The impact of political conservatism is apparent in Allen's question of whether feminism should be rejected by nursing. Baumgart's affirmation of feminism is supported by Smoyak, who notes the relaxation of traditionalism at home and work, despite the backlash against women. To Vance, the "uneasy alliance" between nursing and feminism is resolved by affirming the importance of feminist influence in power, politics in nursing, and in adjusting economic inequities. Nursing's lack of power, political conservatism, and resistance to proactive determination is evident in McCarthy's critique of the National League for Nursing's refusal to change convention sites scheduled in non-ERA states. Membership reactions to the NLN's lack of social consciousness condemned the organization's lack of leadership and responsiveness to issues critical to women.

Indeed, such conservatism and uncertainty about one's own values and the values basic to women's culture lead one to conclude that nurses' learned helplessness, oppression, and powerlessness have not undergone radical change over the decades of this century. As Muff, Vance, and Smoyak particularly have recognized, unity of nurses among themselves and unity of nurses with other women's groups are imperative if nursing is to achieve its goal of power, autonomy, and independence in the next century.

Chapter 9

Where Will Nurses'
Militancy Lead?

Power and powerlessness, a constant motif of feminist theory and research for many years, became a familiar topic in the nursing literature during the 1980s. And efforts to explain power and politics to nurses to increase their political sophistication have continued in the 1990s. These efforts are designed to involve nurses in political analyses, policies, and actions—both inside and outside nursing. But, to many nurses, politics is perceived as a corrupting form of male behavior that often interferes with their legitimate interaction with patients. Frequently, writers point to nurses' political naivete about the process of authority, to the fear of questioning and controversy, which sustains the lack of nursing control over the welfare of patients. Similarly, tokenism, the selection of a few nursing leaders by non-nursing individuals or communities, sustains the negation of women's values.

Why do nurses, who have tremendous power in numbers, continue to believe in the myth of powerlessness? Do nurses fear power? Are nurses oppressed because they are women, or because they are professionally subordinated to medicine? Are they still so afraid of male medical and hospital authority? In a patriarchy, are these fears well-founded? Are strong, independent women reluctant to enter nursing, or, if in nursing, do they simply leave, refusing to accept subordination because they are unable to achieve social change in health-care systems and are unwilling to support the oppression of women as patients and professionals? What accounts for the professional disunity of nurses? Is it the result of medical interventions into the profession? Or of a distance between women leaders and the rank and file of nurses? Or of the relative powerlessness of a women's profession? Answers to these questions and whether nurses can achieve unity and power have been the concern of several nurse authors in very different analyses.

THE DYNAMICS OF OPPRESSION
UNDERLYING NURSING AND FEMALE LEADERSHIP

The subordination of women leaders and their followers creates very special analytic problems. No group is totally powerless, but Nancy Greenleaf (1982) recognizes that initial inequality between power holders and power seekers makes efforts to achieve power difficult. Dominant groups, such as physicians and hospital administrators, control resources and access to them—money, media attention, and public opinion. As examples, Greenleaf contrasts the differences between press coverage of medical and nursing news and of the unequal allocation of federal funds for medical and nursing research. More important, dominant groups not only define themselves, but situations and other groups as well. Subjugated groups may accept or reject such definitions; however, "when medicine is defined as encompassing all health care, any challenge to nursing to define its own uniqueness is a futile effort" (p. 91).

Essential to any theory of power is an understanding of the politics of self-esteem. Greenleaf postulates that enabling power involves energy and vigor in action, which can be directed positively or negatively. If self-esteem is high, more energy or enabling power is produced. If a woman (nurse) feels good about herself, and if she has skills, then her competence leads to confidence that enhances her self-esteem. When women (nurses) cannot see things clearly and work hard but get nowhere, *confusion constrains energy*. Taking risks means vulnerability and fear of failure stops risk taking, even when it produces self-respect. Thus, *fear consumes energy*. When women (nurses) are stopped from doing what they want or getting what they need, anger is experienced, but it often cannot be openly expressed. Thus, *oppression consumes energy*. Suppressed anger becomes rage, but when oppression is understood, women (nurses) find sources of energy of which they may have been unaware. Thus, "The rage becomes outrage and we will no longer acquiesce to the oppression" (p. 100). *Focused anger produces energy*. Greenleaf believes that as more women (nurses) are permanent wage earners, they are more likely to reject the female submissiveness basic to the hierarchical organization of the system. She states: "Increased awareness of past economic exploitation and oppression is leading to a sense of entitlement, a right to participate fully. Above all, nurses are understanding the politics of self-esteem" (p. 100).

From a different perspective, Susan Jo Roberts (1983; 1994) also looks at the implications of oppressed group behavior for nursing. She notes that analysts of nursing leadership have long believed that the dearth of strong feminist nursing leaders is because the profession lacks persons with initiative, high self-esteem, and assertiveness. Reversing this individual-centered explanation, Roberts claims that "the style of leadership within nursing has evolved because nurses, like other groups throughout history, are an oppressed group, which is controlled by societal forces that have determined its leadership behavior" (p. 21). She stresses that the dynamics underlying leadership must be understood in order to develop strategies that can produce more effective leaders.

In accord with critical theorists in nursing education, Roberts turns to Paulo Freire's theory, which asserts that dominant groups identify their own norms and values as correct and force them on those who look and act differently. In this process, the subordinate group is negatively valued and this valuation becomes internalized in both the dominator and oppressed groups; thus, the status quo is sustained through interior colonization. To escape low valuation, the oppressed may try to assimilate, becoming like the oppressor in order to achieve goals that cannot be attained by identification with the subordinated group. However, it is exceedingly difficult, if not impossible, to pass as a member of the dominant group if the biological distinctions are obvious (black skin, penis, breasts). Those who are successful in assimilating achieve a marginal position; unable to fully leave one group or enter the other, they are without clear cultural identity. Internalization and marginality produce low self-esteem, even self-hatred, since subordinates must reject their own characteristics because they are not valued by those in power. This sustains the cycle of subordination; lack of assertiveness in the face of injustice leads to loss of self-respect, which in turn reduces the likelihood of self-assertion.

Unable to express aggression openly, the oppressed will express submissiveness, albeit reluctantly. Furthermore, states Roberts, if authentic feelings cannot be expressed, horizontal violence among the oppressed may occur. This leads to further negative stereotyping (women are their own worst enemies, for example). The learned fear of aggression against the oppressor is the mechanism that sustains the status quo. Thus, battered women come to internalize their presumed inadequacies to the point that they feel it is impossible to escape their batterer. According to Roberts, the basis of the fear is very real; they and any other woman could be destroyed by men. Roberts points to a secondary fear—that of change itself. Without freedom, women cannot exist authentically, but authentic existence is feared because they feel inadequate to live it. Having little faith in their ability, revolt is rejected, even when, as in nursing, there are sufficient numbers to create a successful revolution.

The maintenance of oppression is based on the premise that the powerful have the best possible characteristics; usually more myth than reality, this idea is reinforced through education that supports the dominator's values. Rewards are given for behaviors that express these values, even if derogatory to one's own group. Leaders of oppressed groups share characteristics and beliefs similar to the dominant culture. In the past, they have been called Uncle Toms, Aunt Thomasinas, or Queen Bees. Tokenism involves appointment of oppressed group members to committees or public offices. In these positions, they may criticize their own kind and blunt their own feelings; and they are only allowed if they maintain their dependency on the dominant group. According to Roberts, controlling, coercive, and rigid behavior may emerge from low self-esteem, dislike of their own kind, and a desire to be like the oppressors.

Applying the oppressed group behavior model to nursing, Roberts claims the profession itself is oppressed in its lack of autonomy, accountability, and control. In agreement with Ehrenreich and English (1972), Roberts argues that nurses were once an autonomous group but became oppressed by societal forces in the past century. She recognizes that this is difficult to accept because of nurses' acculturation to the existing structure, but she agrees with Cleland (1971) who said that dominance is most complete when it is not even recognized. Obtaining the characteristics of professionals will not bring power and autonomy either since such traits are simply a description by the powerful of their own "correct" values. Furthermore, Roberts argues that the advice of Marlene Kramer (1974) to become bicultural is an admonishment to be marginal, to adjust as a worker to hospital culture after being socialized in a nursing education program to be a professional.

Oppression of nurses may produce self-hatred and dislike for other nurses; divisiveness and lack of cohesion; and low participation in professional organizations, which reflects a lack of pride and a desire to be disassociated from other oppressed and powerless persons. The horizontal violence in struggles between nurses is a safe way to express aggression, which is actually meant for the oppressor. According to this model, says Roberts, "Unity is doubtful . . . unless the group is willing to make a change in the power alignment with the dominant group" (p. 27).

Nurses have internalized the mechanistic medical model so much, Roberts claims, that they have been unable, until recently, to retain or even discuss their own cultural heritage in nursing. Lack of identity is clear in the confusion over definitions of what nursing is. Another characteristic of oppression, the submissive-aggressive syndrome, is also obvious: though nurses may complain about physicians to each other, they rarely complain directly to the physicians. Roberts rejects the usual criticism of nurses by nurses who write on this syndrome; instead, she sees this behavior as symptomatic of the oppressed situation in which women have been forced to be dependent and submissive in order to deal with domination by a powerful group of men.

What can nurses learn from other oppressed groups? Roberts stresses that nursing leaders must recognize oppression as arising from a culture that does not value women. Again, she does not see nurses' characteristics as individually created, but as culturally produced behaviors. She demands that nursing leaders demythologize, exposing the reality of dominate-subordinate relationships in the system. Furthermore, leaders must emerge from the grassroots through dialogue among nurses who will shift their priorities from the values of the dominator groups and select leaders who focus on unity among women. Finally, leaders must continue to rediscover the cultural heritage of nursing and, we might add, women. In this process, the rights of physicians and hospital administrators to control the health industry becomes highly questionable.

Roberts' thoughtful analysis provides needed emphasis to system-wide explanations and solutions. But it is not clear whether she sees nurses as just another oppressed occupational group or as a subgroup of women whose oppression is prototypic of all other forms of oppression. Her reliance on some male theorists (e.g., Freire), who barely acknowledge the gendered basis of oppression, raises some interpretive problems. Furthermore, the concept of oppression itself has been and continues to be debated among feminist theorists.

POLITICAL ACTION, VERTICAL AND HORIZONTAL CONFLICTS: THE SEARCH FOR NURSES' VALUES

Though the subject of power has become the focus of entire books, such as *Politics of Nursing* (Kalisch & Kalisch, 1982), they often lack a consistent and *systemic* analysis of the gender-stratified nature of power. In the Kalisches' book, for example, gender stratification is not consistently explicated. And even the book cover unintentionally provides an example of nonverbal subordination of a woman nurse; she stands with her head tilted upward, smiling at a male politician who stands several steps above her in front of a public building. From the 1970s on considerable research on the politics of nonverbal communication provides sufficient evidence that the book cover gives a message of powerlessness, contrary to the authors' intent.

Nevertheless, even without overt feminist consciousness, the primer is replete with examples of women contesting male power. The sections on political conflict and mobilization are particularly useful examples of recent efforts by nurses to increase their political sophistication, but in traditional terms and without a feminist perspective. Politics, for example, is defined traditionally by the Kalisches as the authoritative allocation of scarce resources by those who make binding decisions in a system that contains rules for implementation. The central assumptions of competition and scarcity are, of course, male-defined, lacking the feminist emphasis on cooperation or the socialist concern with equitable distribution. Furthermore, scarcity, beyond the most fundamental human requirements, is primarily determined by what men in power have valued. Values transformation, in Wilma Scott Heide's terms, is the essence of feminism; thus, the conception of scarcity and most other ideas about the political process must be subject to critical analysis. To educate nurses about masculist power systems is important, but it is also necessary to analyze patriarchal values so that women can decide what changes their participation in power may cause. For example, the assertion by the Kalisches that politics and science are different would not be acceptable to women's studies scholars, who have studied the manner in which science has been used to sustain sexist values and maintain the political subjugation of women.

Political conflict, according to the Kalisches, is caused by differing values, but what are women's or nurses' values in relation to power processes? This remains unclear in both vertical and horizontal conflicts. Physicians, hospital administrators, and health insurers—all in superordinate relation to nurses—may engage in vertical conflict with them. The Kalisches provide an example of vertical conflict from the May 22, 1980 issue of the *Houston Chronicle*, which describes nurse-physician conflict over what constitutes legal nursing in Texas. To them, the news article depicts an "elite" telling a "nonelite" what to do. But, it is more than this if one analyzes the conflict from a gender perspective.

Paraphrased, the newspaper article begins with a male physician telling female nurses he will not have them telling him what to do. The physician, W. A. Godfrey, goes on to state that government cannot legislate health care. This amazing assertion ignores the American Medical Association's historical efforts to influence legislation on health care. Representing the male-controlled judicial system, Attorney John Hill ruled that nurses could not administer medicines without physician supervision. The nurses rejected this ruling because it would jeopardize what they were already doing in public health clinics. In turn, the Texas Medical Association (male-dominated) rejected the interpretation of the Texas Nurses Association (female-dominated). The state senate subcommittee, another male-dominated political elite, considered the nurses' request for approval for specific activities of advanced nurse practitioners, but still under the supervisory protocols of physicians. Yet even this modified female subservience was unacceptable to the men. Godfrey told a male state senator that the women were telling physicians what to do.

In the first 10 paragraphs of the newspaper article, no woman is specifically mentioned or named. Eventually, in the final two sentences, Deanna Sebestyen, president of the Texas Nurses Association, defines the women's position, explaining that nurses (women) should know what to expect from the physicians (men) supervising them. By inserting gender into the news article, the gender-stratification system becomes obvious, particularly in the overt bias of the news report toward men's words. Equally obvious is the women's attempt to escape from men's control while maintaining a semblance of patriarchal authority. While the Kalisches do not discuss the gendered basis of power and political systems, it is obvious as one analyzes not only this particular reported conflict from their book but others as well.

Horizontal conflicts, too common among nurses, often leave little time to resolve successfully their vertical conflicts with men in power. The divide and conquer strategy is successful: women set against each other will expend their energy fighting each other, rather than challenging their male superordinates. As an example of horizontal conflict, the Kalisches refer to a news article in the *New York Herald Statesman*, which reports nurses fighting over the New York State Nurses Association's 1985 resolution, requiring bachelor's degrees for registered nurses and associate degrees for licensed practical nurses. Once again the gendered basis of the conflict is missing: physicians and hospital administrators watch nurses fight over a problem that the men initially helped create, manipulating for over a century the educational levels and categories of women caregivers. What the newspaper reports is an oppressed group fighting among themselves. What is ignored is the historical gendered grounds for the conflict.

The Kalisches also discuss the Wright State Nursing School disaster, reported in the May 22, 1980 issue of the *Dayton Journal Herald*. The "compromise" reached in the nursing school-medical school controversy was artificial. The medical faculty got what they wanted by swallowing up the nursing school and dictating educational requirements. They forced the nurses to be physicians' assistants, not independent health professionals. Clearly, the men forced the women into submission, but this aspect of gendered life is missing in the Kalisches' analysis. However, in the final paragraph of one section of their book, they do recognize the gender-stratification system: "Upon reflection it is clear how pervasive the sexist double standard has been and how a particular act, done by a nurse, still carries a very different meaning from the same act done by a physician" (p. 51).

Relying on conflict theorists, the Kalisches assume that the differential distribution of power, even to define and implement values, is the source of conflict and change. What happens, however, when power itself is differentially construed by women, who may learn as mothers that masculist dominance and child rearing are incompatible, and men, who learn that actual or symbolic muscle flexing is legitimate? If the quantity of power is the male issue, is the quality of power the women's issue? The California newspaper, *Press-Enterprise* (June 29, 1980), recounts the actions of nurses to contest male power in "male" terms by striking over salaries and pension benefits; refusing to assist in late-term abortions; and carrying signs and distributing leaflets during a labor dispute. According to the reporter, nurses linked their increased activism to a number of things: the women's movement, increased levels of education, the teaching of independence in nursing schools, specialized units for intensive care and the ethical questions they pose. One nurse stated it succinctly: " 'Women know their own worth more than they did 25 years ago' " (p. 444).

A fundamental value of feminism is consciousness-raising of women as a group, and the Kalisches claim that the sense of shared deprivation and discrimination by nurses as women is strongly associated with political action. But so is a sense of shared pride. For example, in Colorado, 1,000 nurses marched to the capitol building to protest a bill; half the nursing staff at one hospital stayed home to protest inadequate staffing and scheduling problems; 100 nurses at another hospital marched to protest the firing of one male nurse; at another hospital 718 nurses withheld services over grievances; nurses picketed a Catholic hospital over scheduling problems; and union petitions were filed at five Denver area hospitals. All of these actions by women unified by grievances led one Denver reporter to ask: "Where will nurses' militancy lead?" (p. 445).

Interestingly, these examples of assertive actions by women in nursing lead the Kalisches to refer to the Black civil rights movement, not the women's movement, as an example of successful group consciousness. Yet the belief that women have the ability to change the status quo is directly related to the refusal by some nurses to be stereotypically weak and dependent and to take strong action. Thus, while some nurses focused on change internal to health-care institutions, others worked on political actions external to hospitals and agencies.

As noted in Chapter 2, some nurses (e.g., Wilma Scott Heide) were early participants in women's organizations, such as the National Organization for Women. Susan W. Talbott and Connie N. Vance (1981) describe the processes they used to become involved in a feminist leadership conference: "When the National Organization of Women's (NOW) Legal Defense and Education Fund held its national convocation on 'New Leadership in the Public Interest' in late 1980, nurses were neither involved nor invited. Yet, six months later, when the second part of the convocation met in New York, not only were nurses invited to attend, but one nursing leader was asked to be a workshop panelist" (p. 592). The authors note that some women in NOW were not aware that many of the foremost concerns of the organization, such as sexism in equal pay and in educational and job discrimination, were also nursing issues. Talbott and Vance claim that nurses had to educate the feminists about nursing's connection to the women's movement and they used the political process to ensure nurses' participation in the conference. "We learned that such political endeavors are powerful ways of increasing nursing's visibility and creating new coalitions" (p. 595). While the actions of Talbott and Vance are commendable, they did not acknowledge previous efforts by nurses in NOW, dating from the early 1970s.

Group solidarity or cohesion derives from unity. Common commitment to goals and leadership are needed to achieve a critical mass of power. How can this be achieved when feminism is not credited by analysts for influencing nurses? How does support for feminism occur if the media has mislabeled it as "man-hating" or "lesbianism"? How do nurses assert themselves without the underlying value system of feminism that legitimatizes assertion for all women? Proselytizing is necessary, but how will that work in the absence of group consciousness of nurses as women? As the Kalisches note, "Masses of apathetic and unmotivated nurses . . . reduce the potential for political mobilization" (Kalisch & Kalisch, 1982, p. 450). Certainly, intensity, single-minded awareness, and capacity for risk taking all require commitment. The financial resources of the have nots, the women's groups, can be offset by mass membership and skillful manipulation for maximum advantage. Only if the group is well organized, however, with a clear ideology and a goal for which people will sacrifice, will the superior numbers in nursing provide the base for power. How this will be accomplished by women who accept their subordination remains uncertain. If recent and basically sound books on politics for nurses do not provide them with an analysis of their status as women, the effects on female and nursing power are also less than certain.

GRASSROOTS POLITICAL INVOLVEMENT:
A NEW MODEL OF NURSE ACTIVISM?

Lack of cohesion and unity among nurses can have negative consequences for those nurses who are willing to commit themselves to political activism. Nurse Theresa Chalich and her campaign manager Lorraine Smith discuss Chalich's candidacy for the Pennsylvania General Assembly. Running as a nurse on a health-care rights platform, she lost but successfully raised issues of nursing care and health-care reform. However, "Despite Chalich's excellent visibility in the campaign, Smith and other volunteers were surprised that few nurses were willing to be actively involved in her pursuit for office. Questions such as 'Don't nurses care about these issues?' and 'Don't nurses see the nursing profession will be more respected if we become more connected to politics?' were raised" (Chalich & Smith, 1992, p. 242).

Chalich and Smith ask why nurses, the most qualified group to articulate national health-care problems, are not more influential in legislative and policy-making positions. Representing one million registered voters, why do nurses not use their voting power to elect nurses to office? If nurses are responsible and compassionate providers of primary care, why do they not act to deal with the national health-care problems? Is it because of insecurity of the profession in which care is undervalued, not easily measured in quantitative terms? Or is it that caring itself does not mesh with a competitive work ethic? Trying to battle low wages and long hours, while being told their work ranks low in economic value, are nurses too insecure or is their educational preparation too task-oriented and linear in thought processes to produce risk-takers who are supported by nurse leaders? To Chalich and Smith, even a secure nurse finds that many leadership skills are not rewarded and only her commitment to caring keeps her in the profession. In a discriminatory health-care system, nurses may fight other nurses or other health-care providers, rather than uniting to reform the system. On the other hand, nurses may withdraw, but take on community, social, and environmental problems instead.

Perhaps, say Chalich and Smith, the emphasis on political involvement overlooks nurse activism in grassroots activities rather than in the more formal two-party system. For example, in their own area, one nurse was a national leader in exposing the risks of lawn pesticides. Another nurse was working long hours to fight the construction of a hazardous waste incinerator. Still another nurse had received national recognition for her efforts in the PTA to reduce pesticides in local schools. Another organized her urban community to get rid of drug dealers and prostitutes on the streets. Chalich herself had organized senior citizens on health-care issues. The work of these nurses and others was at the forefront of grassroots movements that resulted in national lobbying organizations that now vie to get their support for legislative changes, and that nurses, in turn, use to build their causes. They do not align themselves with only one group and this maximizes their influence and prevents their being taken for granted.

Given this evidence of activism, perhaps a different model of nurses and social change is needed. Chalich and Smith propose a ladder model of increasing political sophistication for nurses: at rung 1, *civic involvement* is recommended (for example, working in the PTA, children's activities, and neighborhood groups); rung 2 involves *advocacy* in letter writing to public officials and newspapers, and organized visits to officials on local issues; at rung 3, *organizing* on local issues and networking with other citizens' groups are suggested; and rung 4 focuses on *long-term wielding of power* in campaigning, local government planning, and setting agendas. Only at the fourth level would partisan politics appear; and, perhaps, under traditional analyses of political involvement, nurses' activities at the other three levels might be discounted. Nevertheless, involvement in levels 1 through 3 afford opportunities at the grassroots level that could lead nurses to greater political influence later on.

NETWORKING: A CASE OF COVERT EMOTIONAL NEPOTISM?

Nurses' increasing political sophistication has led some analysts to wonder if nurses, hoping to win acceptance and integration, would simultaneously incorporate some of the weaker organizational practices of the political system. Evelyn R. Barritt (1984), for example, fears that the old boys' network, overtly elitist, might be copied by nurses in an old girls' network, based on "covert emotional nepotism." She claims that women do not want leaders who make decisions on needs, resources, and professional standards, but "rather look to their leaders for nurture and support . . . not for *professional* growth, but for personal, emotional support" (p. 803). This often leads to infighting, says Barritt, which is useful to those outside nursing: without a unified power structure, nursing cannot threaten the patriarchal status quo.

Networking among nurses, however, need not be seen as a negative carbon copy of elitist old boy networks. Kathleen A. Christy (1987) values networking as a technique for sharing information and knowledge; for contacting mentors, role models, and kindred spirits; and for creating channels to solve common problems and enhance professional collegiality. To her, networks emerge when formal hierarchies fail to produce results.

Certainly, alienation and loneliness have forced women to create their own networks, which provide support to counteract sex-role stereotypes about career and family demands and intellectual or emotional unsuitability for "male" jobs. Christy delineates four types of networks: first, business connections that cut across organizational and management levels; second, social linkages through affinity, trust, and obligation; third, support relations for physical, mental, or emotional problems; and fourth, professional interconnections for common goals and interests. Regardless of type, Christy stresses that the woman leader has a responsibility to herself and the network to keep contacts circulating, to foster connections, to form a social community of belonging, and to sustain freedom to interact openly. Although nurses have been networking for years through the American Nurses Association (ANA) and other organizations, Christy notes that the newsletter, *Networking*, is now available and perhaps more nurses would become aware of the advantages networking could offer their personal careers as well as nursing as an influence in community life.

GENDER RESOCIALIZATION, ASSERTIVENESS, AND RISK

Acknowledging that individual, group, and institutional changes are needed to overcome centuries-old patriarchal attitudes and structures, some nurses throughout the 1980s and into the 1990s urged that special efforts be made to reeducate nurses to be assertive. Janet Milauskas (1985), for example, cites Vance's (1979) survey of 71 leaders in nursing who were asked to list the disadvantages of belonging to a predominantly female profession. They responded most frequently with four answers: gender stereotyping; discrimination in income, status, and education; self-image problems (low self-esteem and self-confidence, insecurity, passivity, nonassertiveness); and isolation from the male perspective.

Milauskas recognizes that patriarchal culture inevitably suggests some type of female submissiveness, with less acceptance of strong, assertive, powerful women. She reviewed 86 articles since 1975 on nursing and assertiveness, usually conceptualized as a way to deal with the burnout common in "women's work" and in nursing, the epitome of female stereotypes. Even clinicians, as in the feminist, classical study by Broverman, Broverman, Clarkson, Rosenkrantz, and Vogel (1970), were more likely to describe the healthy woman as more submissive, less independent, less adventurous, more easily influenced, less aggressive and competitive, more excitable in minor crises, more emotional, and less objective than a healthy man. This peculiar version of "health" is, according to the authors, similar to the burnout-prone individual—weak, unassertive, submissive, anxious, fearful of involvement—who is unable to exert control over a situation, passively yielding and becoming emotionally burdened and exhausted from constant adaptation and acquiescence.

To escape from the unhealthy implications of sexism, Milauskas advocates assertiveness training for women in nursing; they must learn to stand up for their rights, to communicate, verbally and nonverbally, honest, direct and appropriate expressions of feelings, beliefs, and opinions. As nurses are urged to become change agents, patient advocates, and political activists, Milauskas very correctly asks, "How well can nurses function in these roles as well as in expanded roles . . . if the majority of them are socialized to be passive and submissive?" (p. 5). That nurses have tried to get rid of passivity through assertiveness training is apparent in reviewing the literature: one to four articles each year in the mid-1970s, a peak of 22 in 1979, and about 10 each year in the 1980s. Most of these have been how-to-do-it articles on assertiveness training or how-it-can-help-nursing statements. For example, a series of articles by Gloria Donnelly presented a nurses' assertiveness workshop, which was published in *RN* magazine and a two-part programmed instruction that appeared in the *American Journal of Nursing*.

What research had nurse scholars conducted on assertiveness training? Milauskas could find only seven studies, five of these on nurses teaching patients assertiveness. There was only one study of nurses themselves; in San Francisco and Houston, nurses were compared and the results showed that higher assertiveness was related to collegiate education, political activism, and collective bargaining. In another study on the control of hospital-induced infections, nurses' assertive practices were found to be the best predictor of high-quality patient-care practices.

What are the risks of being assertive? Several nurses have reported the risks are relatively high. Those who refuse unreasonable requests are seen as effective, but less polite or kind and more hostile. Assertive women are more negatively evaluated than men; thus, the support of other women is critical. The risk that physicians will report assertive nurses is recognized and requires courage. And how will nurses retain compassion? Milauskas advocates assertiveness *plus* empathy, an interesting androgynous suggestion.

What has been done in a methodical way to increase assertiveness by *organized* nursing? Evidently very little. Milauskas recommends national conferences on assertiveness; required assertiveness training for students in degree programs to offset double sex-stereotyped socialization; a coast-to-coast series of workshops, initially for nursing leaders; conflict-resolution and bargaining workshops that incorporate assertiveness; nursing research on gender and assertiveness; and a national newsletter and columns on assertive nurses in journals.

SOLIDARITY AND MENTORING:
ONE MORE FAD FOR NURSES TO LATCH ONTO?

If assertiveness training has been so unsystematically used in nursing, can older nurses successfully mentor younger nurses and thus provide a different model of women's power and leadership? By the latter 1980s continued questioning of female solidarity was apparent in the reappraisal of mentoring as an expression of leadership. Bonnie Hagerty (1986), for example, takes a "second look" at mentoring, reviewing the major theories, and concludes that authors are describing different phenomenon or, minimally, different facets of a broader theory. There is no agreed-upon definition of the concept of mentoring, no construct validity, and much confusion over persons, processes, and purposes. The cause-effect relation between mentoring and career success is not established. The assumption that everyone should "succeed" by moving upward in the hierarchy also negates development *within* a role. The further assumption that mentoring is the same across organizations, professions, and work settings is impossible to sustain in nursing, which is tightly controlled with work clearly delineated. And to also assume that the absence of mentoring prevents women from advancing in their careers overlooks the fact that a stratification system cannot be simply overcome by dyadic mentoring. Research by Fagan and Fagan (1983) and Vance (1979) refute the claim that nurses do no mentoring, showing 84% rates, higher than those found in business, teaching, and police work. If mentoring moves women upward, why is it that so few nurses have moved into the top echelons of power?

In apparent agreement with Barritt (1984), Hagerty asks what exclusive, nondemocratic, personality-based, intense, and emotional mentoring dyads are going to produce. "Is nursing indeed promoting an old girl network based on personality rather than expertise, the very male-oriented style we condemn?" (p. 19). To her, parent-child, intensely emotional bonds promote the perception of the emotionally insecure female. It is more helpful to ask, What is it about a stimulating, adult-to-adult relationship that promotes learning and leads to career achievement? According to Spengler's (1982) research, independent self-starters do not have mentors. Hagerty postulates that perhaps nurse mentors actually *promote* avoidance of risks and dependency and fears that mentoring is just another fad for nursing to latch onto. She does not analyze the effects of female solidarity on change, but calls for reform of broad societal problems. Based on the shift from feminism in the 1920s to social action for others in the 1930s, it is clear that women lost heavily when they did not focus on their own issues. Similarly, women in nursing are not likely to change the status quo if their own powerlessness is not changed first. But can it be changed by mentoring?

ADAPTING, RATHER THAN ADOPTING, MALE NORMS OF MENTORING

Nancy Campbell-Heider (1986) specifically examines the influence of gender socialization on mentoring, a process presumably adapted from male culture and experience. She claims that nurses have developed a variety of sponsorship activities that have proven to be more useful to a practice-oriented profession than are traditional mentoring relationships. But despite research suggesting widespread female mentoring, Campbell-Heider claims that female mentors are underutilized and few women are in the high-level positions in which power can be exerted on behalf of trainees.

Campbell-Heider differentiates male and female mentoring, claiming that men in their 20s and 30s are facilitated by male career models, who help them through developmental transitions. After 40, men actively mentor, using age differentials to negate competition with younger men, sharing information by crossing some generational barriers, and, thus, assuring support from the younger men. On the other hand, the male model poses problems for female protégés and their male mentors. Mentor-protégé relations involve power-dependency interactions, and since females are already culturally accorded less social status, reinforcement of stereotypes can occur in which "women give up their own female normative and belief systems to fit into the male work domain. In such situations female protégés risk being alienated from other women" (p. 111). In the absence of women in powerful positions, women may have to seek out men, incorporating their values and norms. For example, research on women administrators by Hennig and Jardim (1976) confirms that "all of the upper-level managers had had male mentors . . . [however] relationships were frequently overshadowed by paternalistic and sexual themes" (cited in Campbell-Heider, 1986, p. 111). Caught in an atmosphere of sexual ambiguity, the women tried to resolve the dilemma by either refusing sexual innuendos, and consequently facing accusations of "unfemininity," or by accepting sexual relations with their male mentors, and subsequently being perceived as sex-objects. Females are socialized to expect support, to separate career and personal goals, to see risk as negative, to emphasize current, not future performance. All these give rise to a perception that does not fit the male orientation to work.

Given these complexities, should nurses apply traditional male models to nursing? Campbell-Heider thinks not and claims that the variety of sponsorship activities that nurses have developed reflects the unique needs of women and the realities of clinical practice. In clinical situations, apprenticeship learning and mentoring continue to create a transitional system in which professional values are internalized and integrated. In hospital settings where nurses have been exploited and their autonomy blocked, career guides, who can explain the oppressive hospital systems, can assist nurses to take appropriate risks and develop means to strengthen professional identities.

Women aspiring to administrative or academic positions need mentoring that on the surface appears more like the male model, but even here there are differences: nurses have more multiple mentors, many of these outside of nursing; more have female mentors and more of these are work supervisors. There is less organizational separation between female mentors and protégés than between men, but many similarities in the processes of advising, guiding, promoting, role-modeling, stimulating intellect, and inspiring. Admitting a definitional quagmire, Campbell-Heider supports Hagerty's concern that women's mentorship may reflect different dimensions of a broader theory. However, she sees the changes as indicating that "Nurses, like professional women in other settings, now seem much more willing to adapt rather than adopt male norms on a variety of work and social issues" (p. 113).

GENDERED VERBAL AND NONVERBAL COMMUNICATION: IMPLICATIONS FOR NURSES' LEADERSHIP

Gender-based differences in networking and mentoring styles extend to communication patterns as well. By the early 1990s communication differences by gender had been well-researched, and a review of the literature on this issue led Joellen B. Edwards and Cynthia L. Lenz (1990) to recommend different interaction strategies, particularly for female nurse leaders. Attempting to provide a general overview, Edwards and Lenz reviewed 35 sources, but none of these specifically on research from nursing journals. It is astonishing that a profession so involved in intimate touch and physical contact would be so tardy in applying, let alone creating, the extensive literature on gender and verbal and nonverbal communication and on the politics of touch, the unspoken language of the power dimensions between the sexes.

What did the social science literature suggest that might be useful to nurses? In interaction, men talk more, faster, and longer than women, and interrupt more frequently. Women use language differently, expressing themselves with more adjectives and adverbs that connote triviality and expletives less powerful, at least by male standards. Qualifying their communication and using intensifiers and tag questions, women may be seen as less powerful, but men, when using these forms, are simply seen as more polite. Compared to men, women are often more attentive, perceptive, personally involved, and person-centered in their conversations. They are also more likely to share personal information, to be involved in self-disclosure, and to be concerned about the characteristics of the person with whom they are speaking.

Given such gendered differences, what is the impact on women leaders? Leadership involves communication to attain goals and is often focused on tasks and relationships, a mix of these two elements being necessary to the effective exercise of power. To Edwards and Lenz, research on group interactions has indicated that despite societal endorsement of both sexes in leadership positions, the socially acceptable communicative behaviors still constrain women's implementation of leadership roles, even though numerous studies have found no differences in leadership ability, time taken to reach decisions, or group productivity levels between groups led by women and groups led by men. Indeed, female leaders were frequently found to be more open-minded, more likely to emphasize group harmony, to lead without being unfriendly to group members, and to be more person-oriented in their enactment of the leadership role. Edwards and Lenz note: "The problem is not leadership ability, but the pervasive subtle perception that women are not leaders. A leader has no power unless both subordinates and superiors recognize it" (p. 51).

Several studies indicate that people continue to refuse to recognize female leaders. For example, when viewing slides of professional people seated around a rectangular table, women were seen as leaders when seated at the head of the table *only* in all-female groups, but not in all-male or even mixed-gender groups. Such deeply rooted biases are evident in a study of hiring practices of chairpersons of university psychology departments, who rated identical descriptive paragraphs of eight PhDs, four with male and four with female names, and consistently ranked the women as less desirable and lower than their male counterparts. In the business world, when insurance midlevel managers in 1973 described characteristics of men, women, and leaders in general, the male and general leader characteristics matched, but the women's did not.

On the other hand, in a 1979 study women with warm and person-oriented leadership styles had the most satisfied followers. And, in a 1980 study, using *both* warmth and task-orientation, women leaders produced the best ratings, "although males argued significantly more with female leaders" (p. 52). With the right strategies, women leaders can be accepted and highly rated. Edwards and Lenz recommend that nurse leaders develop strategies that not only focus on the task and relations, but on the image conveyed. Are unintentional messages of submissiveness or inferiority being conveyed through body language or voice tone? Head position, eye contact, and other nonverbal cues must be consistent with verbal messages. Indeed, the former are more powerful than the latter.

To avoid the male tendency to interrupt, a woman leader should resist interruptions and refuse to relinquish the floor to another speaker until she completes her statements. Leaders need to take control of the content, pace, and process of interchange. Do nurse leaders meet on their own turf or in a neutral area? Do they arrange seating to their own advantage? Do they try to add new responses that replace stereotypically feminine or low-power interchanges? Do they invest in junior leaders? Do they identify successful leaders and analyze their communication patterns? Do they maximize their effectiveness by using both the "feminine" qualities of warmth and person-orientation and "masculine" qualities of task-orientation and competence? Do they ensure that others perceive and recognize their achievements? These cannot be left to chance. Gender socialization promotes neglect of female achievement; therefore, nurses' accomplishments are often unrecognized because of the profession's association with "femaleness." Edwards and Lenz conclude that nurse leaders should use gender-related tendencies when they help, but replace these patterns when they hinder communication, confronting conflict head on if necessary.

IT IS THE SYSTEM, NOT JUST THE INDIVIDUAL, WHICH NEEDS CHANGING

Although individual and interpersonal solutions to gender-based problems of power and leadership are emphasized to a much greater extent than are organizational and institutional approaches, some writers have focused on gender-typed structural variables and offered various theoretical models as solutions to gendered inequalities. For example, Janelle C. Krueger (1980) is concerned with incorporating women into power positions in *preexisting* patriarchal structures. She asks, What are the barriers to women in top management? Male sponsorship systems, female attitudes toward work, and the values assigned to women's work continue to halt women's movement upward. The critical factor, however, is understanding the rules for corporate politics that govern the goal of money and power. The men's game involves conforming to rules, knowing and playing your position on the team, not fighting with other players, not talking back to the coach, taking defeat in stride, accepting the fact that everyone makes mistakes, realizing that competition is the reward. In short, the competitive team model from sports, such as football, largely unfamiliar to women as participants, depends on paternalistic sponsorship.

Krueger believes that some women do role model successfully; women mentoring other women, infiltration of women apprentices, and "old girls" networks—all these suggest increased potential for upward mobility. However, women still have to be more knowledgeable; they often get sidetracked from the prestigious line positions and fail to obtain management experience; they engage in unpaid management in social organizations, experience that will not count; all these continue their subordination. In addition, the unequal and illogical assignment of value of work, especially with regard to salary and status, creates a lower limit for women in the hierarchy. For example, job ratings in the federal government's *Dictionary of Occupational Titles* illustrate that jobs derived from homemaking and mothering, including nursing, still do not count for much.

Krueger believes that few nurses are prepared to assume high-level, policy-making positions. In agreement with feminist sociologist R. M. Kanter (1979),

Krueger claims that the many one- to three-day workshops for women are really panaceas that "reinforce the idea that women need to remedy something within themselves in order to compete with men. Usually, it is the system rather than the person that needs changing" (p. 377). In this, Krueger shifts to a systemic analysis, using Kanter's structural determinants of opportunity, power, and relative numbers. Types of opportunity include promotion rates, organizational ladders, and access to rewards. Power is defined by formal job characteristics and individual informal alliances. Relative numbers refers to the proportion of gender and ethnic groups in similar work positions.

What can women do to affect these aspects of systemic discrimination? Work-planning and review meetings can be used to identify job competencies; redesign dead-end jobs; balance numbers by gender and race; and create autonomous work groups. Access to the formal power structure can be facilitated by flattening the hierarchy and distributing decision-making powers. Informal power can be increased by opening information and communication channels and fostering joint participation in training programs. Women's support networks can help, but becoming the female equivalent of the "old boys" is rejected by Krueger, who agrees with Sargent's (1979) advocacy of androgynous leaders. Interestingly, Krueger finds that, with one exception, all the authored citations in her article represent the studies or ideas of feminist women. Are they, she asks, the *only* ones looking into the situation?

HEALTH CARE—A THOROUGHLY POLITICAL BUSINESS

One can now answer "No" to Krueger's question. Throughout the 1980s, an increasing number of nurses were interested in the structural aspect of power and nursing's role in politics. Jenniece Larsen (1982), for example, claims a growing interest among Canadian nurses to influence government decisions and institutional policies that affected them, often without their participation. Larsen uses a single definition of power: the ability to get and use whatever resources are needed to achieve nursing goals. While political power is influence on government at all levels and organizational power involves decision making in health-care institutions and is needed by nurses to influence work conditions, personal power is essential to acquire and use power in any context. The personal is political (the basic axiom of feminism) and the transformation of values (an essential tenet of the women's movement) are both incorporated into Larsen's thought.

Political resources must be seen as valuable to others, and Larsen claims that the most valuable resource in health care is nursing; nurses keep the system running. Even though some nurses still believe that nursing and health care are not related to politics, Larsen claims that health care is a thoroughly political business, and urges nursing pressure groups to influence public policy making.

Organizational behavior of women is supposedly marked by lower career aspirations, less personal investment in work, and more passive work styles. But Larsen notes that these assertions are not supported by research, which indicates that apparent gender differences are actually influenced by structural conditions, particularly the organizational hierarchy and the opportunity and power structures. Larsen clearly understands the gender-stratification system as an inherent part of the health system. Health organizations, particularly those employing large numbers of women, provide few structural opportunities for women to become influential practitioners of nursing. With limited opportunities for growth, nurses may suppress their ambition. All that is necessary to keep nursing powerless is to retain the current opportunity structure.

The structural variable of power also works against women, who are assumed to make ineffective leaders. The capacity to mobilize resources, to make things happen, is the characteristic of effective leaders; but how much power do nurse managers really have? Assigning formal authority to a person does not ensure access to power. It is hard to make things happen when the nurse administrator's influence at top decision-making levels is blocked because she has no informal connections with sponsors. Lacking resources, she may rely on conformity to procedures; lacking mobility, she may block the deviant, the educated, or the innovative nurse. To overcome these problems, Larsen stresses that nurses themselves must design and monitor structural changes in health-care institutions.

Recognizing that organizational strategies for empowering nurse leaders and staff are sorely needed, Gail Wiscarz Stuart (1986) uses a theory of strategic contingencies to provide another political perspective on how nurses could unite within organizations and challenge existing power structures. While she does not interconnect gender theory, such as oppressed group behavior, as detailed by Roberts (1983; 1994), her article does focus on empowerment of women. Stuart stresses, first, the need to decide professional issues in relation to the corporate structures in which most nurses work; and, second, to develop ways to negotiate power on professional issues within these organizations. She notes that there has been little research on how nurses can negotiate to attain power; the nursing literature either focuses on vertical, interpersonal power, describing ways to maximize individual influence, or recommends changes in the profession in relation to education, national organizations, knowledge, or socialization. Research is needed that emphasizes structural sources of power, rather than personal psychological attributes.

Strategic-contingencies theory (Hickson, Hinings, Lee, Schneck, & Pennings, 1971) postulates that the power of a subunit is determined by its centrality or degree of interdependence with other subunits; substitutability or degree of replacement by others; and the capacity to develop mechanisms to deal with unpredictable happenings or critical problems and uncertainties, arising either internally or externally. Such organizational strategies require nurses to identify, trust, and pledge loyalty to other nurses. Though unity is essential, Stuart claims that nursing is too often fractured by internal alienation and conflict between roles and units. Nevertheless, Stuart recommends that nurses use four principles of subunit action: first, increase interconnections to establish a higher level of organizational pervasiveness; second, establish irreplaceability by controlling who does nursing, refusing to assume non-nursing functions, and controlling the numbers of nursing graduates; third, demonstrate nursing assets by shifting others' perceptions of nurses as revenue producers and taking over areas of future uncertainty—for example, in areas related to technological changes and population shifts; and fourth, participate in high-level decision making by demanding representation and voting privileges in powerful institutional bodies.

By varying emphasis on these principles, different strategies would be used for different subunits, but all the varied paths should lead to organizational empowerment. Though Stuart's theoretical approach provides a shift from individual to group tactics, she does not analyze gender barriers to these strategies. Given the gender stratification of power in health-care institutions, how would men in power treat women who insist on their centrality as nurses? Would women leaders and even staff nurses who initiate change simply be fired? Women's contingencies must be built into any model for change: The same tactics used by women and men may produce different results.

REVIEWING THE RESEARCH ON WOMEN ADMINISTRATORS: A DISMALLY SMALL NUMBER AT THE TOP!

Given the gender-related problems women must deal with as leaders in patriarchal organizations, how effective have they been in moving into top leadership positions? How many female leaders are able to influence women's environment and enhance nurses' sharing and unity? Mary Wakefield-Fisher (1983) reports that despite increasing numbers of women in higher education and in work outside the home, "a dismally small percentage of administrative positions in industry and education are occupied by women" (p. 3). Reviewing the literature to obtain reasons for these disparities, she found that research on women administrators was fragmented and incomplete. Before the reemergence of feminism and prior to the 1970s, there were infrequent references to females in management leadership. Studies during the 1970s were often based on opinion and sometimes derived from research on men. Specific studies of women were usually conducted in private business settings and in traditionally male-dominated professions. Furthermore, the number of studies that focused on women administrators was insignificant, compared to those on male administrators. Thus, factors affecting women have been neglected and generalizations on women are difficult to make from male samples.

How the women's movement has affected women's support of female leaders is not analyzed by Wakefield-Fisher. Instead, she emphasizes the particularly debilitating effects of discrimination on female-dominated disciplines. For example, women are still socialized to believe that men are more capable leaders. Because of exclusion from power, women may lack role models. They also experience insufficient encouragement, and receive prejudicial evaluations and pay discrepancies. These experiences produce self-doubt or, in Greenleaf's terms, lowered self-esteem.

According to Wakefield-Fisher, differential motivations may characterize nursing administrators. Relying on 1960s research on achievement or affiliative needs, she notes that women were more likely to be motivated by the latter, which may interfere with making decisions in the best interest of organizations as opposed to specific individuals or groups. Successful male managers had high need for achievement, but a low need for affiliation. Instead of seeing something problematic with such male needs, Wakefield-Fisher suggests that women leaders may need to become more like men. But research on women "bosses" in business and academia has shown that they are twice as accessible to their subordinates and more likely to encourage their staffs to seek them out than male "bosses" (Josefowitz, 1982). Wakefield-Fisher does not acknowledge that women, as mothers and wives, are supposed to be constantly available; if these behaviors are transferred to work, a systemic transposition of family dynamics may occur. On the other hand, women's availability and openness as leaders may be a better model; the male model of control and dominance may be, as Sargent (1979) noted, an improper mode of authority in the future. Furthermore, high levels of male achievement motivation, for example, in the early work of David McClelland (1953), reflected the systematic exclusion of females from the research because women did not behave as hypothesized. Whether achievement motivation is even cross-culturally generalizable to non-Western males is questionable since the achievement pattern was not consistently evident.

Wakefield-Fisher claims that the need to avoid failure is presumably higher in females, but she does not discuss the varied findings in the complex research on fear of failure and fear of success. Thus, she finds it difficult to reconcile these presumed fears with women's actual higher levels of achievement, for example, in their high-school records or in the 1970s research finding that women executives had higher needs for achievement or power. Nevertheless, Wakefield-Fisher remains concerned that nursing administrators may be more motivated by a desire to work with people and less by needs for power, authority, and influence. She seems to advocate a better balance of motivations; however, her thinking remains partially within the male-defined model of leadership and her emphasis is on female behavioral change.

RESEARCH ON POLITICAL BEHAVIORS
OF NURSE ADMINISTRATORS

Until recently, there has been little research on nurses' involvement in political processes and few nursing programs have helped nurses prepare for political action. In 1981, however, Sarah Ellen Archer and Patricia A. Goehner provided data from nursing administrators on the types of their political participation; their perceptions and reasons for nurses' failure to be politically active; the resources and organizations that facilitate nurses' political preparation; the successful and unsuccessful political strategies used by nurse leaders; and the ways they help staff, faculty, and students be more politically active.

Archer and Goehner sent questionnaires to 1,086 nurse administrators in a wide variety of settings, receiving responses from 98% of the female directors in hospitals and agencies. Of these, only 9% had less than a BS degree; 58% held master's degrees; and 11% had doctorates. The researchers found that 93% of the nurse administrators voted regularly and 83% wrote to legislators. Fewer were involved on national boards and commissions, although many held posts at the state or local level. Not many indicated active party involvement. There was almost unanimous agreement (94%) that nurses were not as politically active as they should be. This was attributed to lack of preparation (28%), apathy (24%), and failure to realize the importance of such activity (22%).

Few leaders engaged in active protests or took actions beyond the usual letter writing and lobbying of officials. Their resources were the media and community organizations, but the organizations they relied on were mostly state and national nursing groups; thus, the potential for interconnecting with women's groups or other associations dedicated to change seemed less likely. However, since Archer and Goehner did not focus on gender, nursing leaders' actual efforts to interconnect with other women's political and pressure groups are unclear. It appeared that the administrators were less influenced by national nursing and health organizations; schools of nursing also provided little political assistance. However, consumer coalition building was one of the most frequently cited successful strategies; thus, although specific organizations were not named, some nurse leaders had moved toward networking for broader-based, grassroots political support. As noted earlier, this phenomenon was also acknowledged by Chalich and Smith (1992).

Archer and Goehner stressed that many of the successful political actions taken by the nurse leaders required considerable preparation and coalition building. In addition, the administrators also developed long-term relations with legislators and policy makers and spent considerable time educating nurses and getting them involved in political action. The nurse leaders reported that they continued to advocate against passive dependence on others to look after nurses' own interests. Nevertheless, a number of political actions reported, such as posting information, were relatively passive. Although aware of the legal strictures on political activities in public agencies, as prohibited by the conservative Hatch Amendment, the researchers encouraged nurse leaders to find out what activities were not restricted. Archer and Goehner concluded that "Greater emphasis is still needed to overcome many of the residual affects of the socialization of women and nurses into passive roles, to dispel the fear and negativity that have hampered nurses' political development, and to help nurses achieve their goal of becoming skilled and effective protagonists in a variety of political forms" (p. 54).

NURSES' POLITICAL PARTICIPATION VERSUS OTHER PROFESSIONAL WOMEN

Were many nurses networking or participating in political activities outside of nursing? How did their political activism compare to that of other women professionals? Barbara E. Hanley (1987) compared nurses' political participation with that of professional women in teaching and engineering. Since nursing reflects many of the problems women face in a male-dominated society, comparisons with women in other professions would, said Hanley, provide "baseline data on which to develop political strategies and to analyze nurses in the broader context of professional women" (p. 179). Increased politicization of women, following the revitalization of the women's movement, has forced political scientists to acknowledge their biases, particularly as the gender gap in political participation closes. Feminist political scientists assert that traditional explanations of disparities in participation by oppressed groups have sustained the status quo. Reanalysis of the same data, controlling for higher education, for example, has found equal numbers of women and men voting since 1962. Indeed, participation in political campaigns increased first among professional and White college women and this change then diffused to blue-collar women. Thus, it is clear that education and employment do affect female political behavior.

Hanley asked, Would women in disciplines predominantly female, such as nursing, differ from mixed-gender fields, such as teaching, or male-dominated ones, such as engineering? Would gender dominance with differing qualitative experience of work environments affect voting, campaign activities, and community efforts? Voting, a passive activity, has steadily increased among women since suffrage was attained in 1920; over 53% of voters are women— this, despite women's lower scores on measures of political interest, orientation, and efficacy, and their higher scores on political trust. Only 4% to 8% of citizens engage in campaign activities, but by 1970 college women had tripled their participation rates while men's rates had doubled. Given the trend toward baccalaureate education in nursing, Hanley speculated on the influence of higher education on nurses' political activity.

Compared to other women professionals, Hanley found that nurses had a lower educational attainment: 29% had less than BA or BS degrees; 42% held BS degrees; and 25% had master's degrees. All respondents were members of professional organizations; but nurses were significantly *less* active than teachers or engineers. "Nearly half of the nurses did not even attend meetings of their professional organizations, in contrast to 20% of the teachers and 33% of the engineers" (p. 183). According to Hanley, nurses also belonged to significantly fewer organizations; 70% of nurses, 58% of teachers, and 56% of engineers belonged to only one or two organizations. In contrast, 40% of female engineers and teachers, but only 30% of nurses, belonged to three or more organizations.

The mean political participation scores for all factors was not significantly different for all three groups, but nurses had a significantly *lower* voting score due to their lower turnout in local and state elections. Women in all three groups did not engage in campaigning, but the engineers had the highest mean score. For communal activities, all three groups were similar, participating only occasionally. Protest activity was similar for nurses and teachers, but when the item on striking was excluded, no significant difference was found among the groups.

Nurses' political participation increased with age, and those unemployed had higher participation rates. The number of children had a positive significant effect on both nurses' and teachers' political action levels. Family socialization and mothers' political interest were positively related to nurses' participation. Both nurses and teachers, but not engineers, were affected by politicization during professional socialization.

Hanley was particularly concerned about the difference between diploma and associate degree nurses, who voted significantly less in local and state elections than more highly educated nurses, teachers, and engineers. She argued for the inclusion of political education in all nursing and continuing education programs. All women professionals had common economic concerns: comparable worth, day care, and pregnancy leaves. Hanley concluded that nurses must join other professional women to assume political leadership to protect their interests as women and professionals and to enhance their effectiveness as consumer advocates.

WHO SUPPORTS NURSE LEADERS?

The need for unity among women's groups and within nursing is particularly obvious when the treatment of women leaders is analyzed. In 1988 Christina G. Weaver studied the causes of turnover among nurse executives, who appear to be far more vulnerable than authors such as Roberts (1983; 1994) had indicated. Indeed, the picture painted by Weaver is *not* one of Queen Bees, but one of women deans and administrators being dismissed at increasing rates. As they exert themselves and stick out their necks, their throats are being slit according to Thelma Schorr (1981). Weaver focused specifically on *involuntary* departures of women discharged in the previous two years. She used open-ended questions in interviews to explore this seldom-studied problem. The first shock comes from two studies conducted by the American Organization of Nurse Executives, which found that 63.5% of the nurse executives in 1982 and 64.4% in 1985 had held their positions for only one to five years.

Clearly, women leaders do not stay long in one power position. Only about one-third cited personal and family reasons for departure. Less than 2% admitted being dismissed. But in a study by Freund (1985) of 250 university and affiliated hospitals, these institutions averaged 2.5 nursing directors in each hospital in a ten-year period. "Termination and requested resignation were cited by 40% as the most common reason for turnover" (p. 283). This occurred despite the fact that 97.6% of those terminated reported a positive relationship with their chief executive officers. In an informal study of members of one eastern state's organization of nurse executives, 53 members held administrative posts in the state's 110 hospitals; 24 or 45% had left their positions between 1985 and 1987. Of these, 50% had been terminated or left under pressure. Weaver asserted, "Many of those individuals had played not only leadership roles in their hospitals but also in their professional organizations and state hierarchies. They were and several remain acknowledged spokepersons for nursing" (p. 283).

Weaver interviewed a small number of former executives, all women, with master's degrees, and in nursing from 18 to 26 years and in their former positions from 2 to 10 years. The attack by men in power on assertive women leaders is clear. Most nurses cited disagreement with administration as the immediate cause of their departure. The nursing leaders claimed that administrators refused to back them but sided instead with physicians, who "perceived staff nurses as becoming too independent in their practice and not available enough to assist them" (p. 284). The nursing leaders also cited philosophical differences between the administrators, who believed in the "old ways," and the nurse executives, who were trying to initiate innovative programs. Furthermore, increased power of women leaders, when they were invited to attend board of directors' meetings, caused insecurity among other administrators. The nurse executives also had conflict over staff nurses' dissatisfaction with administration, nursing shortages, and inadequate support services. In this regard, administrators, mostly male, supported the physicians, mostly male, in their demands to open more beds in opposition to the nurse executives, who claimed that patient care would be jeopardized due to lack of qualified staff.

Weaver reported that the one phrase that appeared most frequently in the women's reasons for their departure was lack of power. Some of the leaders knew for up to a year that their departure was likely, but to some their firing came as a complete surprise: "One nurse executive had even received a '25 percent raise for outstanding performance' 6 months before being asked to resign" (p. 284). About one-third were told to leave immediately with no time for closure or for organizing women's support. The rest officially resigned, but stayed up to four months, maintaining the "act." One even helped find her own replacement!

No out-placement services were provided. Indeed, Weaver said that the burden fell on each woman *alone* to negotiate a separation agreement, deal with her loss, and move on. The grief process involved initial feelings of being overwhelmed, devastated, upset, and angry, coupled with feelings of worthlessness, frustration, and depression. These feelings continued throughout the first year, particularly when the woman realized how hard it was to get an equivalent position. Only two women moved within six months to an equal or better position; the rest did not; two even left nursing entirely. Several could not even get references from the hospital administrators; indeed, the women were advised that the old boys' network would exclude them for consideration for other positions. That the male power network was effective is clear: three women were not fully employed until one year after termination and two others were still seeking jobs at the time of Weaver's interviews.

What was the nurse executives' advice to others? Focusing more on individual rather than group action, they warned others not to be complacent, to demand a yearly written performance appraisal, and to set aside precautionary savings from earnings. The women recommended developing a hospital policy and program for out-placement services. They urged active networks and contacts with former associates and advised nurses to contact colleagues who had lost jobs, and provide, if possible, temporary or part-time employment. At no point did these leaders recommend political action against the men who fired them. Nor did they seem to look to other nurses to organize on their behalf; nor to demand greater security for future leaders; nor to establish procedures to deal with physicians who pressure nurses to increase patient care without additional sources of support. Indeed, the comment of one leader to those facing termination was this admonition: "Remember, most of our nation's leaders have been fired at least once. You are in good company and can hold your head high" (p. 286).

Weaver noted that nurse executives are the most visible to staff nurses. "They walk a tight rope each day in balancing the needs of patients, the aspirations of the nursing profession, and the realities of the hospital political climate" (p. 286). She did not acknowledge, however, that most nurse leaders are women caught at the interface between male power and female demands for power, between masculist values and feminist concerns. Their departures are not simply a loss to nurses; they are also casualties in the war between the sexes and, as such, they deserve the attention and support of women *external* to nursing. One wonders if any of the terminated leaders turned for support to feminist or women's organizations or even to government agencies working on legal aspects of sex discrimination. No woman leader should be left alone, terminated, and without support for her efforts to help other women and their patients.

THE IMPACT OF MULTIHOSPITAL SYSTEMS ON NURSE EXECUTIVES

The situation may, in fact, be deteriorating for nurse executives. Reporting on a study of chief nurse executives in multihospital systems, Janet K. Harrison and Patricia A. Roth (1987) recognize that many hospitals are joining or forming multi-institutional systems or existing with varying degrees of autonomy within multicorporate structures. By 1995 it is expected that 50% of the hospitals in the United States will be owned, leased, or managed by multihospital systems. Thus, Harrison and Roth, supporting Stuart's (1986) model, emphasize the need for nurses to participate in decision making at all levels, including the corporate. But to what extent are chief nurse executives actually participating in such decision making?

Distributing a questionnaire to 206 nursing leaders across the nation, the researchers found that the chief nurse executive respondent was generally a director of nursing who was between 30 and 49 years old, relatively new to her current position, holding a baccalaureate or higher degree, and with less than 10 years of administrative experience. The women worked at various types of hospitals, some within the military hospital system. Whether any male nurse executives were studied was not reported.

Harrison and Roth found lower involvement in decisions related to hospital operation; for example, women leaders had minimal or no actual involvement in the appointment and performance appraisals of the men, who were predominantly chief executive officers of the entire hospital. The women wanted moderate to maximum involvement, but did not have it. Seventy-two percent reported that they were moderately or maximally involved in hospital strategic plans, but 97% preferred a higher degree of involvement. Even on decisions about patient care, 98% wanted involvement, but only 85% had moderate to maximal influence.

Given the predicted trends toward multihospital systems, the most troubling finding was that "system size was inversely related to the actual degree of involvement of chief nurse executives in those decision areas related to hospital operations" (p. 74). A countervailing trend to high-level titles, such as vice president for patient services, may suggest broader power than director of nursing, or this may simply be a sop since the majority of women still had little power to influence or evaluate the top administrators. The youthful ages may, as the researchers suggest, indicate earlier career planning, but it may also suggest, given the greater discrepancy between actual and preferred involvement with increased age, a revolving door policy for women leaders.

Normally, as age and experience increase so do power and influence. If the assertive nurses are fired, the age would remain relatively low and so would power to create change or even to maintain a unified group of staff nurses. Because of disparities in reports of involuntary dismissals, these factors need much more attention.

If token women are supported and Queen Bees are valued, as Roberts (1983; 1994) asserts, then age and length of time in position should be older and longer. If assertive, relatively liberated, more feminist women are arising from the grassroots, their tenure in office could be shorter. None of these factors are clearly known, but Weaver's exploratory work provides some initial suggestions. It is, of course, equally probable that women leaders are simply worn out by the war of attrition. Tired of struggling for empowerment of themselves and their staffs, they may simply resign from the exhausting and often depressing battle. Others may be forced to leave by nurses themselves, because their leaders are perceived as too militant or too weak. The leaders may have moved with strength only to find themselves "out on a limb," with no support from apathetic or apolitical or fearful women in the ranks. At this time, any or all of these explanations are possible, particularly when interconnected with the trend toward greater centralization of control in hospital conglomerates.

FEMALE NATIONAL HEALTH INDUSTRY ADMINISTRATORS: FORESHADOWING FUTURE ROLES FOR WOMEN?

On a more optimistic note, Helen J. Muller and Carolyn Cocotas (1988), say the health industry may be the prototype for changing gender roles among administrators since the majority of midlevel managers are now female. They conducted an exploratory study of prominent women leaders in Washington, DC, during the 1980s, who were at the forefront in changing national health policy. They found that the women's leadership styles differed from traditional male styles and, although they experienced role conflict in their rise to power, these women may foreshadow the roles of new leaders in the health industry in the 1990s.

During the 1980s women executives were centrally involved in the Health Care Financing Administration (HCFA), in major private national health organizations, and as key congressional committee staff. In 1981 Margaret Heckler, then secretary of the U.S. Department of Health and Human Services, appointed nurse Carolyne Davis as chief executive of HCFA. She followed three male administrators whose average tenure was 14 months. Davis stayed four years. The importance of HCFA to women and children is clear: administration of Medicare and Medicaid programs represented 23% of $458 million spent in 1986 for health care; 60% of aged Medicare enrollees were female, and 75% of Medicaid recipients were women and children under six years of age. Therefore, the inner circle of women executives formulating policy was important to other women.

Muller and Cocotas interviewed 16 of the most frequently mentioned female executives, who were willing to share their personal experiences and were interested in learning about their peers. Most were in their 40's, some in their 30's, and only three were over 50, suggesting that older women had not risen beyond midlevel management positions. Two-thirds held master's or higher degrees. Only one woman, a hospital diploma educated RN, held no degree, but three other RNs held additional higher degrees. It is important to stress that one-fourth of the top executives interviewed were nurses. Half of the 16 woman interviewed were single and of these, three were divorcées whose husbands could not deal with their wives' careers. In general, most male corporate executives (96%) are married, but only 59% of comparable females. Among the married women, husbands were noted as critical to their wives' careers.

All the women began working in their 20s and continued without major interruptions; each had, according to the researchers, a fascinating success story. "One woman's career began when she responded to an advertisement for health service representatives in the 'men only' section of a local newspaper" (p. 73). The researchers noted that most of the women were among the first to deliberate on national health policy in Washington and to rise steadily to prominence. The paucity of women mentors was clear, since most mentioned husbands, male mentors, or national male leaders as influential: "Only 3 of the 16 women attributed their success in part to female mentors" (p. 73). It is unclear if the women executives recognized the influence of the women's movement in forcing open upper-echelon leadership positions. Certainly, several executives saw themselves as trailblazers for other women. They all worked very hard, 12- to 14-hour days and weekends, but the majority expected to be in different jobs within one year.

The overwhelming majority of these women described their management styles as participatory and person-oriented. One said her style was seen as "soft" and she was perceived as someone who did not know what she wanted. But subordinates adjusted and changed their perception as their freedom and authority to make their own decisions were enhanced. The women executives were demanding task masters, expecting high-quality performance. Peculiarly, they did not see their management as gender specific, but, at the same time, saw themselves as role models for other women. Indeed, several mentioned being supportive of individual employees' needs and one even said that management requires caring for people.

Several women thought there was more resistance from men in the private than in the public sector; all thought that power was male-dominated; however, "this did not interfere with women's ability to move ahead to the same degree that it had a decade earlier" (p. 75). Indeed, most felt there were now fewer negative gender issues, but more resistance to their health policies.

Whether this resistance is also gender related was not addressed. However, the researchers found that "Most of the women in the study cited examples of outright discrimination and overt sexist comments that they had encountered in previous jobs" (p. 75). Despite these earlier problems, the women experienced fewer sexist problems in their current positions. This perception is questionable, however, since most of the women reported that they were working twice as hard as their male equivalents. Their competence had to be proven; they had to earn respect rather than getting it by virtue of position; they had to have an unusually thorough knowledge of facts and issues and could not afford to make many mistakes.

Muller and Cocotas noted that about half of the executives said that women bring a value system to the making of health policy that is different from men's value system. Women were more aware of the impact of national policy on local communities and individuals, more sensitive to issues affecting women, children, and the elderly. The nurses believed that their training made them more sensitive to the problems of delivering health services. Two women could not see value differences at all, and others said there were insufficient numbers of women in power to determine any differences.

Paradoxically, many of the women were in agreement that the Reagan administration placed a high value on economic issues, but had little regard for the health problems of varied groups. In fact, said Muller and Cocotas, "the presence of key women in top-level government positions (some of them women in our study) helped to forestall even larger budget cuts in health programs for the elderly and the poor" (p. 77). However, the executives were not as optimistic about influencing positive solutions to the health problems of women and children. One even said that it would be *career suicide to advocate any programs for women*. The researchers believed that this was a widely held opinion because of the dominance of fiscal matters and the fact that at least half of the women were leaving their jobs. This finding did not bode well for the future. If women can attain power only if they act as though they are not specifically interested in women's issues, then change in value systems and in gender segregation cannot be openly espoused. Furthermore, power that is this contingent on male approval can hardly be considered power in any full sense. The movement of half of the women executives to other jobs does not suggest power sufficient to affect public policy over many years. Most of the women executives, however, were more optimistic, predicting that female influence on national health policy would increase as more women attained top leadership roles.

Muller and Cocotas raised several questions: Are the women executives anomalies or the beginning of a trend? If a trend, what are the implications for changing traditional male power structures in the health-care industry? How do male peers of women leaders perceive them? Are the men learning new styles of management from the women? Is the health-care industry different from other corporations in pushing women away from top positions?

Are the kinds of policies developed by women at the top different? Will there be more humanistic strategies and solutions? Will women executives be able to espouse openly feminist strategies and solutions? Will a more adaptable leadership style replace or modify the traditional male modes? The researchers concluded that unless organizational barriers loosen, women will continue to be the exceptions as leaders. And while current women executives may be the "forerunners" of leaders in the health-care industry in the future, unless they can more openly espouse change for women, what kind of forerunners will they be?

THE MATURING OF NURSING'S POLITICAL INFLUENCE AND ACTIVISM

While many individual leaders in nursing and other women executives are still struggling to enhance and secure their political and organizational power and influence, it is clear that organized bodies of nurses—nursing's professional associations—have made significant strides in achieving influence and control since 1985. Nursing's increased awareness of women's subordinate status in society and the negative influences this has had on nurses, coupled with recent strenuous efforts to improve the public image of nurses, have made a positive impact on nursing's political achievements since the late 1980s. Indeed, nursing's traditional pattern of reacting to proposals for change is now shifting to proactive efforts to influence and create system changes in health-care delivery.

Perhaps criticisms of nurses' passivity and lack of influence in affecting the implementation of Diagnostic Related Groups (DRGs) for Medicare provided a turning point, a catalyst for subsequent proactive behavior. For example, critics such as Faye G. Abdullah, former deputy surgeon general, U.S. Public Health Service, deplored nursing's powerlessness to influence DRG parameters, pointing to the exclusion of nursing service as a component of *all* 467 Diagnostic Related Groups. She noted: "not one of these included a nursing service component with related predetermined costs" (Abdullah; cited in Kippinbrock, 1992, p. 211). As a result of DRGs, patients have been discharged home sooner; they are much sicker, and often are sent home needing multiple supports and complex technical equipment. Abdullah stated, "To have included a nursing cost component for each of the DRGs initially would have changed the entire future of nursing practice and education. Outcome measures and cost components would have been identified—we are just now catching up" (p. 211).

Another effect of establishing DRGs was the reduction in the total number of RNs on hospital staffs. To lower costs, nursing budgets were cut first, even though hospitals with a higher proportion of registered nurses have been shown to provide better quality care, measured by lower mortality rates. Thus, the exclusion of professional nurses and the overreliance on physicians and inadequately trained auxiliary personnel lead to poor coverage and inadequate care of patients.

On the other hand, the creation of the Community Health Accreditation Program (CHAP) is another story, providing some evidence of nursing's ability to influence the health-care delivery system. In 1986 the American Bar Association prepared a report on home-care delivery, detailing poor care and even criminal behaviors toward patients. This opened the door for action by the National League for Nursing (NLN), which, in the 1960s, had originally set up accreditation processes for nursing education programs. By the 1980s cost-cutting measures had led to a 50% increase in home-care agencies, many becoming business-oriented. In 1986 the NLN accreditation program, after strong political activism, successfully passed a government review process and created the subsidiary corporation, CHAP, which included a stronger consumer and purchaser presence. This distinguished the nurses' accrediting body from others, most notably the physician-dominated Joint Commission on Accreditation of Health Care Organizations (JCAHO), which opposed the inclusion of consumers on its policy-making boards.

CHAP was a unique alliance of consumers and purchasers of home health-care services, which struggled for four years to change the status quo, the closed system in which accreditation was set by the health-care industry and government regulators. Essential information about the quality of home-care organizations had rarely been released to the public, depriving consumers of vital data from which informed selections among providers could be made. The resistance to releasing information to consumers, for example, on hospital mortality rates, is well known, but controlling the quality of home care has been even more difficult. CHAP has conducted on-site visits in homes, telephoned clients, and demanded that agencies conduct surveys on their clients' degree of satisfaction with services. Basic information about services, or even full accreditation reports on agencies, are now available to consumers, who can rely on the CHAP process to identify the highest quality and most cost-effective providers of home-care services.

CHAP challenges the tradition that accreditation of health-care organizations should be established and controlled by the medical profession, rather than by consumers or nurses, and that results of accreditation should not be open to public scrutiny. Achieving deemed status required those in CHAP to overcome layers of bureaucratic inaction, complacency, waste of resources, and limited access to care. Risking both economic and moral failures, if CHAP had not succeeded, it would have been a severe setback for nursing's role in defining standards of care in community home-care agencies. But organized nursing did not fail in this instance, and their success pointed the way for future reforms.

The CHAP board of governors confronted the issue of public disclosure of hospital mortality data, which had been demanded for years by the American

Association of Retired Persons (AARP). When the data were finally released, a profound power shift occurred. CHAP became the embodiment of current trends, but even then Congress approved stringent quality controls for agencies involved with the Medicare program and a moratorium on deemed status for six months. This designation would level the playing field with the physicians' organization that wanted to control nonhospital care, where the largest growth in health care was taking place.

The W. K. Kellogg Foundation awarded a $1.2 million grant to CHAP to develop consumer-oriented outcome measures. At the same time, in a raw power play, the physicians' group, JCAHO, told home-care agencies that if they accepted referrals from JCAHO-accredited hospitals, the agencies must also be accredited by JCAHO. Physician Dennis O'Leary, director of JCAHO, promised CHAP that these "blackmailing" tactics would stop, but in a true feminist spirit, the nurses demanded that he put this promise in writing! The letter was never received. In the meantime, JCAHO was attacked for lax accreditation procedures by the *Wall Street Journal* which hardened the nurses' resolve to protect the public's health and welfare.

Continuing to work with the AARP, the upcoming elections caused what seemed like an endless waiting game. Finally, in 1991, a new HCFA administrator, Gail Wilensky, signed on the deemed status. The physicians' group then engaged in aggressive lobbying to delay action until they could catch up with the nurses. But finally CHAP's proposal appeared in the *Federal Register* and comments in a flood of letters were sent by nurses to HCFA. The General Accounting Office, after reviewing the proposals, confirmed that CHAP's standards were fully comparable to those of Medicare. In 1992 deemed status was obtained. Certainly, there were many days when the nurses and consumers doubted victory, but they were convinced that the health-care system needed major changes, consumers' needs must be met, and nursing's voice must be heard. In this instance, organized nurses and sophisticated leaders, joining with powerful consumer groups, could and did take on the powerful medical lobby and were successful.

This happy ending has been marred, however, by recent NLN allegations that the CHAP board of governors took inappropriate, unilateral actions in 1993 to distance itself from their parent organization (Lindeman & Moccia, 1994). Claiming that CHAP had moved precipitously to establish their own bank account, enter into separate employment contracts with CHAP officers and staff, and seek alternative office space, the NLN board of governors moved to freeze all CHAP account funds, ordered the return of all CHAP property, and demanded a meeting of all parties involved. The CHAP Board was dismissed and the chief officer was terminated. Subsequently, a new board and chief officer were appointed. Whether the strong differences of opinion and internal organizational conflicts will be settled satisfactorily remains to be seen. Certainly, nursing needs no additional examples of infighting and disunity to erode an image that has only recently gained in power and influence among the public.

Organized nursing's intention to emerge as a major force in influencing the nation's health-care delivery system is best exemplified by the profession's role in developing a national health-care reform proposal, leading to the current Clinton administration's Health Security Act. While a national system for health care has been opposed for decades by the American Medical Association, as it earlier opposed maternal and child health program and even Social Security, Medicaid, and Medicare, the American Nurses Association and other organized groups of nurses have, over several decades, consistently supported such social legislation.

In 1991 American nurses issued a national health-care proposal, *Nursing's Agenda for Health Care Reform*, developed by the National League for Nursing, the American Nurses Association, and the American Association of Colleges of Nursing. The plan was built on the existing system, but rearranged existing caregivers, positioning nurses as primary caregivers, providing new incentives to cut costs, decreasing the emphasis on in-patient acute care, and increasing emphasis on prevention, primary care, and long-term care. Approved by 18 nursing groups, the plan included a federally defined standard package of essential health-care benefits available to all citizens financed through a mix of public and private sources but with federal enforcement. The nurses further advocated improving consumer access by delivering primary care services in convenient settings, such as schools, homes, and the work place. They recommended the control of health-care costs through managed care in which there would be incentives for cost control for both consumers and providers; freedom of choice for types of providers, settings, and delivery arrangements; reduced administrative costs through simplified bureaucratic controls and governance procedures; and payment policies connected to the treatment effectiveness determined by outcomes research.

Clearly, nurses had taken significant action in designing a health-care reform package for the nation, but who would support it outside of nursing? In a fortunate event of timing, the 1992 presidential election was nearing and health-care reform emerged as a primary issue in Clinton's campaign. After being elected, Clinton quickly moved to establish his National Health Reform Task Force, chaired by Hilary Rodham Clinton. Nursing's insistence that it be represented on the task force, and its subsequent inclusion in task force deliberations, was a major political victory for nurses' activism. At the same time, by 1993, the AMA, with 300,000 members, was no longer trying to block sweeping changes in health care, but was striving instead to shape and direct them. Publishing their own blueprint for revamping health care, the AMA organized thousands of physicians who descended on Washington in a massive lobbying effort. It is this powerful group that killed efforts to overhaul reform in health care in the 1970s. But in 1993 the AMA was compelled to complain in a formal letter about their lack of access to Clinton's Health Reform Task

Force. This led to meetings with task force advisors and closer agreement on the principle of a "managed-competition" model that retained the patient's choice of a physician, did away with unnecessary regulatory requirements, and promoted liability reform (*Syracuse Herald-Journal*, 1993).

Though organized nursing groups were satisfied with the influence they had wielded in contributing to the task force recommendations for reform, they were concerned when they saw the health-care reform bill as it was sent to Congress in late October 1993. It was evident that several important components of reform and health-care provision had not been included in the legislative language of the new Health Security Act. ANA representatives quickly met with senior White House staff to insist that critical nursing issues be reinstated and included in an "errata document" to be sent to Congress. ANA President Virginia Trotter Betts stated that the "draft legislation did not adequately address some elements agreed upon by the Administration and nursing in negotiations prior to the release of the legislation" (*The American Nurse*, 1993, p. 1). The ANA specifically wanted the proposed bill to include services of Advanced Practice Nurses (APNs) as a covered benefit for consumers; use of Graduate Medical Education (GME) funds for nursing education; stronger language on preempting state regulatory barriers to nursing practice; clarification of the term "health professional"; and broader criteria for provider participation on the National Health Board.

The Clinton administration approved of the nurses' demands and the redesigned Health Security Act bill now included nurses as "essential community providers" of health care, allowing APNs to be reimbursed directly for their services as primary care professionals. The act essentially overrides state regulatory barriers to reimbursement of several primary health-care professionals. As might be expected, the AMA immediately moved to oppose this action. In December 1993 the AMA House of Delegates released a report that opposes autonomy for APNs, as well as for psychologists, social workers, chiropractors, and podiatrists. AMA opposition to greater use of APNs also includes clinical nurse specialists, certified nurse midwives, and certified registered nurse anesthetists. Exhibiting commendable political sophistication, organized nursing, through the ANA, quickly responded and accused physicians of contributing to the nation's health-care crisis (*The Nation's Health*, 1994). Furthermore, the ANA questioned why the AMA would oppose greater use of primary health-care providers, such as APNs, at a time when there is a shortage of qualified caregivers, due in part to physicians' abandonment of primary care work. ANA President Betts criticized the AMA for attacking the credibility of other health-care providers and claimed: "'The issue is control, especially control of dollars. The AMA wants physician supervision because then the physician gets the first dollar'" (Meehan, 1994, p. 3).

The sustained actions by organized nursing to significantly influence health-care reform in the United States has clearly demonstrated nurses' ability to engage in assertive, political activism. Never before in nursing's history has the political sophistication of the profession been greater. It appears that nurses are now willing to utilize the power of their sheer numbers to demand and effect change. Florence Nightingale, Clara Barton, Lavinia Dock, and other early leaders in nursing would be proud of the actions and achievements of these nurses. Whether such political activism will be sustained depends on women's refusal to maintain their subordinate roles in nursing and in society as a whole.

TRENDS IN NURSING'S POWER AND POLITICAL ACTIVISM

Over time, what trends in power and nursing have emerged from the 1960s to the 1990s? One clear shift is the increasingly open demand for power. Although the interrelations among gender, power, leadership, and internal and external politics are yet to be fully integrated, it is certain that the feminist legitimization of female power has been incorporated in varying degrees into the thinking and writing about nursing. The presumed negative personal characteristics of women leaders have been replaced by a more sophisticated analysis, for example, in Larsen's work, on the effects of subordinate organizational status on nurses and their leaders and in Roberts' work on the dynamics of oppression underlying female leadership roles. Although the mostly positive findings from feminist research on women managers or administrators are not systematically incorporated, there is at least greater clarity on the influence of female socialization for powerlessness on both personal and professional attitudes and behaviors. Whether nursing education has continued the socialization for subordination or has prepared higher-degree nurses for an independence that is not yet fully possible in actual work situations continues to be debated. Similarly, the question of whether nurses in power have sustained subordination, as Queen Bees by identifying with men, or tried to support and protect nurses as women, or retreated to bureaucratic rigidity in the face of overwhelming demands, also continues to be debated. Indeed, Wakefield-Fisher found that there are still dismally small numbers of women administrators in top-level positions, citing a lack of role models, lack of support, and poor self-esteem as major contributing factors. Furthermore, Weaver found nurse executives to be especially vulnerable, being attacked by men in power and fired at increasing rates. This situation is apparent also from the research conducted by Harrison and Roth. In a parallel manner, the issue of nurses as individuals or followers is still debated: Have they left their leaders out on a limb with no support for strong leadership efforts to change the status quo? Or have nurses retreated, fearing power is "unprofessional"? Have they stereotyped strong nurses as "mannish" or lesbians? Or have nurses integrated change only to be blocked by their own women leaders?

How do women achieve a public image of power when men continue to take credit for nurses' accomplishments? The reconstitution of nursing history is necessary to reclaim the achievements of women; for example, in establishing public health measures, which physicians have subsequently credited to themselves rather than to the nurses and women who initiated these reforms. Some nursing leaders name the oppressors as physicians and hospital administrators; if so, nurses have had to collaborate with and advocate *for* their oppressors! With collaboration and advocacy of medical and hospital men, nurses constantly react to outside influences; they are not proactive in promulgating their own group and their own system of values. Thus, nurses did not initiate expanded roles, but reacted negatively to physicians' ideas of physicians' assistants. The vicious cycle of reactive behavior leads to nurses' conformity and to disunity among their leaders, who are caught between the old model of conforming to the establishment and the new order of confrontation and negotiation. With the increasing size and complexity of organizations, nurses may feel "competitive shock," since they are not prepared to develop the institutional strategies needed for change.

The key problem to several writers is the issue of values in patriarchal versus matriarchal systems. For example, Krueger and Weaver recognize the differences between medicine's values and nursing's values in their positions on health care and social programs: nurses stress humane, caring values while the economic value of competition is generally espoused by physicians. Nursing may well be the only remaining profession that stands for the protection of a value system that stresses the holistic and the humane in a health-delivery system dominated by masculist ideology and practice. What stands in the way of implementing women's values? Some believe that nurses' perceptions of political action as unprofessional or unwomanly—the lack of feminist consciousness of the personal as political—are to blame, leaving nurses' power unchecked and unharnessed.

What solutions are suggested? Some nurses support N-CAP (Nurses Coalition for Action in Politics); Talbott and Vance focus on NURSES NOW; others point to the CHAP alliance; and many nurses support various Political Action Committees (PACs). All warn, however, that gender resocialization of women is critical to full colleagueship with physicians. To these and other writers, nurses cannot continue to extend the same behavior used with patients to medical co-workers, who are not sick people, but rather physicians who may be afraid of nurses as severe economic threats. Edwards and Lenz focus on gender-based interaction patterns and recommend strategies for nurse leaders that would combine the best of "feminine" and "masculine" communication behaviors. Harrison and Roth prove the system is hostile to women in power, since they remain one or two levels below chief medical officers in hospitals. The continued rejection of women in power beyond midlevel hospital management is consistent with the same trend in other societal institutions. In an effort to focus on the empowerment of women,

Stuart embraces a theory of strategic contingencies, helping nurses unite to challenge existing power structures.

Many authors continue to urge resocialization to help nurses see the reality that power is a simple requirement for personal and professional lives. Greenleaf, for example, proposes a model that links self-esteem and enabling power. The trend to resocialize nurses to men's politics may, however, as noted by Muller and Cocotas, leave women's version of reality unacknowledged.

How can nurses achieve consistency? To what extent should women's groups incorporate male group processes? Values fusion between women's inner and men's outer approaches to power through the model of the androgynous manager may bring together the male norms of achievement and competition and the female norms of affiliation and cooperation. Women should not simply learn male politics, but insist on power that is characterized by symmetry and openness. The place of work in life, the role of intimacy, and the conceptions of time and success must be reconfigured to progress beyond the crossed interactions that confuse women managers with mothers, instead of adult problem solvers with parental nurturance and child spontaneity. The shift from proving that women's leadership is as "good" as men's to whether men's processes should be used at all represents a significant strategy change.

How will female-defined power, the androgynous synthesis, be incorporated, given the historical reality of medical politics? No simple fusion is possible without a reintegration and reconstitution of historical reality. How will nurses integrate their own values with those of physicians when the AMA has historically fought progressive social changes, sometimes sustaining an oppressor consciousness in which human beings have been reduced to the status of objects to be used for the goal of profit? Nurses must break their silence on physicians' unquestioned right to coerce and manipulate both nurses and patients. That organized nursing is becoming more assertive in confronting physicians is clear from their actions related to the proposed Health Security Act. Whether individual nurses will be as assertive is not as certain.

Some authors, such as Campbell-Heider, analyze power in feminist terms; others, such as the Kalisches, in terms with no clear explication of sex-stratification systems. An integration of a new gendered model of power has yet to emerge in the 1990s. The civil libertarian position, now mixed with women's cultural values, continues as an *implicit* model in institutional analyses. Krueger focuses on the rules of corporate politics, money and power, and questions nurse-physician team analogues as unequal, illogical, and asymmetrical in values. The system needs changing; nurses need new innovative strategies, and nurses are joining feminists in critically looking into the situation.

The negative critique of nurses' power continues. Muller and Cocotas claim that nurses do not understand organizational pyramids of power; still isolated, ambivalent, and lacking career commitment, they are often led by Queen Bee women, whose antifeminist attitudes counter militancy, emphasize institutional allegiance, and foster personal, not professional, identities. By the 1980s it was still necessary for writers to decry military protocols, urging the use of corporate structures by women instead of relying on men to solve the problems of women in nursing. The analytic advance is seen in the shift from primarily individual solutions to organizational analyses. Muller and Cocotas envision increasing congruence between feminist and futurist visions, which would predict that rigid hierarchy and patriarchal control will give way to more horizontal, flexible, and power-sharing models, more consonant with androgynous and feminist expectations. To what extent have such futurist and feminist models emerged? Evidently, not very frequently. During the 1980s health-policy changes emerged from Reagan's decrease in government support, an increased emphasis on presumed competition and "better" business practices. Instead of decentralization, institutional managers have achieved greater control through trade-offs between cost control and quantity of services and increased monitoring of health professionals, particularly since the introduction of the prospective payment system.

Whether the masses of apathetic and unmotivated nurses, as the Kalisches describe them, can mobilize politically is still the critical issue. Often lacking gender analyses, books on power for nurses, nevertheless, appear as adaptations of traditional political science, almost educational primers, rallying naive nurses to action. The success of these mobilization efforts, however, are uncertain, evidenced by Hanley's finding that nurses' political participation is less than that of non-nurses, such as teachers and engineers. Still, the fundamental issue of unity continues, for example, in Larsen's questions: What does organized nursing *want* to change? What is the role of the nurse? Relying on feminist research, Larsen questions the traditional views of women's organizational and political behavior, focusing instead on the structural conditions that shape women; the opportunity structures that create generalists, interchangeable entities, whose dead-end positions create rationales and values to justify staying in nursing. To Larsen and Harrison and Roth, nursing leaders are caught in structures that in reality give them little real power. Lacking power, they may deny innovation and turn to procedures they can control. Lacking unity in definition, purpose, and action, they may turn to male nurses, whose socialization for power is supposedly going to help more passive women, or to male physicians, whose power may be used to resolve women's rights.

Calls for increasing nurses' political sophistication have emphasized mentoring and assertiveness training. Derived from feminist and organizational scholars, mentoring is espoused by Campbell-Heider and others; but in the absence of a career ladder, the adaptation of the process seems problematic. Even lateral communication among nurses may be limited by structural arrangement. To Barritt, the emulation of male structure and style may, on adaptation, lead to covert emotional nepotism and continued reliance on men for conflict resolution. The different values in women's culture may lead nurses to look to their leaders for nurturance, not professional growth. Infighting among subordinates and membership in an oppressed group, as noted by Roberts, may make it impossible for nurses to coalesce into a viable power structure. Hagerty reviews the work on mentoring, questioning whether, in dyadic relations, mentoring can change the gender-stratification system. She fears that emotion-laden mentoring will prepare nurses for avoidance of risks as women, rather than resocialize them for independence. Campbell-Heider questions whether women can actually hold high-level positions of power from which mentoring for power can occur. Will mentoring with women reinforce traditional dependency? If with men, will it alienate nurses from female value systems? Different sponsorship models for women are needed; adaptation, not adoption, of male organizational behaviors is recommended. Christy agrees, but values networking strategies when formal processes fail to provide sufficient opportunities for upward movement. The trend toward resolving the conflicts between female and male cultures has sustained over several decades.

Still another trend is the mixture of individual, group, organizational, institutional, and societal analyses of power. Individual change, derived from the feminist adaptation of assertiveness in the 1970s, enabled nurses in the 1980s to review a large number of articles on assertiveness as a means of combating submissiveness and sexism, and of assuming more independent and expanded roles, an approach espoused by Milauskas. The individual solutions are not systematically intermeshed with the organizational solutions. The Kalisches, for example, deplore the lack of organizational membership among nurses, but even a few organized nurses can effect political change in legislation and expanded roles. Chalich and Smith, on the other hand, postulate that nurses' greatest political efforts may be at the grassroots level and support these efforts as leading to a new model of nurse activism. Archer and Goehner express dismay, however, over nurse administrators' general lack of political involvement and activism. Thus, by the 1990s, it is clear that the risks of being assertive are still high. On the other hand, while organized nursing has yet to move to system-wide gender resocialization and has not yet worked out processes to protect women as they became more assertive, it has established itself as a respected political force and certainly a leader in health-care reform.

TOWARD THE 21ST CENTURY

This book has examined from a historical perspective the multiple connections between the subordinated status of women and of women in the nursing profession. Of particular concern has been the effect of feminism on nurses and nursing, and whether nurses themselves espoused feminist principles. The deep resources women nurses have called on to overcome their subordination must now be met by the elimination of sexist structures that sustain a pseudosuperiority in the face of contradictory evidence. Feminist nurses envision a time when all women unite to change the structures of hospitals and agencies so that divide-and-conquer tactics will no longer prevail. Ultimately, the basic struggle will be accomplished when women's values are translated by nurses into organizational contexts that force a change from patriarchal structures to ones that value the human in all people. Until the historical subjugation of women is reversed and women in nursing control their own profession and a values transformation occurs, there will continue to be nursing shortages, professional disunity, and lack of autonomy.

If the services of nurses are essential, then they must be given the authority to do their jobs, the respect and recognition for what they really do, the freedom to do all they can do, and the economic support that rewards them fairly. The alternative is the present system of enforced and subordinated silence in which physicians overcharge for what nurses can do instead, take credit for what nurses actually do, and deny patients access to nurses' expertise; a system in which hospital administrators demand more and more competence from nurses and increase their responsibilities, but expect nurses to do their work without full authority or the economic rewards to make it worthwhile. By the same token, nurses must solidify recent gains in their positions of power and use feminist strategies of networking and political activism to gain the professional autonomy they deserve. If this is not done, nurses and their public will continue to suffer the consequences of a gender-stratified system that cannot give the best patient care.

As we saw in the early chapters of this book, our feminist foremothers clearly understood the need for nurses, and indeed all women, to develop strategies of networking and political activism. Florence Nightingale's phenomenal efforts to establish nursing as a respectable profession for women and to effect military and sanitation reforms, Clara Barton's lifelong commitment to and support of women's rights, Lavinia Dock's fight for women's suffrage and her admonition to nursing to involve itself in the "urgent social claims" of the day, and Lillian Wald's crusade for public health reform were all early models of political activism in nursing. Most important, they, and others such as Margaret Sanger and Emma Goldman, understood the relationship between the status of nursing and women's status in a patriarchal society. Let not the ideals of these women be lost. And, as nursing enters the 21st century, we would do well to remember Nightingale's warning: "Let us take care not to be left behind," crying "'Forward, Forward,' every two minutes . . . ," and never stirring a step.

References

Abbott, L. (1909). The assault on womanhood. *American Journal of Nursing, 9*(8), 566–573.

Adams, G. W. (1952). *Doctors in blue: The medical history of the Union Army in the Civil War.* New York: Henry Schuman.

Allen, D. (1986). Nursing and oppression: "The family" in nursing texts. *Feminist Teacher, 2*(1), 14–20.

Allen, D. R. (1975, Summer). Florence Nightingale: Toward a psychohistorical explanation. *Journal of Interdisciplinary History, 8*, 33.

Allen, M. (1985). Women, nursing and feminism: An interview with Alice J. Baumgart, RN, PhD. *The Canadian Nurse, 81*(1), 20–22.

AMA swaps sides on health-care plan. (1993, March 31). *Syracuse Herald-Journal,* p. A6.

Amenta, M. M. (1977). NURSES NOW: A model of worksite organizing. *Nursing Forum, 16*(3/4), 343–345.

American Journal of Nursing. (1908, February). Editorial comment: Progress and reaction, *8*(5), 333–335.

American Journal of Nursing. (1911a, November). Editorial, *11*, 595–596.

American Journal of Nursing. (1911b, November). Editorial, *11*, 777.

American Journal of Nursing. (1975, October). Nurses and Nursing's Issues, *75*(10), 1848–1859.

The American Nurse. (1993, November/December). Working to advance health care reform, *25*(10), 1, 3.

Appelbaum, A. L. (1975). Women in health care administration. *Hospitals, 49*(16), 52–59.

Archer, S. E., & Goehner, P. A. (1981). Acquiring political clout: Guidelines for nurse administrators. *Journal of Nursing Administration, 11*(11/12), 49–55.

Ashley, J. A. (1973). This I believe about power in nursing. *Nursing Outlook*, *21*(10), 637–641.

Ashley, J. A. (1975). Nurses in American history: Nursing and early feminism. *American Journal of Nursing*, *75*(9), 1465–1467.

Ashley, J. A. (1976). *Hospitals, paternalism and the role of the nurse*. New York: Teachers College Press.

Ashley, J. A. (1980, April). Power in structured misogyny: Implications for the politics of care. *Advances in Nursing Science*, *2*, 3–22.

Associated Press, *Salt Lake City Tribune*. (1991, June 12), p. A12.

Austin, A. L. (1975). Nurses in American history: Wartime volunteers, 1861–1865. *American Journal of Nursing*, *75*(5), 816–818.

Austin, J. K., Champion, V. L., & Tzeng, O. C. S. (1985). Crosscultural comparison on nursing image. *International Journal of Nursing Studies*, *22*(3), 231–239.

Backer, B. A. (1993, March). Lillian Wald: Connecting caring with activism. *Nursing and Health Care*, *14*(3), 122–129.

Bakunina, E. (1898, March). Vospominanija sestry miloserdija Krestovozdvizhenskoj obshchiny, 1854–1860. *Vestnik Evropy*. CXC, #3, 134, #4 (April), 518–520.

Baly, M. E. (1973). *Nursing and social change*. London: Heinemann Medical.

Barritt, E. R. (1984). Inbreeding, infighting, and impotence. *American Journal of Nursing*, *84*(6), 803–804.

Belenky, M. F. (1988). *Women's ways of knowing: Development of self, voice, and mind*. New York: Basic Books.

Benson, E. R. (1991, Winter). Some thoughts on F. B. Smith's *Florence Nightingale: Reputation and power*. *Bulletin: American Association for the History of Nursing*, *29*, 6–7.

Benson, E. R. (1992, Spring). On the other side of the battle: Russian nurses in the Crimean War. *Image: Journal of Nursing Scholarship*, *24*(1), 65–68.

Benson, E. R., & Selekman, J. (1992, December). Jewish women and nursing: An overview of early history. *Journal of the New York State Nurses Association*, *23*(4), 16–19.

Bille, D. (1972, October). *Anatomy—destiny or damnation?* Unpublished term paper, University of Wisconsin, Madison.

Bird, C. (1968). *Born female*. New York: David McKay Co.

Birdwhistell, R. L. (1949). Social science and nursing education; Some tentative suggestions. *Fifty-Fifth Annual Report of the National League of Nursing Education* (pp. 316–328). New York: Livingston Press.

Blancett, S. S. (1989, December). Editorial. She is a man: Avoiding sexist language. *Journal of Nursing Administration*, *19*(12), 5.

Blassingame, W. (1967). *Combat nurses of World War II*. New York: Random House.

Blum, L. C. (1989–90, Winter). The story of the Vietnam Women's Memorial. *Professional Nurses Quarterly, 4*(4), 1, 6, 9, 12.

Boyd, L. C. (1908, November). The suffrage—another view. *American Journal of Nursing, 9,* 135–136.

Boyd, N. (1982). *Three Victorian women who changed their world: Josephine Butler, Octavia Hill, Florence Nightingale.* New York: Oxford University Press.

Brand, K. L., & Glass, L. K. (1975). Perils and parallels of women and nursing. *Nursing Forum, 14*(2), 160–174.

Brittain, V. (1947). *Testament of friendship: The story of Winifred Holtby.* London: Macmillan.

Brook, M. J. (1990). Some thoughts and reflections on the life of Florence Nightingale from a twentieth century perspective. In V. Bullough, B. Bullough, & M. P. Stanton (Eds.), *Florence Nightingale and her era: A collection of new scholarship* (pp. 23–39). New York: Garland Publishing, Inc.

Broverman, I. K., Broverman, D. M., Clarkson, F. E., Rosenkrantz, P. S., & Vogel, S. R. (1970). Sex role stereotypes and clinical judgments of mental health professionals. *Journal of Consulting and Clinical Psychology, 34*(1), 1–7.

Bullough, B. (1976). Nurses in American history: The lasting impact of World War II on nursing. *American Journal of Nursing, 76*(1), 118–120.

Bullough, V. (1983–1984, Winter). Nurses who had a significant impact upon society: Emma Goldman. *Bulletin: American Association for the History of Nursing, 4,* 4.

Bullough, V., & Bullough, B. (1978). *The care of the sick: The emergence of modern nursing.* New York: Prodist.

Bullough, V., & Bullough, B. (1984). *History, trends, and politics of nursing.* Norwalk, CN: Appleton-Century-Crofts.

Bullough, V., Bullough, B., & Stanton, M. P. (Eds.). (1990). *Florence Nightingale and her era: A collection of new scholarship.* New York: Garland Publishing, Inc.

Calhoun, J. (1993, March). The Nightingale Pledge: A commitment that survives the passage of time. *Nursing and Health Care, 14*(3), 130–136.

Campbell, J. (1981). Misogyny and homicide of women. *Advances in Nursing Science, 3*(2), 67–85.

Campbell, M. A. (1974). *Why should a girl go into medicine?* Old Westbury, NY: The Feminist Press.

Campbell-Heider, N. (1986). Do nurses need mentors? *Image, 18*(3), 110–113.

Carnegie, M. E. (1962). The path we tread. *International Nursing Review, 9*(5), 25–33.

Chalich, T., & Smith, L. (1992, April). Nursing at the grassroots. *Nursing & Health Care, 13*(5), 242–244.

Chinn, P. L. (1985). Historical roots: Female nurses and political action. *Journal of the New York State Nurses Association, 16*(2), 29–37.

Chinn, P. L., & Wheeler, C. E. (1983). Report of the gathering. *Cassandra: Radical Feminist Nurses News Journal, 1*(3), 4–11.

Chinn, P. L., & Wheeler, C. E. (1985). Feminism and nursing. *Nursing Outlook, 33*(2), 74–77.

Christy, K. A. (1987, April). Networks: Forming "Old Girl" connections among nurses. *Nursing Management, 18*(4), 73–75.

Christy, M. (1987, Spring). Letter from a World War I nurse, 1919. *Bulletin of the American Association for the History of Nursing,* (14), 7–8.

Christy, T. E. (1969). Portrait of a leader: Lavinia Lloyd Dock. *Nursing Outlook, 17*(6), 72–75.

Christy, T. E. (1969). Portrait of a leader: M. Adelaide Nutting. *Nursing Outlook, 17*(1), 20–24.

Christy, T. E. (1970). Portrait of a leader: Lillian D. Wald. *Nursing Outlook, 18*(3), 50–54.

Christy, T. E. (1971). Equal rights for women: Voices from the past. *American Journal of Nursing, 71*(2), 288–293.

Christy, T. E., Stein, L. I., & Wolf, C. (1972). AORN Congress Presentation —Liberation movement: Impact on nursing. *AORN Journal, 15*(4), 67–85.

Cleland, V. S. (1971). Sex discrimination: Nursing's most pervasive problem. *American Journal of Nursing, 71*(8), 1542–1547.

Cleland, V. S. (1974). To end sex discrimination. *Nursing Clinics of North America, 9*(3), 563–571.

Clemons, B. (1971). Women's liberation and nursing: Historic interplay. *Journal of the Association of Operating Room Nurses, 13*(6), 71–72, 74, 77–78.

Cominos, P. T. (1972). Innocent femina sensualis in unconscious conflict. In *Suffer and be still* (pp. 163–164). Bloomington: Indiana University Press.

Cook, B. W. (1977). Female support networks and political activism: Lillian Wald, Crystal Eastman, Emma Goldman. *Chrysalis, 3,* 43–61.

Cook, E. (1913–1914). *A short life of Florence Nightingale.* London: Macmillan. `

Cooper, P. (1946). *Navy nurse.* New York: McGraw-Hill.

Cordua, G. D., McGraw, K. O., & Drabman, R. S. (1978, March). *Preschool children's perceptions of atypical sex roles.* Paper presented at the meeting of the Southwestern Society for Human Development, Dallas, TX.

Cordua, G. D., McGraw, K. O., & Drabman, R. S. (1979). Doctor or nurse: Children's perception of sex typed occupations. *Child Development, 50,* 590–593.

Corea, G. (1985). *The hidden malpractice: How American medicine mistreats women.* New York: Harper & Row.

Coss, C. (Ed.). (1989). *Lillian D. Wald: Progressive activist*. New York: The Feminist Press at the City University of New York.

Cowan, B. (1977). *Women's health care*. Ann Arbor, MI: Anshen.

Coyle, B. J. (1989, April). Women on the front lines. *Proceedings*, 37–40.

Creighton, H. (1971, November). The expensive practice of sex discrimination. *Supervisor Nurse, 71*(11), 14–15.

Curtis, A. (1836). *Lectures on midwifery and forms of disease peculiar to women and children*. Delivered to the members of the Botanico-Medical School at Columbus, OH. Columbus, OH: Jonathan Phillips.

Curtiss, J. S. (1966). Russian Sisters of Mercy in the Crimea, 1854–1855. *Slavic Review, 25*(1), 84–100.

Curtiss, J. S. (1968). Russian Nightingale. *American Journal of Nursing, 68*(5), 1029–1031.

Dains, J. E. (Ed.). (1984). An act of betrayal. *Update, 10*(3), 20A–21A.

Daly, M. (1980). *Woman, church and state: The original exposé of male collaboration against the female sex.* Watertown, MA: Persephone Press.

Daniels, D. (1976). *Lillian D. Wald: The progressive woman and feminism*. Unpublished doctoral dissertation, The City University of New York, New York.

Daniels, D. (1989). *Always a sister: The feminism of Lillian D. Wald*. New York: The Feminist Press at the City University of New York.

David, O. D. (1962). Anticipating the future for students and teachers in nursing: Concepts about women are changing. *American Journal of Nursing, 62*(12), 82–84.

de Castillejo, I. C. (1973). *Knowing women: A feminine psychology*. New York: Harper & Row.

Dickson, B. L. (1909). The suffrage (President Roosevelt's letter). *American Journal of Nursing, 9*(5), 360–361.

Dixon, M. B. (1908a, October). A criticism of the editor. *American Journal of Nursing, 9*, 48–49.

Dixon, M. B. (1908b, October). "Votes for women." *Nurses' Journal of the Pacific Coast, 4*, 442–447.

Dock, L. L. (1904). The duty of this society in public work. In *Proceedings of the Tenth Annual Convention of the American Society of Superintendents of Training Schools*, October 7–9, 1903. Baltimore: J. H. Furst Co.

Dock, L. L. (1907, August). Some urgent social claims. *American Journal of Nursing, 7*, 895–905.

Dock, L. L. (1908a, August). The suffrage question. *American Journal of Nursing, 8*, 925–926.

Dock, L. L. (1908b, August). A letter to the editor. *Nurses' Journal of the Pacific Coast, 366*.

Dock, L. L. (1909, May). The relation of the nursing profession to the woman movement. *Nurses' Journal of the Pacific Coast, 5*, 197–201.

Dock, L. L. (1915). The Foreign Department: A woman's peace party. *American Journal of Nursing, 15*, 665–667.

Dock, L. L. (1916, October). The Foreign Department: War and nurses. *American Journal of Nursing, 17*, 58–59.

Dock, L. L. (1922, December). The Foreign Department: War and nurses. *American Journal of Nursing, 23*, 209.

Dock, L. L. (1923, March). The Foreign Department: War and nurses. *American Journal of Nursing, 23*, 493.

Dock, L. L. (1924). Equal rights. *American Journal of Nursing, 24*(10), 834.

Dock, L. L. (1929, July). Editorial: 1899–July 1929. *The ICN, 4*(3), 14.

Dock, L. L. (1977). Lavinia L. Dock: Self-portrait—July 6, 1932. *Nursing Outlook, 25*(1), 22–26.

Doering, L. (1992). Power and knowledge in nursing: A feminist poststructuralist view. *Advances in Nursing Science, 14*(4), 24–33.

Drabman, R. S., Robertson, S., Cordua, G., Jarvie, G. J., & Hammer, D. (1977, May). *Children's perception of media portrayed sex roles*. Paper presented at the meeting of the Southeastern Psychological Association, Hollywood, FL.

Duffus, R. L. (1938). *Lillian Wald: Neighbor and crusader*. New York: Macmillan.

Earley, P. (1982). Nurses haunted by memories of service in Vietnam. *The American Nurse, 14*(2), 8.

East, C. (1969). What do women want? *The Catholic Nurse, 18*(1), 38–45, 60.

Edelstein, R. G. (1971). Equal rights for women: Perspectives. *American Journal of Nursing, 71*(2), 294–298.

Editor. (1909, January). Again the "woman question." *Nurses' Journal of the Pacific Coast, 5*, 2–4.

Editorial. (1971). Letter to probationers by Florence Nightingale. *International Nursing Review, 18*(1), 3–5.

Editorial. (1988, January/February). Forgotten soldiers. *AD Nurse, 3*(1), 6–8.

Editorial Comment. (1913). Isabel McIsaac, nurses in suffrage parade. *American Journal of Nursing, 13*(7), 489–497.

Editors. (1924). The Lucretia Mott Amendment. *Public Health Nurse, 16*(3), 135–136.

Edwards, J. B., & Lenz, C. L. (1990, Fall). The influence of gender on communication for nurse leaders. *Nursing Administration Quarterly, 15*(1), 49–55.

Ehrenreich, B., & English, D. (1972). *Witches, midwives, and nurses*. Old Westbury, NY: The Feminist Press.

Ehrenreich, B., & English, D. (1973). *Complaints and disorders: The sexual politics of sickness*. Old Westbury, NY: The Feminist Press.

Ehrenreich, B., & English, D. (1978). *For her own good: 150 years of the experts' advice to women*. Garden City, NY: Anchor Press/Doubleday.

Elmore, J. A. (1976). Black nurses: Their service and their struggle. *American Journal of Nursing, 76*(3), 435–437.

Enloe, C. (1983). *Does khaki become you? The militarization of women's lives.* Boston: South End Press.

Evans, D. (1989–90, Winter). Memorial project founder addresses its healing power. *Professional Nurses Quarterly, 4*(4), 2.

Fagan, M. M., & Fagan, P. D. (1983, February). Mentoring among nurses. *Nursing & Health Care, 4,* 77–82.

Fagin, C. M. (1975). Nurses' rights. *American Journal of Nursing, 75*(1), 82–85.

Fagin, C. M. (1978, December). Knowledge is power—professional and political. *Journal of the New York State Nurses Association, 9*(4), 10–16.

Fagin, C. M. (1981). *Nursing's pivotal role in achieving competition in health care.* Keynote address: American Academy of Nursing, September 21, 1981. Washington, DC.

Fagin, C. M., & Diers, D. (1983). Nursing as metaphor. *The New England Journal of Medicine, 309*(2), 116–117.

Faludi, S. (1991). *Backlash: The undeclared war against American women.* New York: Crown.

Fee, E. (1983). *Women and health: The politics of sex in medicine.* Farmingdale, NY: Baywood.

Feinman, C. (1992). *The criminalization of a woman's body.* Binghamton, NY: The Haworth Press.

Fenwick, E. G. (1917). Congratulations to our American cousins. *British Journal of Nursing, 59*(1,547), 342, 344.

Fenwick, E. G. (1918). The King's assent. *British Journal of Nursing, 60*(1,559), 107.

Firestone, S. (1971). *Dialectic of sex: The case for feminist revolution.* New York: Bantam Books.

Fisher, S. (1986). *In the patient's best interest.* New Brunswick, NJ: Rutgers University Press.

Fishwick, M. W. (1966). *Illustrious Americans: Clara Barton.* Morristown, NJ: Silver Burdett Co.

Forsythe, P. (1971, November). Letter to the editor. *American Journal of Nursing, 71*(11), 2112.

Frankfort, E. (1972). *Vaginal politics.* New York: Quadrangle.

Freidan, B. (1963). *The feminine mystique.* New York: W. W. Norton.

Freund, C. (1985). The tenure of nursing service administrators. *Journal of Nursing Administration, 15*(2), 11–15.

Gage, M. J. (1896). *Woman, church and state.* Chicago: Charles H. Kerr & Co.

Gass, G. Z. (1967). Identity: A contemporary problem for women. *The university in motion: Status of women,* Bevier Lecture Series, 1967. Urbana, IL: University of Illinois Press.

Gerbner, G., Gross, L., Morgan, M., & Signorielli, N. (1981). Health and medicine on television. *New England Journal of Medicine, 305*(15), 901–904.

Gerds, G. (1963). The status of women today and its effect on nursing. *American Journal of Nursing, 63*(11), 70–73.

Gilgannon, Sr. M. M. (1962). *The Sisters of Mercy as Crimean War nurses.* Unpublished doctoral dissertation, University of Notre Dame, Notre Dame, IN.

Golick, T. (1971). The amendment: Do women need it? *American Journal of Nursing, 71*(2), 285–287.

Greenleaf, N. P. (1982). The politics of self-esteem. In E. C. Hein & M. J. Nicholson (Eds.), *Contemporary leadership behavior: Selected readings* (pp. 91–102). Boston: Little, Brown & Co. (reprinted from *Nursing Digest, 6*(3), 1978).

Greer, G. (1971). *The female eunuch.* New York: McGraw-Hill.

Grissum, M. (1976). How you can become a risk taker and a role breaker. *Nursing '76, 6*(11), 89–98.

Grissum, M., & Spengler, C. (1976). *Womanpower and health care.* Boston: Little, Brown & Co.

Group, T. M., & Roberts, J. I. *Nurses as caregivers at work and at home.* Publication pending.

Guyot, H. (1962). The nurse in Civil War literature. *Nursing Outlook, 10*(5), 311–314.

Hagell, E. I. (1989). Nursing knowledge: Women's knowledge. A sociological perspective. *Journal of Advanced Nursing, 14,* 226–233.

Hagerty, B. (1986). A second look at mentors. *Nursing Outlook, 34*(1), 16–24.

Halperin, J. (1980). Eminent Victorians and history. *The Virginia Quarterly Review,* 433–441.

Hanley, B. E. (1987). Political participation: How do nurses compare with other professional women? *Nursing Economics, 5*(4), 179–188.

Harrison, J. K., & Roth, P. A. (1987). Empowering nursing in multihospital systems. *Nursing Economics, 5*(2), 70–76.

Harty, M. B. (1976). Change by design rather than by default. *American Journal of Medical Technology, 43*(2), 173–176.

Hawkins, J. W., & Matthews, I. (1991, Fall). "Tugboat Annie": Nursing's hero of Pearl Harbor—Grace Lally (1897–1983). *Image: Journal of Nursing Scholarship, 23*(3), 183–185.

Heide, W. S. (1971, May/June). Women's liberation means putting nurses and nursing in its place! *Imprint, 18,* 4–5, 16.

Heide, W. S. (1973, May). Nursing and women's liberation: A parallel. *American Journal of Nursing, 73,* 824–827.

Heide, W. S. (1983). Personal letter to Joan I. Roberts.

Henderson, E. (1988, July/August). Interview: Dr. Peggy Chinn. *Newsletter, Alberta Association of Registered Nurses, 44*(7), 7–9.

Henle, E. L. (1978). Clara Barton, soldier or pacifist? *Civil War History, 24,* 152–160.

Hennig, M., & Jardim, A. (1976). *The managerial woman.* New York: Doubleday & Co.

Henry, S. (1992, Summer). Exclusive *Revolution* interview with Susan Faludi. *Revolution, 2*(2), 39–45, 134.

Hickson, D., Hinings, C., Lee, C., Schneck, R., & Pennings, J. (1971). A strategic contingencies' theory of organizational power. *Administrative Science Quarterly, 16,* 216–229.

Hine, D. C. (1988). "They Shall Mount Up With Wings as Eagles": Historical images of black nurses, 1890–1950. In A. H. Jones (Ed.), *Images of nurses: Perspectives from history, art, and literature* (pp. 177–195). Philadelphia: University of Pennsylvania Press.

Hoffman, M. S. (1970). The modern woman and the modern world. *Occupational Health Nursing, 18*(12), 16–17.

Holman, N. K. (1908, November). The suffrage. *American Journal of Nursing, 9,* 135.

Holroyd, M. (1980). *Lytton Strachey: A biography.* Middlesex, England: Penguin Books.

Horner, M. (1969, November). Why women want to fail. *Psychology Today, 6,* 36–38, 62.

Hott, J. R. (1976). The struggles inside nursing's body politic. *Nursing Forum, 15*(4), 325–340.

Hott, J. R. (1984). To see ourselves as others see us. *Imprint, 31*(1), 45–48.

Howe, J. W. (1909). Woman and the suffrage. *American Journal of Nursing, 9*(8), 559–566.

Hughes, L. (1980). The public image of the nurse. *Advances in Nursing Science, 2*(3), 55–72.

Hughes, L. (1982). Little girls grow up to be wives and mommies: Nursing as a stopgap to marriage. In J. Muff (Ed.), *Socialization, sexism, and stereotyping: Women's issues in nursing.* St. Louis: C. V. Mosby.

Iafolla, M. C. (1965). The dilemma of women leaders. *Nursing Forum, 4*(2), 54–67.

James, J. W. (1985). Biographical introduction. In J. W. James (Ed.), *A Lavinia Dock reader* (pp. vii–xix). New York: Garland Publishers, Inc.

Jezierski, M. (1987, March/April). Vietnam Women's Memorial project: Donna Marie Boulay highlights women's wartime roles. *Journal of Emergency Nursing, 13*(2), 122–124.

Johnston, M. (1911). The reason why. *American Journal of Nursing, 12*(1), 76–77.

Jolly, E. R. (1927). *Nuns of the battlefield*. Providence, RI: Providence Visitor Press.

Josefowitz, N. (1982). Management men and women: Closed vs. open doors. In D. Hampton (Ed.), *Organizational behavior and the practice of management* (pp. 223–227). Glenview, IL: Scott Foresman & Co.

Kaler, S. R., Levy, D. A., & Schall, M. (1989). Stereotypes of professional roles. *Image, 21*(2), 9, 85–89.

Kalisch, B. J., & Kalisch, P. A. (1976). A discourse on the politics of nursing. *Journal of Nursing Administration, 6*(3), 29–34.

Kalisch, B. J., & Kalisch, P. A. (1976). Nurses in American history: The Cadet Nurse Corps—in World War II. *American Journal of Nursing, 76*(2), 240–242.

Kalisch, B. J., & Kalisch, P. A. (1980). Perspectives on improving nursing's public image. *Nursing and Health Care, 1*(1), 10–15.

Kalisch, B. J., & Kalisch, P. A. (1982). *Politics of nursing*. Philadelphia: J. B. Lippincott.

Kalisch, B. J., & Kalisch, P. A. (1982a). Nurses on prime time television. *American Journal of Nursing, 82*(2), 264–279.

Kalisch, B. J., & Kalisch, P. A. (1982b). *The image of the nurse in the mass media*. Paper presented at the Region Five Assembly, Sigma Theta Tau, Garden City, NY.

Kalisch, B. J., & Kalisch, P. A. (1983a, April). Heroine out of focus: Media images of Florence Nightingale, Part 1. *Nursing and Health Care*, 181–187.

Kalisch, B. J., & Kalisch, P. A. (1983b, May). Heroine out of focus: Media images of Florence Nightingale, Part 2. *Nursing and Health Care*, 270–278.

Kalisch, B. J., & Kalisch, P. A. (1983c). Improving the image of nursing. *American Journal of Nursing, 83*(1), 48–52.

Kalisch, B. J., & Kalisch, P. A. (1983d). *Images of nurses on television*. New York: Springer Publishing.

Kalisch, B. J., Kalisch, P. A., & McHugh, M. L. (1982). The nurse as a sex object in motion pictures, 1930 to 1980. *Research in Nursing and Health, 5*, 147–154.

Kalisch, B. J., Kalisch, P. A., & Scoby, M. (1981). Reflections on a television image. *Nursing and Health Care, 2*(5), 248–255.

Kalisch, P. A. (1975). Heroines of '98: Female army nurses in the Spanish-American War. *Nursing Research, 24*(6), 411–429.

Kalisch, P. A. (1976). How army nurses became officers. *Nursing Research, 25*(3), 164–177.

Kanter, R. M. (1979). *Men and women of the corporation*. New York: Basic Books.

Kelly, D. N. (Ed.). (1963). The status of women. *The Catholic Nurse, 12*(2), 16–17.

Kelly, D. N. (Ed.). (1965). Women—Our favorite subject. *The Catholic Nurse, 13*(3), 16–17.

Kelly, L. Y. (1976). Our nursing heritage: Have we renounced it? *Image, 8,* 43–48.

Kippinbrock, T. A. (1992, April). Wish I'd been there: A sense of nursing history. *Nursing & Health Care, 12*(4), 208–212.

Kirkland-Casgrain, C. (1965). Women must be worthy of their freedom. *The Canadian Nurse, 61*(7), 527–528.

Kjervik, D. K., & Martinson, I. M. (1979). *Women in stress.* New York: Appleton-Century-Crofts.

Kjervik, D. K., & Martinson, I. M. (1986). *Women in health and illness.* Philadelphia, PA: Saunders.

Kramer, M. (1974). *Reality shock: Why nurses leave nursing.* St. Louis: C. V. Mosby.

Kritek, P. B. (1991). Editorial. *Nursing Forum, 26*(4), 3–4.

Krueger, J. C. (1980). Women in management: An assessment. *Nursing Outlook, 28*(6), 374–378.

Lamb, K. T. (1973). Freedom for our sister, freedom for ourselves: Nursing confronts social change. *Nursing Forum, 12*(4), 328–351.

Larsen, J. (1982). Nurse power for the 1980s. *Nursing Administration Quarterly, 6*(4), 74–82.

Leininger, M. (1974). The leadership crisis in nursing. *Journal of Nursing Administration, 4*(2), 29–34.

Leininger, M. (1981). Woman's role in society in the 1980s. *Issues in Health Care of Women, 3*(4), 203–215.

Leone, L. P. (1987). The U.S. Cadet Nurse Corps: Nursing's answer to World War II demands. *NSNA/Imprint, 34*(5), 46–48.

Leopard, D. (1984, Spring). The Army Nurse Corps and women in the military: World War II. *Bulletin: American Association for the History of Nursing, 5,* 4.

Letters to the Editor. (1988). *Image: Journal of Nursing Scholarship, 20*(3), 176–177.

Lewenson, S. B. (1990). The woman's nursing and suffrage movement, 1893–1920. In V. Bullough, B. Bullough, & M. P. Stanton (Eds.), *Florence Nightingale and her era: A collection of new scholarship* (pp. 123–137). New York: Garland Publishing, Inc.

Lewenson, S. B. (1991, Summer). Historian's corner: Lavinia Dock's T. C. connection. *Courier,* (58), 10–11.

Lewin, E. (1985). *Women, health, and healing.* London: Tavistock.

Lindabury, V. A. (Ed.). (1971). A look at the Francis Report on the status of women in Canada. *The Canadian Nurse, 67*(2), 25–26.

Lindeman, C., & Moccia, P. (1994, January). President's message: To the members and friends of the National League for Nursing. *Nursing & Health Care, 15*(1), 39–40.

Livingston, J. A., & Rankin, J. M. (1986). Propping up the patriarchy: The silenced soldiering of military nurses. In a woman's recovery from the trauma of war. *Women and Therapy*, *5*(1), 107–119.

Lopate, C. (1968). *Women in medicine*. Maryland: The Johns Hopkins Press.

Lorber, J. (1984). *Women physicians: Careers, status, and power*. New York: Tavistock Publications.

Mapanga, M. (1985). Women and the media. *Nursing Mirror*, *161*(8), 1, 6–7.

Marieskind, H. I. (1980). *Women in the health delivery system: Patients, providers and programs*. St. Louis: C. V. Mosby.

Marshall, M. L. (1957, July). Nurse heroines of the Confederacy. *Bulletin of the Medical Library Association*, *45*, 334–335.

McBride, A., Diers, D., Slavinsky, A., Schlotfeldt, R., Christman, L., & Kibrick, A. (1972). Leadership: Problems and possibilities in nursing. *American Journal of Nursing*, *72*(8), 1445–1456.

McCarthy, P. A. (1981, June). Old Vegas and other anachronisms. *Nursing Outlook*, *347*.

McClelland, D. (1953). *The achievement motive*. New York: Appleton-Century-Crofts.

McVicker, S. J. (1985). Invisible veterans: The women who served in Vietnam. *Journal of Psychosocial Nursing*, *23*(10), 13–19.

Meehan, J. (1994, January). *The American Nurse*, *26*(1), 1, 3.

Melosh, B. (1983). Doctors, patients, and "big nurse": Work and gender in the postwar hospital. In E. C. Lagemann (Ed.), *Nursing history: New perspectives, new possibilities* (pp. 164–179). New York: Teachers College Press.

Mendelsohn, R. S. (1982). *Malepractice: How doctors manipulate women*. Chicago: Contemporary Books.

Milauskas, J. (1985). Will nursing assert itself? *Nursing Administration Quarterly*, *9*(3), 1–15.

Mill, H. T. (1851, July). Enfranchisement of women. *Westminster Review*, *60*, 150–161.

Mill, J. S. (1869). *The subjection of women*. Bungay, Suffolk: Richard Clay, Ltd.

Millett, K. (1970). *Sexual politics*. New York: Doubleday & Co.

Monteiro, L. A. (1978). Lavinia L. Dock (1947) on nurses and the Cold War. *Nursing Forum*, *17*(1), 46–54.

Monteiro, L. A. (1984). On separate roads: Florence Nightingale and Elizabeth Blackwell. *Signs: Journal of Women in Culture and Society*, *9*(3), 520–533.

Monteiro, L. A. (1990). Nightingale and her correspondents: Portrait of the era. In V. Bullough, B. Bullough, & M. P. Stanton (Eds.), *Florence Nightingale and her era: A collection of new scholarship* (pp. 40–59). New York: Garland Publishing, Inc.

Monteiro, L. A. (1991, Winter). The Nightingale myth continues. *Bulletin: American Association for the History of Nursing, 29*, 5–6.

More, M. T. (1971). A woman's right to nag—inalienable and essential. *The Canadian Nurse, 67*(9), 38–40.

Muff, J. (1982). Handmaiden, battle-ax, whore: An exploration into the fantasies, myths, and stereotypes about nurses. In J. Muff (Ed.), *Socialization, sexism, and stereotyping: Women's issues in nursing*. St. Louis: C. V. Mosby.

Muff, J. (1982). *Socialization, sexism, and stereotyping: Women's issues in nursing*. St. Louis: C. V. Mosby.

Muff, J. (1984). A look at images in nursing. *Imprint, 31*(1), 41–44.

Muff, J. (1988). Of images and ideals: A look at socialization and sexism in nursing. In A. H. Jones (Ed.), *Images of nurses: Perspectives from history, art and literature* (pp. 197–220). Philadelphia: University of Pennsylvania Press.

Mullane, M. K. (1970). Women and their role in shaping society. *Occupational Health Nursing, 18*(6), 7–9.

Muller, H. J., & Cocotas, C. (1988). Women in power: New leadership in the health industry. *Health Care for Women International, 9*(2), 63–82.

The Nation's Health. (1994, January). Essential providers gain seat at health reform table, 1, 12.

National Park Service. (1987). *Clara Barton*. Washington, DC: U.S. Government Printing Office.

Nauright, L. (1984). Politics and power: A new look at Florence Nightingale. *Nursing Forum, 21*(1), 5–8.

Nelson, J. (1976). Florence, the legend. *Nursing Mirror, 142*(20), 40–41.

Newcomb, E. (1945). *Brave nurse*. New York: Appleton-Century-Crofts.

Newton, L. H. (1981). In defense of the traditional nurse. *Nursing Outlook, 29*, 348–354.

Nightingale, F. (1858). *Subsidiary notes as to the introduction of female nursing into military hospitals in peace and war*. London: Harrison & Sons.

Nightingale, F. (1860). *Suggestions for thought to seekers after religious truth*. Privately printed by Eyre & Spottiswoode, London.

Nightingale, F. (1871). *Introductory notes on lying-in institutions. Together with a proposal for organizing an institution for training midwives and midwifery nurses*. London: Longmans, Green.

Nightingale, F. (1888, May 16). Letter to the probationer nurses in the Nightingale Fund School at St. Thomas' Hospital. London. Reprinted in *International Nursing Review*, 1971, p. 4.

Nightingale, F. (1928). Cassandra. In R. Strachey (Ed.), *"The cause": A short history of the women's movement in Great Britain* (pp. 395–418). London: G. Bell & Sons, Ltd.

Nightingale, F. (1980). Concluding thoughts. In F. Nightingale, *Notes on nursing: What it is and what it is not* (pp. 108–112). Edinburgh, London, & New York: Churchill Livingstone. (First published London: Harrison & Sons, 1859).

NLN Public Policy Bulletin. (1991).

Nursing Outlook. (1981, September). Letters to the editor. Storm over Old Vegas, 492–493.

Nutting, M. A. (1908, November). The suffrage. *American Journal of Nursing*, 9, 134–135.

Nutting, M. A., & Dock, L. L. (1907). *A history of nursing*, Vols. 1–4. New York: Putnam.

O'Connor, L. (1968, June). Women: Their own worst enemies. *The Catholic Nurse*, 16, 26–35, 68–69.

On Campus with Women. (1986, Spring). 15(4).

Palmer, I. S. (1976). Florence Nightingale and the Salisbury Incident. *Nursing Research*, 25(5), 370–377.

Palmer, I. S. (1983a). Nightingale revisited. *Nursing Outlook*, 31(4), 229–233.

Palmer, I. S. (1983b). Florence Nightingale: The myth and the reality. *Nursing Times*, Occasional Papers, 79(20), 40–42.

Palmer, S. F. (1908, October). Editor's response. *American Journal of Nursing*, 9, 49–50.

Parsons, M. E. (1983). Mothers and matrons. *Nursing Outlook*, 31(5), 274–278.

Pearce, E. C. (1954, April). The influence of Florence Nightingale on the spirit of nursing. *International Nursing Review*, 1, 20–22.

Peplau, H. E. (1976). A time to stand up and be counted. In L. Flanagan (Ed.), *One strong voice: The story of the American Nurses' Association* (pp. 589–592). Kansas City, MO: American Nurses' Association.

Petersen, A. (1942, August). The nurse's fight for military rank. *The Trained Nurse and Hospital Review*, 98–100.

Phelps, E. S. (1897). *Chapters from a life*. Boston & New York: Ayer Co., Publishers.

Pickering, G. (1974). *Creative malady*. New York: Dell Publishing Co.

Pogrebin, L. C. (1987). *Among friends: Who we like, why we like them, and what we do with them*. New York: McGraw-Hill.

Pollard, T. (1989). Profiles: Mother Mary Francis Clare, CSJP. In U. Stepsis & D. Liptak (Eds.), *Pioneer healers* (pp. 212–217). New York: Crossroad.

Poslusny, S. M. (1989). Feminist friendship: Isabel Hampton Robb, Lavinia Lloyd Dock and Mary Adelaide Nutting. *Image*, 21(2), 64–68.

Powell, D. J. (1976). The struggles outside nursing's body politic. *Nursing Forum*, 15(4), 341–362.

Pryor, E. B. (1987). *Clara Barton: Professional angel*. Philadelphia: University of Pennsylvania Press.

Pugh, E. L. (1982). Florence Nightingale and J. S. Mill debate women's rights. *Journal of British Studies*, *21*(2), 118–138.

Raymond, J. (1986). *A passion for friends: Toward a philosophy of female affection*. Boston: Beacon Press.

Reavill, N. (1976). Professionally speaking: Free to be. *Maternal-Child Nursing*, *1*(2), 55–57, 60–62.

Resnick, A. (1974). Lillian Wald: The years at Henry Street (Doctoral dissertation, University of Wisconsin, 1973). *Dissertation Abstracts International*, *35*, 01A, 382A.

Reverby, S. (1987a). A caring dilemma: Womanhood and nursing in historical perspective. *Nursing Research*, *36*(1), 5–11.

Reverby, S. (1987b). *Ordered to care: The dilemma of American nursing, 1850–1945*. Cambridge, MA: Cambridge University Press.

Richter, L., & Richter, E. (1974). Nurses in fiction. *American Journal of Nursing*, *74*(7), 1280–1281.

Riegler, N. N. (1990). Lytton Strachey's biography of Florence Nightingale: A good read, a poor reference. In V. Bullough, B. Bullough, & M. P. Stanton (Eds.), *Florence Nightingale and her era: A collection of new scholarship* (pp. 60–74). New York: Garland Publishing, Inc.

Roberts, H. (1992). *Women's health matters*. New York: Routledge.

Roberts, J. I. (1994). *Leaving visions that transcend what is: A tribute to Wilma Scott Heide, feminist, activist, and nurse*. Unpublished manuscript.

Roberts, J. I., & Group, T. M. *Gender and the nurse-physician game*. Publication pending.

Roberts, J. I., & Group, T. M. *Nursing, physician control, and medical monopoly*. Publication pending.

Roberts, J. I., & Group, T. M. (1973). The women's movement and nursing. *Nursing Forum*, *12*(3), 303–322.

Roberts, M. M. (1956). Lavinia Lloyd Dock—nurse, feminist, internationalist. *American Journal of Nursing*, *56*(2), 176–179.

Roberts, S. J. (1983). Oppressed group behavior: Implications for nursing. *Advances in Nursing Science*, *5*(4), 21–30.

Roberts, S. J. (1994). Oppressed group behavior: Implications for nursing. *Revolution—Journal of Nurse Empowerment*, *4*(3), 28–35.

Rogge, M. M. (1987). Nursing and politics: A forgotten legacy. *Nursing Research*, *36*(1), 26–30.

Rothblum, E. D., & Cole, E. (Eds.). (1986). Ruth: A case description. *Women and Therapy*, *5*(1), 7–11.

Ruffing-Rahal, M. (1986). Margaret Sanger: Nurse and feminist. *Nursing Outlook*, *34*(5), 246–249.

Ruzek, S. B. (1978). *The women's health movement: Feminist alternatives to medical control*. New York: Praeger Publishers.

Safford, A. M. (1909). The suffrage. *American Journal of Nursing*, *9*(5), 359–360.

Safier, G. (1977). *Contemporary American leaders in nursing: An oral history*. New York: McGraw-Hill.

Salvage, J. (1983, January). Distorted images. *Nursing Times*, 13–15.

Sandelowski, M. (1980). *Women, health and choice*. St. Louis: C. V. Mosby.

Sandelowski, M. (1981). Women in nursing. In *Women, health, and choice* (pp. 158–174). Englewood Cliffs, NJ: Prentice Hall.

Sanders, B. H. (1956). Are we equal to our future? *The Canadian Nurse*, *52*(10), 781–785.

Sanger, M. (1920). *Woman and the new race*. New York: Truth Publishing Co.

Sanger, M. (1971). *Margaret Sanger: An autobiography*. New York: Dover Publications, Inc.

Sargent, A. G. (1973). Fourth world issues and beyond. *Supervisor Nurse*, *4*(8), 16–17, 20–21, 25.

Sargent, A. G. (1979, March). The androgynous manager. *Supervisor Nurse*, *10*, 23–30.

Schaefer, M. J. (1973). The political and economic scene in the future of nursing. *American Journal of Public Health*, *63*(10), 887–889.

Schorr, T. (1981). Nursing's leaders: An endangered species. *American Journal of Nursing*, *81*(2), 313.

Schwartz, L. S. (1987). Women and the Vietnam experience. *Image*, *19*(4), 168–173.

Seaman, B. (1972). *Free and female*. New York: Coward.

Seigel, H. (1984). Up the down staircase in nursing education: An analysis of the nurse educator as a professional. *Journal of Nursing Education*, *23*(3), 114–117.

Selavan, I. C. (1975). Nurses in American history: The Revolution. *American Journal of Nursing*, *75*(4), 592–594.

Seltzer, M. (1991, September). A nurse in the sand: Letters home. *Nursing & Health Care*, *12*(7), 372–375.

Shockley, J. S. (1974). Perspectives in femininity: Implications for nursing. *Journal of Obstetric, Gynecologic, and Neonatal Nursing*, *3*(6), 36–40.

Showalter, E. (1981). Florence Nightingale's feminist complaint: Women, religion, and *Suggestions for Thought*. *Signs: Journal of Women in Culture and Society*, *6*(3), 395–412.

Sicherman, B., & Green, C. H. (1981). *Notable American women: The modern period*. Cambridge, MA: Harvard University Press.

Siegel, B. (1983). *Lillian Wald of Henry Street*. New York: Macmillan.

Skeet, M. (1980). *Notes on nursing: The science and the art*. London: Churchill Livingstone.

Slater, V. E. (1994). The educational and philosophical influences on Florence Nightingale, an enlightened conductor. *Nursing History Review*, *2*, 137–152.

Smith, F. A. (1977). Personal and professional objectives for change. *Occupational Health Nursing, 25,* 18–20.

Smith, F. B. (1982). *Florence Nightingale: Reputation and power.* New York: St. Martin's Press.

Smith, F. T. (1981, May). Florence Nightingale: Early feminist. *American Journal of Nursing, 81*(5), 1021–1024.

Smoyak, S. A. (1974). The changing role of nursing today. *Occupational Health Nursing, 22*(10), 9–13.

Smoyak, S. A. (1982). Women/nurses in 1982: How are we doing? *Occupational Health Nursing, 30*(7), 9–13, 45.

Speedy, S. C. (1987). Feminism and the professionalization of nursing. *Australian Journal of Advanced Nursing, 4*(2), 20–28.

Spender, D. (1980). *Man made language.* London: Routledge & Kegan Paul.

Spender, D. (1983). *Women of ideas.* Boston: Routledge & Kegan Paul.

Spengler, C. D. (1982). *Mentor-protege relationships: A study of career development among female nurse doctorates.* Unpublished doctoral dissertation, University of Missouri-Columbia, MO.

Spillane, E. J. (1973). *Contrasting backgrounds and career patterns of hospital administrators and assistant administrators.* Unpublished doctoral dissertation, St. Louis University, St. Louis, MO.

Stanton, M. (1974). Political action and nursing. *Nursing Clinics of North America, 9*(3), 579–585.

Stark, M. (1979). Introduction to Cassandra. In Florence Nightingale, *Cassandra* (pp. 1–23). Reprinted in Old Westbury, NY: The Feminist Press.

Starr, D. S. (1974). Poor baby: The nurse and feminism. *The Canadian Nurse, 70*(3), 20–23.

Steffel, M. L., & Kaczmarek, M. G. (1987, Winter). Women in the military: An historical perspective on the Nursing Corps. *Journal of NAWDAC, 32–38.*

Stein, L. I. (1967). The doctor-nurse game. *Archives of General Psychiatry, 16,* 699–700.

Stepsis, U., & Liptak, D. (Eds.). (1989). *Pioneer healers: The history of women religious in American health care.* New York: Crossroad.

Stimson, J. C. (1924). Equal rights. *American Journal of Nursing, 24*(8), 665–666.

Strachey, L. (1918). *Eminent Victorians.* New York: G. P. Putnam's Sons.

Strachey, R. (1928). *"The cause": A short history of the women's movement in Great Britain.* London: G. Bell & Sons, Ltd.

Stuart, G. W. (1986). An organizational strategy for empowering nursing. *Nursing Economics, 4*(2), 69–73.

Survey of perceived relationships between chief operating officers and directors of nurses. (1977, March/April). *Hospital Topics,* 38–40.

Talbott, S. W., & Vance, C. N. (1981). Involving nursing in a feminist group—NOW. *Nursing Outlook, 29*(10), 592–595.

Tarbox, M. P. (1990). A fierce tenderness: Florence Nightingale encounters the Sisters of Mercy. In V. Bullough, B. Bullough, & M. P. Stanton (Eds.), *Florence Nightingale and her era: A collection of new scholarship* (pp. 274–287). New York: Garland Publishing, Inc.

Thoms, A. (1929). *Pathfinders: A history of the progress of colored graduate nurses.* New York: Ray Printing House.

Todd, A. D. (1989). *Intimate adversaries: Cultural conflict between doctors and women patients.* Philadelphia: The University of Pennsylvania Press.

Turnbull, E. (1986). Nurses respond to NBC over "Accurate Portrayals." *Nursing Science Today, 3*(6), 4–13.

Van Devanter, L. (with C. Morgan). (1983). *Home before morning: The story of an army nurse in Vietnam.* New York: Beaufort Books.

Vance, C. (1979). Women Leaders: Modern day heroines or societal deviants? *Image, 11*(2), 39.

Vance, C., Talbott, S., McBride, A., & Mason, D. (1985). An uneasy alliance: Nursing and the women's movement. *Nursing Outlook, 33*(6), 281–285.

Veith, S. (1990). The recluse: A retrospective health history of Florence Nightingale. In V. Bullough, B. Bullough, & M. P. Stanton (Eds.), *Florence Nightingale and her era: A collection of new scholarship* (pp. 75–89). New York: Garland Publishing, Inc.

Vicinus, M. (1990). What makes a heroine? Girls' Biographies of Florence Nightingale. In V. Bullough, B. Bullough, & M. P. Stanton (Eds.), *Florence Nightingale and her era: A collection of new scholarship* (pp. 90–106). New York: Garland Publishing, Inc.

Wakefield-Fisher, M. (1983). Women in administration. *Nursing Success Today, 3*(3), 3–8.

Wald, L. D. (1976). The business of being a woman: NYSNA proceedings, 14th Annual Meeting, October 20–21, 1915. Reprinted in the *Journal of the New York State Nurses Association, 7*(1), 15–17.

Walsh, M. R. (1977). *Doctors wanted: No women need apply, sexual barriers in the medical profession, 1835–1975.* New Haven & London: Yale University Press.

Weaver, C. G. (1988). Nurse executive turnover. *Nursing Economics, 6*(6), 283–286.

Webb, C. (1983). Words fail me . . . . sexist language in the nursing context. *Nursing Times, 79*(27), 65–66.

Welch, M. (1986, April). Nineteenth-century philosophic influences on Nightingale's concept of the person. *Journal of Nursing History, 1*(2), 3–11.

Wheeler, C. E. (1984, July). Viewpoint: Essay in response to republication of a biography. *Advances in Nursing Science,* 74–79.

Wheeler, C. E. (1985, January). The *American Journal of Nursing* and the socialization of a profession, 1900–1920. *Advances in Nursing Science, 7*(2), 20–34.

Whittaker, E., & Olesen, V. (1964). The faces of Florence Nightingale: Functions of the heroine legend in an occupational sub-culture. *Human Organization, 23*(2), 123–130.

Widerquist, J. (1990). Dearest Rev'd Mother. In V. Bullough, B. Bullough, & M. P. Stanton (Eds.), *Florence Nightingale and her era: A collection of new scholarship* (pp. 288–308). New York: Garland Publishing, Inc.

Wilson, V. (1971). An analysis of femininity in nursing. *American Behavioral Scientist, 15*(2), 213–220.

Winters, D. E. T. (1985, June). Perceptions of occupational status of army nurses and physicians regarding themselves and each other. *Military Medicine, 150*, 297+.

Wolf, C. (1972). Liberation movement: Impact on nursing. *American Operating Room Journal, 15*(4), 79–85.

Wood, A. D. (1972). The war within a war: Women nurses in the Union Army. *Civil War History, 18*, 197–212.

Wood, J. (1981). Sex differences in group communications: Directions for research in speech communications and sociometry. *Journal of Group Psychotherapy, Psychodrama, and Sociometry, 34*, 24–31.

Woodham-Smith, C. (1951). *Florence Nightingale: 1820–1910*. New York & London: McGraw-Hill.

Yates, G. G. (1975). *What women want: The ideas of the movement*. Cambridge, MA: Harvard University Press.

Yeaworth, R. C. (1976). Women and nurses: Evolving roles. *Occupational Health Nursing, 24*(8)), 7–9.

Young, A. (1959). *The women and the crisis: Women of the North in the Civil War*. New York: McDowell, Obolensky.

Zimmerman, A. (1976). ANA: Its record on social issues. *American Journal of Nursing, 76*(4), 588–590.

Index

Abbott, Grace, 78
Abbott, Lyman, 156–157
Abdullah, Faye G., 325
Abstract for Action (ANA), 240
Adams, George W., 112
Addams, Jane, 73, 74, 75, 77, 78, 79, 127, 128
Adelstein, Willa, 140
Alcott, Louisa May, 111, 113
Allen, Donald R., 15
Allen, Margaret, 285, 286
Always a Sister: The Feminism of Lillian D. Wald (Daniels), 70
Amenta, Madelon M., 259
American Association of Colleges of Nursing, 328
American Journal of Nursing (AJN), 9, 80, 152; ERA and, 170; lessons from the past and position of, 162–165; sexism and, 199; suffrage and, 156–157
American Medical Association (AMA), 328–329
American Nurses Association (ANA), 131; ERA and, 194, 203; formation of, 82, 157, 197; national health-care proposal

of, 328, 329; pension benefits for nurses and, 215, 226; research on nursing and education, 240–241; suffrage and, 157, 160, 161
American Red Cross, Barton and, 56, 59, 60–61, 106, 107, 108–109, 118
American Revolutionary War, 102–103, 115, 137
American Sanitary Commission, 112
American Society of Superintendents of Training Schools for Nurses, 160
American Woman's Suffrage Association, 197
Anthony, Susan B., 57, 58–59, 61, 202
Applebaum, Alan, 246–247, 248
Archer, Helen Margaret, 265
Archer, Sarah Ellen, 316–317
Army Nurse Corps, World War II and, 132
Army Reorganization Act (1920), 125
"Art of Biography, The" (Woolf), 7–8

Arthur, Helen, 76
Ashley, Jo Ann, 159, 223–226,
    238–240, 261–263, 269
Assertiveness training, 306
Austin, Anne L., 113
Austin, J. K., 284, 285

Backer, Barbara A., 72–73,
    79–80
Bakunina, Ekaterina M., 104, 105
Baly, Monica E., 104
Banfield, Maud, 160
Barritt, Evelyn R., 304, 307,
    333–334
Barton, Clara: American Red
    Cross and, 56, 59, 60–61, 106,
    107, 108–109, 118; Anthony's
    relationship with, 57, 58–59,
    61; Civil War and, 106,
    109–110, 118; as a feminist,
    56–62; Franco-Prussian War
    and, 107; Nightingale and, 58;
    relationship with other
    feminists/women, 57, 58–59,
    61; Spanish-American War
    and, 107; suffrage and, 58,
    59–60, 61; war and views of,
    106–110
Baumgart, Alice J., 285–286
Beauvoir, Simone de, 179, 237
Belenky, M. F., 24
Bender, Gerald C., 145
Benner, Patricia, 288
Benson, Evelyn R., 41–42, 88,
    104–105
Berkeley, Reginald, 36, 37–38
Berkman, Alexander, 65
Berkman, Sasha, 77
Bickerdyke, Mary Ann, 118
Bille, Donald, 207
Bird, Caroline, 196
Birdwhistell, Raymond, 210
Birth control, feminists' work for,
    64–69, 71–73

Birth Control Review (Sanger), 68
Black women: struggle to become
    nurses, 89–93; in wartime,
    120–121
Blackwell, Alice Stone, 59
Blackwell, Elizabeth, 29, 46–47,
    113, 196, 229
Blakeney, Hazel, 250, 251
Blancett, Suzanne Smith,
    269–270
Blassingame, W., 130
Blum, Leslie C., 146
Bolton, Frances Payne, 131
Boulay, Donna Marie, 145–146
Boyd, Louie Croft, 154
Boyd, Nancy, 19–25, 27
Bracebridge, Selina, 47, 48, 49
Brand, Karen L., 227–230
Brewster, Mary, 69
Bridgeman, Mary Francis, 52
Brittain, Vera, 73
Brontë, Charlotte, 2
Brook, M. J., 32
Brown, Elsa, 263–264
Brown, J. Carter, 146
Bryant, Anita, 75
Buckle, Henry Thomas, 25, 26
Bullough, Bonnie, 32, 94–96, 133,
    163
Bullough, Vern L., 32, 64, 65,
    94–96, 163
Burns, Ken, 104

Cadet Nurse Program, 131
Calhoun, Judith, 53, 54
Call, The, 67
Campbell, J., 267
Campbell-Heider, Nancy,
    308–309, 332, 333, 334
Canada, suffrage and feminism
    in, 176–177, 189–190, 216
Carlson-Evans, Diane, 145
Carnegie, Mary Elizabeth, 90–91

Carter, Hilary Bonham, 12, 25, 45, 47, 48
Cassandra (Nightingale), 2, 11, 15, 16, 29, 30
Cassandra: Radical Feminist Nurses Network, 268
Castillejo, Irene Claremont de, 51
Catheart, H. Robert, 247
Catt, Carrie Chapman, 127, 129, 165, 197–198
Celler, Emanuel, 193
Chalich, Theresa, 303–304, 316, 334
Chantal, Jane Frances de, 23
Children's Bureau, 70, 75
Chinn, Peggy, 81, 268, 288–289
Christman, Luther, 238
Christy, Kathleen A., 304–305
Christy, Mary, 122, 123
Christy, Teresa E., 70, 80, 81, 84–85, 201–203
Cipriano, Pam, 249, 250
Civil War: Barton and, 106, 109–110, 118; gender war within, 114–119; Harvey and, 110–111; impact of, on nursing, 113, 118–119; literature about, 111–112; number of women serving in, 137; relief societies in, 112; Hannah Ropes and, 110
Civil War, The, 104
Clara Barton: Professional Angel (Pryor), 56
Clare, Mary Francis, 62–64
Clarke-Mohl, Mary, 12, 34, 47–48
Cleland, Virginia S., 198–200, 203, 207, 213–215, 249, 250, 251, 298
Clemons, Betty, 197, 198, 228
Clinton, Bill, 328, 329

Cocotas, Carolyn, 322–324, 332–333
Cold War, nursing activism and, 133–136
Cole, Aileen B., 121
Cole, Ellen, 141
Collins, Emily, 202
Cominos, Peter T., 15
Community Health Accreditation Program (CHAP), 326–328
Comprehensive Health Manpower Act (1971), 215
Comte, Auguste, 21, 25, 26
Cook, Blanche Wiesen, 73, 74–75, 76–77, 86
Cook, Edward, 6–7, 36, 50, 81
Cooper, P., 130
Cordua, G. D., 222, 223
Coss, C., 70
Coyle, Barry J., 144
Creative Malady (Pickering), 13
Creighton, Helen, 203
Crimean War, 32, 104–105, 197
Cumming, Kate, 119
Curtis, A., 114
Curtiss, J. S., 104
Cusack, Margaret Anna. *See* Clare, Mary Francis

Daimer, Annie, 160
Dains, Joyce E., 279–280
Daly, Mary, 36, 262
Daniels, Doris, 70–71, 72, 77–78, 79, 165–169
David, Opal D., 175–176
Davis, Frances Elliott, 91–92
Declaration of Sentiments, 151
Delano, Jane, 160
Descartes, Rene, 27
Diagnostic Related Groups (DRGs), 325
Dickson, Bessie Louise, 155
Diers, Donna, 237–238, 277–278, 288

Dieterle, William, 36
Dix, Dorothea, 109, 112–113,
    116, 118, 195
Dixon, Mary Bartlett, 153, 154
Dock, Lavinia Lloyd, 70, 79; Cold
    War and views of, 134–136;
    ERA and, 83, 162, 169, 203; as
    a feminist, 80–84, 86–87,
    152–154, 155–156; importance
    of past nursing history and,
    227, 228; male domination in
    nursing and, 225–226; nursing
    history developed by, 82;
    suffrage and, 83, 152–154, 166,
    229; Wald and, 75, 76; World
    War I and views of war, 83,
    126, 127–128, 129
Doctors in Blue (Adams), 112
Dominica, Frances, 53
Drabman, R. S., 222, 223
Draft laws, ERA and, 194
Duffus, Robert L., 70, 79, 125,
    166
Dunne, Irene, 39

Earley, Pete, 136
East, Catherine, 182–184, 188
Eastman, Crystal, 73–74, 77, 127
Edelstein, Ruth Greenberg, 194–
    197
Education: discrimination in, 195;
    reemergence of feminism in
    the 1960s and, 174–176;
    women's movement and need
    for, 214–215
Education of nurses: for Blacks,
    90–91, 93; Dock and, 83–84;
    equality equated with
    education, 255–257; impact of
    World War II on, 131–132;
    Nightingale and, 13, 14, 45;
    Nutting and, 84–85, 86;
    restriction imposed by, 231

Edwards, Joellen B., 309–311,
    331
Ehrenreich, Barbara, 208, 228,
    233, 262, 298
Elliot, Jo Eleanor, 248, 250, 251
Elmore, Joyce Ann, 89
Eminent Victorians (L. Strachey),
    7, 36
Enfranchisement, Nightingale's
    views on women's, 28–31
English, Deirdre, 208, 228, 233,
    262, 298
Enloe, Cynthia, 141
Equal pay issues: in Canada, 190;
    in the 1980s, 265–266; in the
    United States, 199–200,
    209–212, 265–266
Equal Rights Amendment
    (ERA): attempts at passing,
    171; Dock and, 83, 162, 169,
    203; nurses' debate over, 162,
    169–170, 192–198, 263–264;
    resurrection and debate over in
    the 1970s, 192–198
Erikson, Erik, 213
Etzioni, Amatai, 196
Evans, Diane, 146
Evans, Marianne, 6

Fagan, M. M., 307
Fagan, P. D., 307
Fagin, Claire M., 245–246,
    255–257, 265, 277–278
Family Limitation (Sanger),
    67–68
Feminine Mystique, The
    (Friedan), 173
Feminist/feminism: Barton as a,
    56–62; in Canada, 176–177;
    contemporary feminists in the
    field of nursing, 96–99;
    contribution of nursing to,
    287–289; Dock as a, 80–84,
    86–87, 152–156; effects of

Depression on, 168–169; impact of, on nursing, 285–287; need for activism, 289–292; Nightingale as a, 6, 9–10, 11–15, 44, 195; in the 1960s, 173–185; in the 1970s, 187–219; in the 1980s, 261–294; organization of, in the United States, 151, 165–170; resurrecting the power motif, 187–190; Sanger as a, 65–69; support groups for, 73–80, 85, 87; traditional views of, 237–238; Wald as a, 69–73. *See also* Women's movement; *specific issues*

Feminist Press, 11

Feminist views: of Barton, 57, 58–59, 61; of Nightingale, 43, 195, 201, 228

Fenwick, Ethel Gordon, 82, 158–159, 197, 198

Firestone, Shulamith, 224

Fishwick, Marshall W., 106

Flaherty, Agnes, 249

Flikke, Julia, 132

Florence Nightingale (film), 38

Florence Nightingale: 1820–1910 (Woodham-Smith), 36, 37

Forsythe, Patricia, 203

Francis, Anne, 190

Francis Report, 190, 216

Frank, Rose, 88

Freeman, Ruth, 97

Freire, Paulo, 297

Freud, Sigmund, 182, 262

Friedan, Betty, 173, 218

Frye, Elizabeth, 4

Gabrielson, Rosamond, 203–204, 249, 250

Gaffney, Evangelista, 63, 64

Gage, Matilda Joselyn, 60

Gaskell, Elizabeth, 51

Gass, G. Z., 188–189

Gaynor, Florence, 247

Gender role socialization and struggles: as a barrier to nursing power, 244–245, 309–311; importance of resocialization, 212–219, 305–306; nursing history as a chronology of, 238–240

Gender stereotypes, power of, 223, 282–84

Gerds, Gretchen, 174

Gilgannon, Mary, 52

Gilligan, Carol, 286

Gittings-Reid, Edith, 36, 37

Glass, Laurie K., 227–230

Goehner, Patricia A., 316–317

Goldman, Emma, 64–65, 73–74, 77, 79

Goldmark, Josephine, 88

Goldmark Report, 84–85, 88

Golick, Toby, 192–194

Goodacre, Glenna, 145

Goodrich, Annie, 125, 160

Greeley, Helen Hoy, 122, 124

Green, Carol Hurd, 81

Greenleaf, Nancy, 296, 332

Gretter, Lystra Eggert, 53

Grissum, Marlene, 234–236

Group, Thetis M., 206–209, 227, 228, 233, 283, 290

Guyot, Henrietta, 111, 112, 113

Haener, Dorothy, 193

Hagerty, Bonnie, 307, 334

Halperin, John, 7, 8

Hamilton, Alice, 78, 79

Hampton, Isabel, 82

Hanley, Barbara E., 317–318, 333

Harris, Julie, 39

Harrison, Janet K., 321, 330, 331

Harty, Margaret, 231–232

Harvey, Cordelia, 110–111

Hawkins, Joellen, 130
Health Care Financing
    Administration (HCFA),
    322–323, 327
Health care reform, nurses'
    impact on, 312–314, 325–330
Heide, Wilma Scott, 98–99, 173,
    191–192, 233, 287
Henle, Ellen Langenheim,
    106–107, 108
Henry Street Settlement House,
    69, 70, 72, 73, 82
Herbert, Elizabeth, 47, 48–49
Herbert, Sidney, 49
Hine, Darlene Clark, 91, 92, 93
History of Nursing, A (Dock), 82
Hoffman, Mary, 184
Holman, Nora, 154–155
Holroyd, M., 8
"Holy Terror, The," 37, 39–40
Homeopathy, Nightingale's views
    on, 3–4
Homosexuality: Addams and, 75;
    feminist support groups and,
    79–80; Goldman and, 77;
    Nightingale and, 34–35, 37;
    Wald and, 75, 76
Hoover, Kathleen, 250
Hopkins, Juliet, 111
Horner, Matina, 201
Hospital Sketches (Alcott), 111
Hospitals, 28
Hott, Jacqueline Rose, 253,
    278–279
Howe, Florence, 286
Howe, Julia Ward, 107, 156
Howland, Eliza, 117
Hughes, Linda, 270–271, 290
Hull House, 73
Hygiene and Morality (Dock), 83,
    84

Iafolla, Mary Ann C., 178–179
IMAGE, 140

International Council of Nurses
    (ICN), 82; 1947 conference,
    134–135
*Introductory Notes on Lying-in
    Institutions* (Nightingale), 13

Jacob, Timothy A., 130
Jacobs, Aletta, 128
James, Janet Wilson, 81, 83
Jewish women, role of, 88
Jezierski, Marlene, 145, 146
Johnston, Mary, 157
Joint Commission on
    Accreditation of Health Care
    Organizations (JCAHO), 326,
    327
Jolly, Ellen Ryan, 113
Jordan, Clifford, 249, 250
Jowett, Benjamin, 2, 18, 25

Kaczmarek, Margaret G., 137,
    138
Kaler, S. R., 283–284
Kalisch, Beatrice J., 35–40, 41,
    131, 252–253, 274–276,
    299–302, 332, 333, 334
Kalisch, Philip A., 35–40, 41,
    119, 124, 131, 252–253,
    274–276, 299–302, 332, 333,
    334
Kelley, Florence, 70, 78–79
Kelly, Dorothy, 173–174,
    177–178
Kelly, L. Y., 45
Kibrick, Ann, 238
Kijek, Jean, 264–265
King's College Hospital, Training
    School for Midwives at, 12
Kirkland-Casgrain, Claire,
    176–177
Kittredge, Mabel Hyde, 76
Korean War, 136, 138
Kramer, Marlene, 298

Krueger, Janelle C., 311–312, 331, 332

Lady With a Lamp, The, 36, 38–39
Lally, Grace, 130–131
Lamb, Karen T., 209–212, 288
Larsen, Jenniece, 312–313, 333
Lavinia Dock Reader, A (James), 81
Leadership: androgynous, 257–259, 312; crisis and lack of internal, 240-43; gender communication differences and, 309–311; need for risk-takers and role-breakers, 234–237; in the 1990s, 267; perceptions/treatment of nurse administrators/leaders, 254–255, 318–325; qualities needed for, 248–251; traditional views of, 237–238; upper echelon positions needed to be filled by women, 246–248, 314–315
Leary, Catherine L., 120, 121
Lee, James, 39
Legal/legislation issues: debate over, 213–214; examples of, needed by nurses, 215
Leininger, Madeleine, 242–243, 267–268
Lenz, Cynthia L., 309–311, 331
Leone, Lucile Petry, 131–132
Leopard, Donald, 132
Lewenson, Sandra, 83–84, 159–161
Lewis-Jones-Raker bill, 123–124
Lewisohn, Alice, 75
Lewisohn, Irene, 75–76
Lewis-Raker bill, 122
"Liberation Movement: Impact on Nursing," 201–202

Life of Florence Nightingale, The (Cook), 36
Lillian D. Wald: The Progressive Woman and Feminism (Daniels), 70
Lindabury, Virginia A., 190
Liptak, Dolores, 62
Livingston, Joy A., 141–143, 149
Luc, Marjorie M., 265
Lucretia Mott Amendment, 161–162

Mahoney, Mary, 89
Mapanga, Margo, 284
Marriage: Nightingale's views on, 7, 12, 23; in the 1960s, 176; Wald's views on, 72
Marshall, George, 134, 135
Marshall, Mary Louise, 112
Martineau, Harriet, 6, 29, 47, 49
Materia Medica for Nurses (Dock), 82, 84
Matthews, Irene, 130
Mauksch, Ingeborg, 248–251
Mayne, Michael, 52, 53
McBride, A., 237
McCarthy, Penny A., 263
McCauley (or McKelly), Mary Ludwig Hays, 102
McGovern, James R., 79
McGraw, K. O., 223
McHugh, Mary L., 274–276
McIsaac, Isabel, 157, 160
McVicker, Sara J., 136, 137
Mead, Margaret, 189, 218
Media: portrayals of Nightingale, 35–40; portrayals of nurses, 274–277
Melosh, Barbara, 271–272
Mentoring, role of, 307–309
Merton, Robert, 94
Milauskas, Janet, 305, 334
Military rank, nurses' fight for, 122–125, 133, 138

Mill, John Stuart, 6, 13, 21, 25, 26, 28, 29–30, 31
Millett, Kate, 191
Misery, 276
Mohl, Mary. *See* Clarke-Mohl, Mary
Monteiro, Lois A., 46–49, 52, 53, 134–136
Moore, Georgiana, 50
Moore, Mary Clare, 50–51
More, M. Thomas, 189–190
Morgenthau, Rita, 75, 76
Mott, Lucretia, 197
Muff, Janet, 280–281, 289–292
Mullane, Mary Kelly, 97–98, 187–189
Muller, Helen J., 322–324, 332–333
Murphy, Ruth, 236
Murtha, Rena, 236

Nathan, Maud, 88
National Association of Coloured Graduate Nurses, 90, 160, 161
National Association of Nurse Alumnae (NANA): name change, 157; suffrage and, 152, 153–155
National Birth Control League, 67
National Black Nurses Association, 94
National Labor Relations Act, 215
National League for Nursing (NLN), 160, 197, 326, 327; convention held in non-ERA states, debate over, 263–265; national health-care proposal of, 328
National League of Nursing Education, 160, 161
National Organization for Public Health Nursing, 161

National Organization for Women (NOW), 246, 253, 276, 286, 302; NURSES NOW, 259, 293, 331
National Society for Woman's Suffrage, 13, 28
National Women Suffrage Association, 58
Nauright, Lynda, 45–46
Nelson, Jean, 11
Networking, 304–305
Newcomb, E., 130
Newton, Lisa H., 282–283
Nicholson, Hannah, 23
Nicholson, Henry, 50
Nicholson, Marianne, 12, 34
Nightingale, Florence: Barton and, 58; changing views of, 5–15, 44–46; Crimean War and, 32, 104, 197; drug taking and, 33, 34; as a feminist, 6, 9–10, 11–15, 44, 195; feminist views of, 43, 195, 201, 228; health and physical condition of, 32–34; homosexuality and, 34–35, 37; influence of philosophers on, 26, 27; media portrayals of, 35–40; memorial service for (1991), 52–53; mystical/spiritual side of, 6–7, 12, 14, 15–27, 50–51; negative images created by biographies, 41–44; reforms and accomplishments of, 11–12; relationship with family, 15–16, 42; relationship with other women, 34–35, 37, 46–52; traditional view of, 10–11;
Nightingale, Florence, views of: on the education of nurses, 13, 14, 45; on female control of the nursing field, 9–10; on marriage, 7, 12, 23; on the medical profession, 29; on the

mystical state, 24; on natural laws and the nature of God and religion, 18, 20–27; on nursing as a profession, 7; on the Roman Catholic Church, 18, 20; on women, 2–5, 13–14, 19, 29, 34, 50; on women's suffrage/enfranchisement, 6, 13, 28–31

Nightingale, Parthenope, 15, 16

Nightingale Pledge, 53–54

Nightingale, William, 15

Norton, Eleanor, 193

Notable American Women: The Modern Period (Sicherman & Green), 81

Notes on Nursing: What It Is, and What It Is Not (Nightingale), 3, 4–5, 25, 28, 29

Nurse Training Amendment Act (1971), 215, 252

Nurses Associated Alumnae, 82

Nurses' Journal of the Pacific Coast (*NJPC*), 154

Nursing, impact of Nightingale movies on, 40

Nursing as a profession: danger of men in, 206; debate in the 1970s over, 196–197, 210; Nightingale's views on, 7; in the 1950s and 1960s, 172–173

Nursing Council on National Defense, 131

Nursing image(s): British stereotyped, 272–273, 284; cross-cultural perceptions of nurses, 284–285; depicted as sex objects, 274–275, 279–280; depicted in greeting cards, 278–279; media portrayals of nurses, 274–277; as a metaphor, 277–278; need for new mythos for, 223–226; need for risk-takers and

role-breakers, 234–237; need to change stereotypes maintained by nurses, 230–234, 262–263; in the 1980s, 270–272; power of gender stereotypes, 223, 282–284; sexist images of nurses, 280–282; traditional images, 221–223, 262; use of historical information for, 227–230. *See also* Leadership

Nursing Outlook, 80

Nursing's Agenda for Health Care Reform, 328

Nutting, Adelaide, 87, 124–125: education of nurses and, 84–85, 86; importance of past nursing history and, 228; military rank for nurses and, 124–125; nursing history developed, 82; suffrage and, 154, 229

O'Connor, Lillian, 179–182

Olesen, Virginia, 10, 11

One Flew Over the Cuckoo's Nest, 273, 276

Oppressed behavior, impact of, 296–299

O'Reilly, Leonora, 82

Osborne, Estelle Massey, 97

Palmer, Irene Sabelberg, 31–35, 45, 104

Palmer, Sophia, 153–154, 163–164

Parsons, Margaret E., 119

Parsons, Sara E., 124

Paul, Alice, 73

Pavlovna, Elena, 105

Pearce, Evelyn C., 10

Pember, Phoebe, 119

Peplau, Hildegard E., 236–237, 245

Perkins, Frances, 78
Persian Gulf War, 147–149
Petersen, Annabelle, 122, 123, 125
Peterson, Esther, 174–175
Peterson, Martha E., 241
Pethick-Lawrence, Emmeline, 127
Petry, Lucile. *See* Leone, Lucile Petry
Phelps, Elizabeth Stuart, 115
Phillips, Ann, 33
Physician-nurse relationships, history of and the need to change, 203–205, 207–209
Pickering, George, 13, 32
Pioneer Healers: The History of Women Religious in American Health Care (Stepsis & Liptak), 62
Pirogov, Nicholas, 105
Pitcher, Molly, 102
Playboy, 279–280
Pogrebin, Lottie, 85
Political action: grassroots type of, 303–304; horizontal and vertical conflicts, 299–303; need for political awareness by nurses, 252–254; nurses' views of, 243–244; research/trends on nurses' participation in, 316–318, 325–335
Politics of Nursing (Kalisch & Kalisch), 299
Pollard, Terri, 62, 63, 64
Porter, Felicia Grundy, 113
Poslusny, Susan M., 80, 85–86, 87
Powell, Diane F., 253–254
Power: barriers to nursing, 244–245, 296–299; horizontal and vertical conflicts, 299–303; motif in the 1970s, resurrection of, 187–190

President's Commission on the Status of Women, 173–175
Pryor, Elizabeth Brown, 56, 57–58, 59–60, 61
Pugh, Evelyn L., 28–31

Rankin, Jeanette, 129
Rankin, Joanna M., 141–143, 149
Raymond, Janice, 289
Reavill, Noreen, 232–233
Religion: Nightingale's views on natural laws and the nature of God and, 18, 20–27; women defined by, 262
Report of the Royal Commission on the Status of Women in Canada, 190
Resnick, A., 70
Resocialization, importance of, 212–219, 305–306
Reverby, Susan, 54, 73, 159
Revolution, The, 57
Richter, Elizabeth, 221–222
Richter, Lucretia, 221–222
Riegler, Natalie N., 49–50
Rights of nurses, 245–246
Rinehart, Mary Roberts, 276
Rivers, Eunice, 92
Robb, Isabel Hampton, 85, 86–87
Roberts, Joan I., 98, 206–209, 227, 228, 233, 283, 290
Roberts, Mary, 80
Roberts, Susan Jo, 296–299, 313, 318, 322
Rogers, Edith Nourse, 132
Rogge, Mary Madeline, 109, 110, 111
Rollins, Clara A., 121
Roosevelt, Eleanor, 92, 173
Ropes, Hannah, 110
Roth, Patricia A., 321, 330, 331
Rothblum, Esther D., 141
Rothstein, Ruth, 247

Rousseau, Jean Jacques, 27
Roy, Adrienne, 289
Ruether, Rosemary, 262
Ruffing-Rahal, Mary-Ann, 65, 69
Rush, Benjamin, 103
Russell, Gail, 140
Russian nurses: in the Crimean
    War, 104–105; International
    Council of Nurses 1947
    conference and, 134–135

Safford, Ada M., 155
Safier, Gwendolyn, 96–97, 98
Sahli, Nancy, 75
St. Angela of Foligno, 23
St. Catherine of Genoa, 24
St. Catherine of Siena, 24
St. Francis of Assisi, 23
St. Joseph Sisters of Peace, 63
St. Teresa of Avila, 23, 24
St. Thomas' Hospital, Nightingale
    School and Home for Nurses
    at, 12
Salvage, Jane, 272–273
Sandelowski, Margaret, 263
Sanders, Byrne Hope, 172–173
Sandler, Bernice, 214
Sanger, Margaret, 65–69, 217,
    235, 236
Sanger, William, 67
Sargent, Alice G., 212–213,
    257–259, 312, 315
Schaefer, Marguerite J., 240–241
Schiff, Jacob, 75, 79
Schlotfeldt, Rosella, 238
Schorr, Thelma, 253, 319
Schwartz, Linda Spoonster, 138,
    139, 140
Schwimmer, Rosika, 127
Scott, Jessie, 250, 251
Seigel, H., 288
Selavan, Ida Cohen, 102–103
Seleckman, Janice, 88
Seltzer, Meta, 147–149

Seneca Falls Convention, 151,
    202
Sex objects, nurses as, 274–275,
    279–280
Sexism: realization of, by nurses
    in the 1970s, 201–209; role of,
    in nursing, 198–201
Sexist terminology, changing,
    269–270
Sexual Politics (Millett), 191
Sheinwold, Marcy, 247
Shippen, William, 103
Shockley, Judith Salmon,
    217–218
Short History of Nursing, A (Dock
    & Stewart), 84
Showalter, Elaine, 14–15, 16, 17,
    18, 19
Sicherman, Barbara, 81
Siegel, Beatrice, 127, 128, 129,
    130
Skeet, Muriel, 13
Slater, Virginia E., 26, 27
Slavinsky, Ann, 238
Smith, F. B., 41–42, 50
Smith, Florence T., 13–14
Smith, Fran A'Hern, 234
Smith, Lorraine, 303–304, 316,
    334
Smith, Mary Rozet, 74, 75
Smoyak, Shirley A., 244–245,
    265–266
Southmayd, F. R., 60
Spanish-American War, 119, 137
Speedy, Sandra, 287, 288
Spender, Dale, 8, 46, 163, 269
Spengler, Carol, 234, 307
Sperry, Almeda, 77
Spillane, Edward J., 248
Stakhovich, Aleksandra Petrovna,
    105
Stanley, D. Elva Mills, 161
Stanton, Elizabeth Cady, 57, 107,
    197, 202

Stanton, Marjorie P., 32, 243–244
Stark, Myra, 11–13, 28
Starr, Dorothy S., 215–216
Staupers, Mabel K., 90, 92
Steffel, Marilyn L., 137, 138
Stein, Leonard I., 204–205, 207
Stephany, Theresa M., 140
Stepsis, Ursula, 62
Stewart, Dugald, 26, 27
Stewart, Isabel, 84, 86, 195, 229
Stimson, Julia, 125, 162
Stone, Lucy, 59, 180, 181, 217
Strachey, Lytton, 7–9, 36, 49–50
Strachey, Ray, 2, 6, 14, 30
Strelnick, E. Gayle, 264
Stuart, Gail Wiscarz, 313–314,
   321, 332
Student Nurses, The, 276
Subjection of Women (Mill), 28,
   30
Suffrage: Abbott (Lyman) and,
   156–157; Barton and, 58,
   59–60, 61; in Canada,
   176–177; debate over National
   Association of Nurse Alumnae
   position on, 152, 153–155;
   Dock and, 83, 152–154, 166,
   229; Howe and, 156; Lucretia
   Mott Amendment, 161–162;
   Nightingale and, 6, 13, 28–31;
   nursing organizations' views on,
   159–161; Nutting and, 154,
   229; Wald and, 70, 158, 165,
   166, 167–168; women urged to
   use the power of voting in the
   1970s, 188–190
Suggestions for Thought to Seekers
   After Religious Truth
   (Nightingale), 15, 16, 18, 25, 28
Szold, Henrietta, 88

Talbott, Susan W., 264, 302, 331
Tarbox, Mary P., 52
Taylor, Harriet, 6, 29

Teachers Insurance and Annuity
   Association (TIAA), 215
Thompkins, Sally, 111
Thoms, Adah, 89, 120, 121, 161
Tocqueville, Alexis de, 188
Truth, Sojourner, 89
Tubman, Harriet, 89
Turnbull, Eleanor, 281–282

Unionism for nurses, 193, 196,
   215
U.S. armed services: draft laws
   and ERA, 194; integration of
   Black nurses in, 90, 92

Vance, Connie N., 264, 286–287,
   302, 305–306, 307, 331
Van Devanter, Lynda, 143
Veith, S., 32, 33
Vicinus, Martha, 42, 43, 44
Vietnam War: impact on nurses,
   136–147; number of women
   serving in, 138; sexual
   harassment, 139
Vietnam Women's Memorial
   Project, 145–147
Vindication of the Rights of
   Woman (Wollstonecraft), 181
Voda, Ann M., 288

Wakefield-Fisher, Mary,
   314–315, 330
Wald, Lillian, 88; as a feminist,
   69–73; Goldman and, 79;
   homosexuality and, 75, 76;
   relations with Black nurses, 93;
   relations with other feminists/
   women, 74, 75–76, 77–80;
   suffrage and, 70, 158, 165, 166,
   167–168; World War I and
   views of war, 125–126, 127,
   128–129
War: Barton's views of, 106–110;
   Dock's views of, 83, 126,

127–128, 129; traditional treatment of women during, 103–106; Wald's views of, 125–126, 127, 128–129. *See also name of*
Washington, Booker T., 92, 93
Washington, George, 103
Washington, Martha, 103
Waters, Mary, 103
Weaver, Christina G., 318–320, 330, 331
Webb, Christine, 269
Weeks v. Southern Bell, 183–184
Welch, Marylouise, 25–26, 27
"What Every Girl Should Know" (Sanger), 67
"What Every Mother Should Know" (Sanger), 67
Wheeler, Charlene Eldridge, 44–45, 162–165, 268, 289
Wheeler, Elizabeth Mathier, 289
Whitbeck, Caroline, 288
White Angel, The, 36, 38
Whittaker, Elvi, 10, 11
Widerquist, JoAnn G., 50, 51, 52
Wilcox, Anna Neagle, 38
Wilcox, Harold, 38
Williams, Daniel Hale, 93
Wilson, Henry, 109–110
Wilson, Victoria, 200–201
Winters, Debbie Tipton, 144–145
Witches, Midwives, and Nurses (Ehrenreich & English), 208
Wittenmeyer, Annie, 118
Wolf, Charlotte, 205–206, 288
Wolfgang, Myra K., 193
Wollstonecraft, Mary, 180, 181, 217, 235–236
Woman and the New Race (Sanger), 68
Woman, Power and Health Care (Grissum & Spengler), 234
Woman Rebel, The, 67

Woman's Christian Temperance Union (WCTU), 60
Woman Suffrage Party, 165
Women and the Crisis, The (Young), 112
Women and Therapy (Rothblum & Cole), 140–141
Women, Church, and State (Gage), 60
"Women Who Went to the Field," 56
Women's Army Auxiliary Corps (WAAC), 132
Women's International League for Peace and Freedom, 73, 141
Women's movement: need for changes in values and social structures in the 1990s, 267–268; realization of, by nurses in the 1970s, 201–209. *See also* Feminist/feminism; Suffrage
Women's Peace Party, 73, 75, 127
Wood, Ann Douglas, 114–118
Woodham-Smith, Cecil, 36, 37, 44
Woolf, Virginia, 7–8
Woolsey, Georgeanna, 109, 117
World War I: Dock and, 126, 127–128, 129; number of women serving in, 137; nurses' fight for military rank, 122–125; Wald and, 125–126, 127, 128–129
World War II: impact on nursing, 130–133; number of women serving in, 137–138
Wright, Frances, 180, 181

Yates, G. G., 266
Yeaworth, Rosalee, 230–231
Young, Agatha, 111–112
Zimmerman, Ann, 169

About the Authors

JOAN I. ROBERTS is Professor Emerita of Child, Family, and Community Studies at Syracuse University. A pioneer in Women's Studies in higher education, she is the author of numerous books and articles on gender issues, discrimination, the anthropology of education, and problems in urban education.

THETIS M. GROUP is Professor Emerita of Nursing at Syracuse University where she was dean of the School of Nursing for 10 years. She has published numerous articles in professional nursing journals.